Chronic Pain

Chronic Pain

A Primary Care Guide to Practical Management

Dawn A. Marcus, MD

Pain Institute, University of Pittsburgh
Pittsburgh, PA

*To another
fast talker -
Dawn Marcus*

HUMANA PRESS ✳ TOTOWA, NEW JERSEY

© 2005 Humana Press Inc.
999 Riverview Drive, Suite 208
Totowa, New Jersey 07512

humanapress.com

Due diligence has been taken by the publishers, editors, and authors of this book to assure the accuracy of the information published and to describe generally accepted practices. The contributors herein have carefully checked to ensure that the drug selections and dosages set forth in this text are accurate and in accord with the standards accepted at the time of publication. Notwithstanding, as new research, changes in government regulations, and knowledge from clinical experience relating to drug therapy and drug reactions constantly occurs, the reader is advised to check the product information provided by the manufacturer of each drug for any change in dosages or for additional warnings and contraindications. This is of utmost importance when the recommended drug herein is a new or infrequently used drug. It is the responsibility of the treating physician to determine dosages and treatment strategies for individual patients. Further it is the responsibility of the health care provider to ascertain the Food and Drug Administration status of each drug or device used in their clinical practice. The publisher, editors, and authors are not responsible for errors or omissions or for any consequences from the application of the information presented in this book and make no warranty, express or implied, with respect to the contents in this publication.

This publication is printed on acid-free paper. ∞
ANSI Z39.48-1984 (American Standards Institute) Permanence of Paper for Printed Library Materials.

Production Editor: Robin B. Weisberg

Cover design by Patricia F. Cleary

For additional copies, pricing for bulk purchases, and/or information about other Humana titles, contact Humana at the above address or at any of the following numbers: Tel.: 973-256-1699; Fax: 973-256-8314; E-mail: humana@humanapr.com, or visit our Website: http://humanapress.com

Printed in the United States of America. 10 9 8 7 6 5 4 3 2 1

eISBN 1-59259-882-X.

Library of Congress Cataloging-in-Publication Data

Marcus, Dawn A.
  Chronic pain : a primary care guide to practical management /
Dawn A. Marcus.
     p. ; cm. -- (Current clinical practice)
  Includes bibliographical references and index.
  ISBN 1-58829-501-X (alk. paper)
  1. Chronic pain. 2. Headache. 3. Analgesia.   I. Title. II.
Series.
  [DNLM: 1. Chronic Disease. 2. Pain--therapy. 3. Headache
--therapy. 4. Pain--psychology. 5. Primary Health Care--methods.
WL 704 M322c 2005]
  RB127.M3855 2005
  616'.0472--dc22

                                                                2004010140

Series Editor's Introduction

"They are and suffer, that is all they do"
—*W. H. Auden*[1]

"Although the world is full of suffering,
it is also full of overcoming it."

—*Helen Keller*[2]

When patients come to us with their pain they present us with a marvelous opportunity—the chance to understand them, to understand how their pain is affecting their lives, the challenge of discovering what is causing their pain, and finally the opportunity to prescribe medications and lifestyle changes to help them gain relief from their pain. *Chronic Pain: A Primary Care Guide to Practical Management* is an important book, offering concrete evidence-based approaches to diagnose and treat myriad causes of chronic pain that we as primary care physicians see in our office every day. It is an ambitious book, covering this large topic in only slightly more than 300 pages. In doing so, the author understands that for this book to be useful to primary care physicians, who are busy and have little time to concern themselves with unnecessary information, it must be practical, clear, evidence-based, and succinct.

Chronic Pain: A Primary Care Guide to Practical Management approaches the discussion of pain management as primary care clinicians approach their patients, first trying to determine—with as much clarity as possible—the etiology of a patient's pain; then discussing the specific treatments and general treatments of the condition that has been diagnosed as well as the pain it causes. All this occurs against a backdrop of general issues relevant to all pain management. Most of the common conditions that lead patients to come into our offices with a pain as their chief complaint are covered. The book presents clear recommendations for treatment and supports those recommendations with useful references. *Chronic Pain: A Primary Care*

---

[1]From Auden, W. H. "Surgical Ward." The Selected Poetry of W. H. Auden. Vintage, New York, NY, 1971.

[2]From http://www.quotationspage.com/quotes.php3?author=Helen+Keller>http://quotations page.com/quotes.php3?author=Helen+Keller. Accessed 9/7/04. Quoted also on <http://www.brainyquote. com/quotes/authors/h/helen_keller.html>http://www.brainyquote.com/quotes/authors/h/helen_keller.html accessed 9/7/04 .

Guide to Practical Management is also filled with excellent easy-to-understand figures, tables, and algorithms.

The *Current Clinical Practice Series*, conceived by a number of editors at Humana Press, has as its mission to create high-quality, evidence-based books for primary care clinicians, with an emphasis on relevance, and providing practical approaches to common problems. The books in the *Current Clinical Practice Series* can be used to gain an updated understanding of common problems and/or can be placed on office shelves and in PDAs to serve as important references when questions come up during the course of patient care. *Chronic Pain: A Primary Care Guide to Practical Management* fulfills the mission of this series—it is practical, useful, and relevant. There is no higher compliment for any book of medicine.

Neil Skolnik, MD
Professor of Family and Community Medicine
Temple University School of Medicine
Associate Director
Family Practice Residency Program
Abington Memorial Hospital

Preface

Thoughts of the busy clinician who picks up the chart for a new visit for a patient with a chief complaint of chronic pain:

I'm already running behind today. Hope the next patient has a straightforward problem. ...Chronic low back pain, failed surgery, out of work for the last 6 months, requesting signature on a disability form, refill of pain medications, and a sleeping pill, refuses to see a psychologist because "it's real pain." How will I ever handle this assessment during a short office visit?

These thoughts have been repeated in some form by most clinicians, easily overwhelmed with the typically complex stories of patients with chronic pain. When confronted with pain patients, it is important to remember that there are three common but false myths about chronic pain:

1. Patients with chronic pain are easy to manage.
2. Chronic pain is easily relieved with just a pill.
3. As pain improves, associated problems (e.g., depression, disability, relationship issues) will spontaneously resolve.

Patients with chronic pain present a unique set of challenges to the primary care physician, who must first recognize and accept the difficult and complex constellation of problems often encountered by these patients.

The clinical management of chronic pain is frequently requested by patients seeing primary care physicians, although most medical schools provide little background for dealing with these often complex patients. Patients with chronic pain often report a variety of complaints, including pain, sleep abnormalities, mood disturbance, and interference with personal, social, and work relationships. Lack of easily identified pathology in patients who report disabling symptoms may result in conflicts between patients and their treating clinicians. In addition, managing chronic pain generally requires assessment and treatment of pain, associated symptoms, and disability.

Developing pain management skills requires listening to patients' stories, becoming invested in their lives, and following the results of prescribed therapy over ensuing months and years. The information and recommendations provided in this book are the result of many instructive hours of listening to patients describe their own pain experiences, both the nociceptive symptoms and the profound impact that their pain had upon many aspects of their lives. I will always be profoundly grateful to those many patients who trusted and shared their lives with me and truly educated me to become a pain doctor.

Dawn A. Marcus, MD

Contents

Continuing Medical Education

RELEASE DATE
December 1, 2004

EXPIRATION DATE
December 1, 2007

ESTIMATED TIME TO COMPLETE
5 hours

ACCREDITATION
This activity has been planned and implemented in accordance with the essential areas and policies of the Accreditation Council for Continuing Medical Education (ACCME) through the joint sponsorship of The American Society of Contemporary Medicine and Surgery and Humana Press/eXtensia. The American Society of Contemporary Medicine and Surgery is accredited by the Accreditation Council for Continuing Medical Education to provide continuing medical education for physicians.

CREDIT DESIGNATION
The American Society of Contemporary Medicine and Surgery designates this educational activity for a maximum of 5 category 1 credits toward the AMA Physician's Recognition Award. Each physician should claim only those credits that he/she actually spent in the activity.

METHOD OF PARTICIPATION AND FEE
The American Society of Contemporary Medicine and Surgery is pleased to award category 1 credit(s) toward the AMA Physician's Recognition Award for this activity. By reading the chapters and completing the CME questions, you are eligible for up to 5 category 1 credits toward the AMA/PRA. Following that, please complete the Answer Sheet and claim the credits. A minimum of 75% correct must be obtained for credit to be awarded. Finally, please complete the Activity Evaluation on the other side of the Answer Sheet. Please submit the Answer Sheet/Activity Evaluation according to the information printed on the top of that page. Your test will be scored within 4 weeks. There is no fee for this activity. You will then be notified of your score with a certificate of credit, or you will receive an additional chance to pass the posttest. Credit for the activity is available until December 1, 2007.

FACULTY AND DISCLOSURE

Faculty for CME activities are expected to disclose to the activity audience any real or apparent conflict(s) of interest related to the content of the material they present. The following relationships have been disclosed:

Dawn A. Marcus, MD
Research Support
Eisai, Pfizer

PROVIDER DISCLOSURE

The American Society of Contemporary Medicine and Surgery is an independent organization that does not endorse specific products of any pharmaceutical concern and therefore has nothing to disclose. Humana Press/eXtensia are independent organizations that do not endorse specific products of any pharmaceutical concern and therefore have nothing to disclose.

INTENDED AUDIENCE

This activity is intended for internal medicine and family physicians, obstetrician/gynecologists, psychiatrists, geriatricians, rheumatologists, physician assistants, and nurse practitioners.

OVERALL GOAL

The overall goal of this activity is to update the knowledge of clinicians on strategies and techniques needed to comprehensively manage patients with chronic pain.

LEARNING OBJECTIVES

After completing this CME activity, participants should have improved their overall knowledge and attitudes in regard to managing chronic pain. Specifically, attendees should be able to:

- Understand the pathogenesis of chronic pain.
- Discuss the prevalence and predictive factors for a variety of chronic pain conditions, as well as how those conditions change when occurring in different age categories or unique medical conditions, such as pregnancy.
- Describe assessment strategies for patients with a variety of common chronic pain conditions.
- Differentiate state-of-the-art treatment techniques for a variety of chronically painful conditions, including both medication and non-medication therapies.
- Assess controversies surrounding use of opioids in chronic pain patients and develop practical strategies for considering supplemental opioids in individual patients.

UNLABELED/ UNAPPROVED USE DISCLOSURE

In accordance with ACCME standards for Commercial Support, the audience is advised that this CME activity may contain references to unlabeled or unapproved uses of drugs or devices.

Value-Added eBook/PDA

This book is accompanied by a value-added CD-ROM that contains an Adobe eBook version of the volume you have just purchased. This eBook can be viewed on your computer, and you can synchronize it to your PDA for viewing on your handheld device. The eBook enables you to view this volume on only one computer and PDA. Once the eBook is installed on your computer, you cannot download, install, or e-mail it to another computer; it resides solely with the computer to which it is installed. The license provided is for only one computer. The eBook can only be read using Adobe® Reader® 6.0 software, which is available free from Adobe Systems Incorporated at www.Adobe.com. You may also view the eBook on your PDA using the Adobe® PDA Reader® software that is also available free from Adobe.com.

You must follow a simple procedure when you install the eBook/PDA that will require you to connect to the Humana Press website in order to receive your license. Please read and follow the instructions below:

1. Download and install Adobe® Reader® 6.0 software
   You can obtain a free copy of Adobe® Reader® 6.0 software at www.adobe.com
   Note: If you already have Adobe® Reader® 6.0 software, you do not need to reinstall it.
2. Launch Adobe® Reader® 6.0 software
3. Install eBook: Insert your eBook CD into your CD-ROM drive
   PC: Click on the "Start" button, then click on "Run"
   At the prompt, type "d:\ebookinstall.pdf" and click "OK"
   Note: If your CD-ROM drive letter is something other than d: change the above command accordingly.
   MAC: Double click on the "eBook CD" that you will see mounted on your desktop.
   Double click "ebookinstall.pdf"
4. Adobe® Reader® 6.0 software will open and you will receive the message "This document is protected by Adobe DRM" Click "OK"
   Note: If you have not already activated Adobe® Reader® 6.0 software, you will be prompted to do so. Simply follow the directions to activate and continue installation.
   Your web browser will open and you will be taken to the Humana Press eBook registration page. Follow the instructions on that page to complete installation. You will need the serial number located on the sticker sealing the envelope containing the CD-ROM.

If you require assistance during the installation, or you would like more information regarding your eBook and PDA installation, please refer to the eBookManual.pdf located on your CD. If you need further assistance, contact Humana Press eBook Support by e-mail at ebooksupport@humanapr.com or by phone at 973-256-1699.

*Adobe and Reader are either registered trademarks or trademarks of Adobe Systems Incorporated in the United States and/or other countries.

xiii

I
Introduction

1

Chronic Pain and Headache

1. CHRONIC PAIN: EPIDEMIOLOGY

Pain is a common chief complaint for patients in primary care, with approximately 10 to 20% reporting chronic pain *(1–3)* (*see* Fig. 1). In a sample of general practices, chronic pain requiring pain medications and treatment was identified in 14% of patients, with 6% of these patients reporting high levels of disability because of pain *(4)*. A World Health Organization survey of patients in primary care in 14 countries revealed that back, head, and joint pain are the three most commonly affected areas *(3)* (Fig. 2). Interestingly, two-thirds of patients reported pain affecting more than one body region.

Pain is even more prevalent in samples of patients in community settings. Musculoskeletal complaints were reported by 80% of 15- to 84-year-olds in a general population survey, with 13% reporting substantial pain *(5)*. The area most commonly affected by musculoskeletal pain is the back *(6)* (Fig. 3). In addition, musculoskeletal conditions (which frequently involve chronic pain) rank as fifth in terms of hospital costs and first in terms of costs related to work absenteeism and disability *(7)*. A survey of health care expenditures for employees showed that among all physical health complaints, mechanical low back pain was the fourth most expensive condition, with other back disorders collectively ranked as the seventh most expensive condition *(8)*.

Patients reporting chronic pain often experience psychological distress and disability in addition to pain (Fig. 4). The significant impact of chronic pain was recently highlighted in a study by Blyth and colleagues *(9)*. Their survey of Australian adults with chronic pain revealed that, although only 29% reported work restrictions owing to pain complaints, 58% reported reduced work effectiveness. Respondents reported working with pain for 84 days during a 6-month period, but only losing 4.5 days from work because of pain. Considering both work absenteeism plus reduced-effectiveness workdays, an average of 16 workday equivalents was lost over 6 months.

Despite frequent patient complaints about chronic pain, a recent survey of primary care physicians noted that only 15% felt comfortable treating patients with chronic pain *(10)*. Primary care physicians were also uncomfortable with

From: *Chronic Pain: A Primary Care Guide to Practical Management*
Edited by: D. A. Marcus © Humana Press, Totowa, NJ

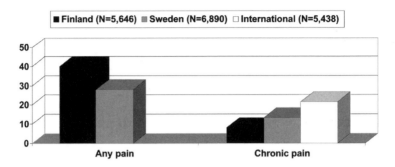

Fig. 1. Prevalence of a chief complaint of any pain and chronic pain in primary care (Based on refs. *1–3.*)

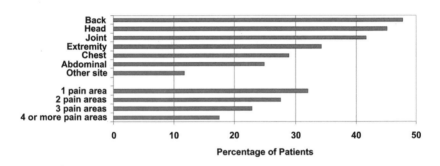

Fig. 2. Pain location reported in international survey of primary care patients. (Based on ref. *3.*)

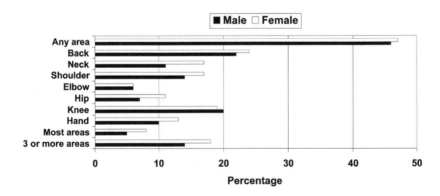

Fig. 3. Musculoskeletal pain prevalence. Percentage of patients from primary care physician practices reporting musculoskeletal pain lasting more than 1 week during the previous month. (Based on ref. *6.*)

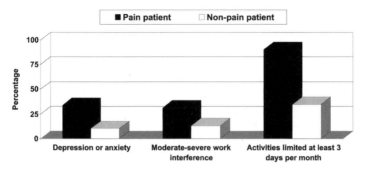

Fig. 4. Chronic pain-associated distress and disability. Based on data derived from the World Health Organization survey of primary care patients in 14 countries. (Based on ref. *3*.)

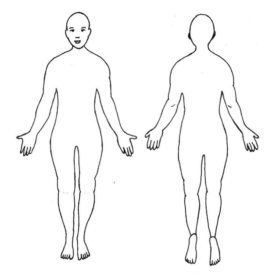

Fig. 5. Pain drawing. Instructions to pain drawing: please shade all painful areas, using the following key: ///// = pain; ::::: = numbness; *** = burning or hypersensitivity to touch.

the expanded need to prescribe opioids to patients with chronic pain; 41% of doctors waited for patients to initiate a request for pain medication.

2. CHRONIC PAIN ASSESSMENT TOOLS

The evaluation of pain begins with identifying pain location. This is most conveniently done by asking patients to complete a simple pain drawing (Fig. 5). This drawing effectively identifies all potentially important pain areas, rather than focusing only on a particular area of immediate concern to the patient.

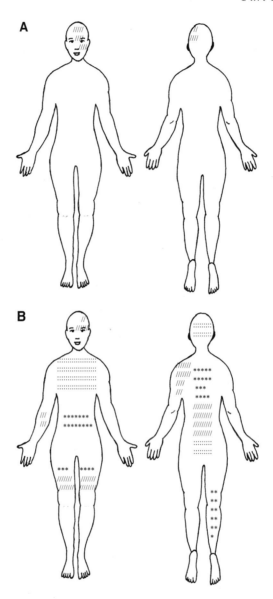

Fig. 6. Chief complaints with sample pain drawings. (**A**) episodic, left-sided, incapacitating headache; (**B**) episodic, left-sided, incapacitating headache; *(continued)*

Although the majority of patients will report more than one active pain area *(3)*,
many patients may only express verbal complaints about the area that is most
troublesome on the day of evaluation or for which the patient believes treatment
is available. For example, patients with fibromyalgia may bring a chief com-

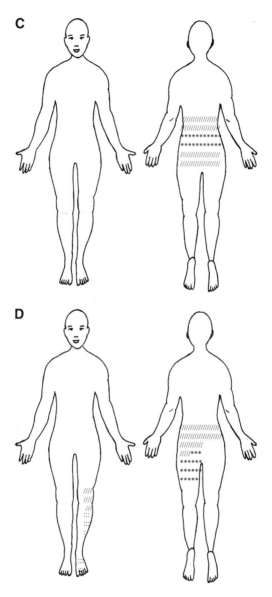

Fig. 6. *(continued)* (**C**) persistent low back pain; (**D**) persistent low back pain. Diagnoses: (**A**) migraine, (**B**) migraine plus fibromyalgia, (**C**) myofascial low back pain, and (**D**) low back pain with radiculopathy.

plaint of headache or low back pain to the doctor, despite having widespread pain areas. Failure to recognize additional pain complaints may result in an incomplete diagnosis and failure to adequately identify all of the patient's disabling complaints. Samples of completed pain drawings are shown in Fig. 6.

Some patients also find it easier to describe pain complaints using a drawing rather than verbally. A study evaluating headache complaints in 226 children showed the diagnostic sensitivity of a pain drawing for evaluating pain in patients with migraine of 93%, a specificity of 83%, and positive predictive value of 87% *(11)*. The findings in a second study were perhaps most significant, because up to half of children with symptoms of migraine failed to endorse the features of migraine that were reported during the initial interview *(12)*. For example, aura was not identified in 46% who were later discovered to have an aura; vomiting was not confirmed by 50%, nausea by 31%, unilateral location by 38%, throbbing quality by 29%, photophobia by 11%, or phonophobia by 11%.

Patients should also be asked to rate the severity of their pain. Verbal rating scales (using selected descriptive adjectives), visual analog scales (marking a severity score on a line scaled from 0 to 100), and numerical rating scales (e.g., 0 = *no pain* and 10 = *excruciating pain*) may all be used. Numerical rating scales ("select a pain severity rating between 0 and 10") are easy for patients, valid, and sensitive to treatment impact *(13)*. Furthermore, recorded numerical pain scores can be easy to use to assess and document the effectiveness of treatment interventions.

3. SUMMARY

Clinicians can gain confidence and comfort with managing chronic pain by becoming more knowledgeable about the causes, diagnoses, and treatment options for patients with chronic pain. This can be achieved with easy-to-use pain assessment strategies and tools. This book is designed to provide practical information about the pathogenesis, diagnosis, and treatment of the most common chronic pain conditions seen in typical patients, as presented in case histories. In addition, patient assessment and educational materials are provided in formats that are easy to use in most busy primary care practices. The practical information provided in this text should improve both the understanding of these conditions and the efficacy of chronic pain management options in primary care. The information and tools provided in this book should help the busy clinician simplify broad patient complaints into manageable problems, with tools for addressing commonly encountered problems.

REFERENCES ·

1. Mantyselka P, Kumpusalo E, Ahonen R, et al. Pain as a reason to visit the doctor: a study in a Finnish primary health care. Pain 2001; 89:175–180.
2. Hasselström J, Liu-Palmgren J, Rasjö-WrååK G. Prevalence of pain in general practice. Eur J Pain 2002; 6:375–385.
3. Guereje O, von Korff M, Simon GE, Gater R. Persistent pain and well-being: a World Health Organization study in primary care. JAMA 1998; 280:147–151.

4. Smith BH, Elliott AM, Chambers WA, et al. The impact of chronic pain in the community. Family Practice 2001; 18:292–299.
5. Ihlebaek C, Eriksen HR, Ursin H. Prevalence of subjective health complaints (SHC) in Norway. Scand J Public Health 2002; 30:20–29.
6. Urwin M, Symmons D, Allison T, et al. Estimating the burden of musculoskeletal disorders in the community: the comparative prevalence of symptoms at different anatomical sites, and the relation to social deprivation. Ann Rheum Dis 1998; 57: 649–655.
7. Van Tulder MW, Koes BW, Bouter LM. A cost-of-illness study of back pain in the Netherlands. Pain 1995; 62:233–240.
8. Goetzel RZ, Hawkins K, Ozminkowski, Wang S. The health and productivity cost burden of the "top 10" physical and mental health conditions affecting six large US employers in 1999. J Occup Environ Med 2003; 45:5–14.
9. Blyth FM, March LM, Nicholas MK, Cousins MJ. Chronic pain, work performance and litigation. Pain 2003; 103:41–47.
10. Potter M, Schafer S, Gonzalez-Mendez E, et al. Opioids for chronic nonmalignant pain: attitudes and practices of primary care physicians in the UCSF/Stanford Collaborative Research Network. J Fam Pract 2001; 50:145–151.
11. Stafstrom CE, Rostasy K, Minster A. The usefulness of children's drawings in the diagnosis of headache. Pediatrics 2002; 109:460–472.
12. Metsähonkala L, Sillanpaa M, Tuominen J. Headache diary in the diagnosis of childhood migraine. Headache 1997; 37:240–244.
13. Von Korff M, Jensen MP, Karoly P. Assessing global pain severity by self-report. TEN 2002; 4:34–39.

2

Summary of Pain Management Issues

Frequent Concerns in Treating Chronic Pain Patients

Chronic pain patients often come to their doctors with a myriad of complaints and expectations. When confronted with the patient with chronic pain, doctors often have their own concerns about the legitimacy of reported pain severity and associated disability, amount of time and resources that may be used by patients to address these concerns, and the inadequate amount of information they received during their medical education and training concerning the management of chronic pain.

This book is designed to fill this knowledge gap for the most common chronic pain conditions and to provide useful clinical tools to facilitate the effective approach to patient complaints in a busy office practice. Several concerns about pain legitimacy, significance, and ability to effectively treat patients with pain are addressed here. Each of these issues is addressed in greater detail in the following chapters.

Do People Really Have Chronic Pain Long After They've Recovered From an Injury?

- Chronic pain is one of the most common reasons for seeing a primary care physician. For example, about one-third of primary care visits are for musculoskeletal pain.
- Studies in laboratory animals consistently show changes in the nervous system in response to old injuries. Increased nerve sensitivity and the rewiring of nerves to activate pain pathways occur after injuries and correspond to demonstrated pain behaviors.
- Complete fabrication of pain symptoms, or malingering, is rare.
- Premorbid depression, work dissatisfaction, poor social support, and smoking increase the risk for a chronic pain complaint.

Isn't It Unusual for Children to Report Chronic Pain?

- Chronic pain complaints are reported by approximately 5 to 15% of children and adolescents.
- The most common chronic pain complaints in pediatric patients s are headache, stomach pain, and musculoskeletal pain.
- Children should not be expected to quickly "outgrow" their pain complaints. For example, chronic musculoskeletal pain persists for at least 1 year in approximately 75% of children.
- Untreated chronic pain in children is associated with significant distress and disability (including school absences) and may predispose children to chronic pain in adulthood.

From: *Chronic Pain: A Primary Care Guide to Practical Management*
Edited by: D. A. Marcus © Humana Press, Totowa, NJ

Aren't Aches and Pain Part of the Normal Aging Process?

- Approximately one-third of elderly patients are affected by chronic pain, often because of arthritis, osteoporosis-associated fractures, and lumbar stenosis. These conditions are treatable and should not be considered part of the normal aging process.
- Untreated chronic pain in elderly patients can result in depression, poor quality of life, and loss of independence.
- The ability to identify and manage pain in elderly patients will become increasingly important in primary care settings because the world population is aging.

I've Heard That You Can't Really Treat Chronic Pain and Patients Just Need to "Learn to Live With" the Pain. Are There Really Any Effective Treatments for Chronic Pain?

- Although it is not necessarily curable, chronic pain is definitely a treatable condition.
- Individual pain conditions often require different treatment modalities.
- Some treatments—e.g., stretching exercises, relaxation techniques, antidepressant therapy, and antiepileptic drugs—are beneficial for a wide variety of chronic pain conditions.

Are Opioids Effective for Patients With Chronic Pain, or Do They Usually Lead to Addiction?

- Opioids can help reduce the severity of pain, but they must be used within the context of a comprehensive pain treatment program.
- Patients with chronic pain who are treated with opioids need to be monitored closely. Approximately 25 to 30% of patients with chronic pain who are treated with opioids will demonstrate medication abuse behavior.
- Opioid misuse and abuse can be minimized by establishing realistic treatment goals, using low doses of medications, and employing strictly followed opioid contracts.

Isn't Caring for Chronic Pain Patients Too Time-Consuming for a Busy Practice?

- Chronic pain patients may have complicated complaints that cannot all be addressed in a single office visit. Patients may present multiple long-term issues to their primary care doctors: pain severity, sleep disturbance, depressed mood, work disability, and family conflicts.
- Office tools, such as pain drawings and other self-assessment tools, can help patients focus on short- and long-term goals that can be addressed with treatment. Helping patients focus on specific goals is also facilitated by using goal assessment and attainment tools. These tools can be completed by most patients with minimal instruction.
- Educational tools, such as written handouts, can reinforce treatment messages and minimize the amount of face-to-face time needed to deliver patient education.

Is It Really Important to Address Chronic Pain? Isn't My Office Time Better Spent Focusing on "Real" Medical Problems, Like Diabetes, Heart Disease, and Hypertension?

- Chronic pain complaints are very common and frequently bring patients to the doctor's office to request information and seek a diagnosis and treatment.
- Untreated chronic pain conditions can exacerbate frustration and psychological distress and result in significant disability, including school absences in children and unemployment or underemployment in adults.

- Chronic pain complaints may also be caused by or aggravated by other medical conditions, such as diabetes-related neuropathy and the aggravation of mechanical joint pain by obesity. Compliance with treatment for the primary medical disorder is often enhanced when that treatment also improves a secondary pain condition.
- Treatment options for patients with chronic pain—including exercise, relaxation skills, stress management, and appropriate use of medication—are also invaluable for maintaining overall good health and maximizing the efficacy of treatment prescribed for other medical conditions.

II

Pathogenesis

3

Pathogenesis of Chronic Pain

CASE HISTORY

Mr. Thompson, a 46-year-old school custodian, has always enjoyed his work and has an excellent work attendance record. While lifting a large bucket of water, he developed excruciating back pain that radiated down his leg and felt that he "couldn't stand up straight." He left work and went home to bed, but noticed numbness in his big toe the next morning, as well as persistent back pain. He was unable to sit up in bed and needed his wife's assistance to get out of bed. Mr. Thompson saw his doctor, who diagnosed a herniated lumbar disc with an L5 radiculopathy. Mr. Thompson proceeded to have surgery and noticed some decrease in numbness postoperatively. He and his wife were told by the surgeon that the surgery was a success. At a follow-up visit with the surgeon 1 month later, Mr. Thompson reported persistent, disabling pain. Physical examination showed good muscle strength and reflexes, and appropriate sensation in his legs. Forward flexion of the back was moderately decreased, and the muscles next to the spine were increased in bulk and tender to gentle palpation. Repeat magnetic resonance imaging and electromyographic testing were unremarkable. The surgeon provided a book showing back exercises and suggested that Mr. Thompson return to work when he felt ready. Three months after surgery, Mr. Thompson saw his family doctor, who read the surgeon's notes of good neurological outcome from the procedure. Mr. Thompson, however, continued to report persistent pain. He reported an inability to do the exercises because of pain and had not returned to work. Mr. Thompson spent the day watching television and had discontinued all household chores. Mr. Thompson noted that his wife was "just an angel," bringing him his meals in bed and helping him dress. He asked the primary care physician (PCP) for a note to continue staying home from work. Mr. Thompson was advised to begin his exercise program and return to work part time. A follow-up appointment was made in 3 months. Six months after surgery, Mr. Thompson continued to report persistent pain, as well as irritability and frustration over continued pain and disability. He remained sedentary throughout the day and had not returned to work. Mr. Thompson came to the appointment with a

From: *Chronic Pain: A Primary Care Guide to Practical Management*
Edited by: D. A. Marcus © Humana Press, Totowa, NJ

disability form and a request for handicapped parking. His wife frequently adjusted pillows behind his back and carried a drink for him. Repeat examination and review of testing again revealed no obvious pathology. The PCP became suspicious of symptom magnification and secondary gain and ordered a psychological evaluation.

* * *

This case illustrates many common features of the course of chronic pain, as well as the common change from effective worker to disabled person. Chronic pain frequently occurs in the absence of identifiable pathology, leading to the frequent misperception that the pain is imaginary or being fabricated to obtain financial benefits or solicitous behavior from others. Current research from animal models, however, clearly demonstrates long-lasting changes in central nervous system (CNS) wiring and activity as a result of an initial painful injury from which the animal has recovered. These studies suggest similar patterns of neural plasticity may be responsible for persistent pain in humans, even after any identifiable pathology has been corrected.

KEY CHAPTER POINTS

- Chronic pain is the consequence of abnormal nerve sensitivity, firing, and connections.
- Pain persisting for 3 months is unlikely to resolve spontaneously.
- Premorbid psychological distress, occupational issues, nicotine use, and a previous pain condition can be used to predict the persistence of pain.
- Complete fabrication of pain complaints or malingering occurs rarely.

Acute pain is a frequent life experience, occurring when stubbing a toe, hitting a finger with a hammer, or falling on an icy sidewalk. Acute pain typically occurs as a consequence of the injury or trauma and may be associated with symptoms of inflammation. A twisted ankle, for example, is hot, red, tender, and swollen, with spasms occurring in the surrounding muscles. These acute changes are beneficial: pain teaches the person to be more careful in the future to avoid additional injury and promotes rest for healing, a muscle spasm provides a natural protective cast, and increased blood flow brings repair cells. Healing occurs over several weeks to months and is generally associated with a reduction of pain, muscle spasm, and inflammation (Fig. 1).

Chronic pain is defined as pain lasting longer than 3 months. Chronic pain may occur as a sequel to an acute injury, as a symptom of a degenerative illness (e.g., rheumatoid arthritis), or insidiously. Chronic pain beginning after trauma is associated with greater pain severity, disability, and psychological distress than nontraumatic pain *(13)*. The link between trauma and emotional distress in patients with chronic pain may be particularly strong in males *(4)*.

Stage I. *Development of acute pain*

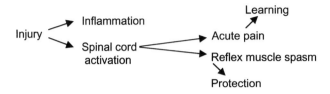

Stage II. *Resolution of acute pain*

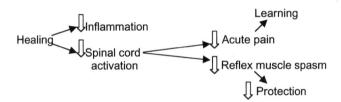

Stage III. *Progression to chronic pain*

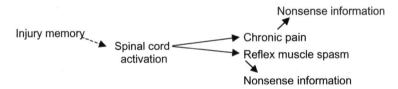

Fig. 1. Pathogenesis of acute and chronic pain. *Stage I:* Acute pain is associated with inflammation and activation of spinal pathways that send instructive pain messages to encourage future injury avoidance and cause protective muscle spasm. *Stage II:* Over ensuing weeks, injured tissues heal, inflammation resolves, and fewer central impulses are sent that can be registered as pain or trigger muscle spasm. *Stage III:* In patients who develop chronic pain, the nervous system continues to send signals for pain and muscle spasm as though in response to an acute injury, even though the injury is only a memory. Therefore, someone with chronic lumbar pain who is sitting in a chair may receive useless information that he or she is being injured and experience pain and muscle spasm, even though no active injury is present.

This association between potentially compensable injury and resultant pain severity often leads to a suspicion that chronic pain is, for the most part, imagined, exaggerated, or feigned for secondary gain (e.g., worker's compensation or disability benefits, reduced household chores, and increased spousal attention).

Why some individuals exposed to an injury will develop acute pain only whereas others develop chronic pain is unknown. Healing appears to occur with both types of pain, but pain signals are reduced with healing in those with acute pain only. In patients who develop chronic pain it is believed that neural connections are rewired and neural stimulus sensitivity changes during the healing process (Fig. 1). These changes in central plasticity have been well defined in rodent models of chronic pain *(5)*.

1. PATHOPHYSIOLOGY OF CHRONIC PAIN

Investigators have identified consistent behavioral and physiological changes in animal studies that occur in response to trauma. These findings have been used to isolate physiology from possible secondary gain issues and help to confirm the veracity of chronic pain complaints for both the health care provider and patient. The most useful findings have been obtained from partial sciatic nerve ligation studies in the rat *(6,7)*. In these studies, a temporary ligature is tied around the exposed sciatic nerve and later removed. Although the nerve regains neurological function, the rats display pain behaviors-they attempt to auto-amputate the affected leg (i.e., commit *autotomy*) by biting it. Autotomy is believed to be the laboratory equivalent of human pain behaviors, such as verbalizing complaints or rubbing the painful back. Autopsy of rats used in these experiments revealed widespread neurological changes, with rewiring of neurons in the dorsal horn, spinal cord, and brain *(8,9)*. Such changes increase neuronal excitation, as well as the risk for abnormal connections from touch nerves to pain pathways.

The most carefully studied area in chronic pain models is the dorsal horn. Evaluations of models of chronic pain rats reveal increased sensitivity of second-order neurons in the dorsal horn, with an increased number of action potentials and spontaneous discharges. These changes result in increased sensitivity to painful stimuli, or hyperalgesia. In addition, central terminals of mechanoreceptors are redistributed within the dorsal horn to connect with pain pathway neurons that would normally be triggered by pain stimuli (Fig. 2). In this case, stimulation with nonpainful tactile stimuli, such as light touch or vibration, will activate pain neurons and the result in a perception of pain or allodynia. The size of the neuronal receptive field also increases in the dorsal horn, resulting in the spread of pain perception to areas that were not originally involved with the injury that induced acute pain.

This model is similar to that of chronic lumbar pain that persists after "successful" herniorrhaphy and discectomy, as occurred with Mr. Thompson. Similar to the rat, the human nerve may recover function while significant physiologic and microscopic neural changes persist (Fig. 3). Patients may express symptoms of neural rewiring, including hyperalgesia, allodynia, and the spread of pain (Table 1).

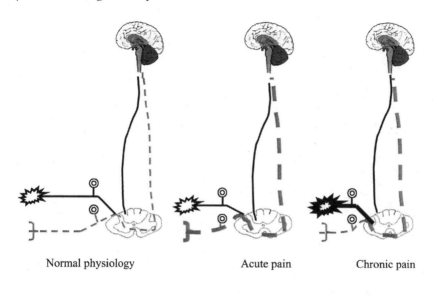

| Normal physiology | Acute pain | Chronic pain |

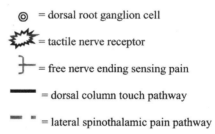

◎ = dorsal root ganglion cell

= tactile nerve receptor

= free nerve ending sensing pain

▬ = dorsal column touch pathway

▬ ▪ = lateral spinothalamic pain pathway

Fig. 2. Pathogenesis of chronic pain. Normally, stimulation of tactile receptors activates the dorsal column pathway and activation of free nerve endings activates the lateral spinothalamic pain pathway. Painful stimuli that are active during acute pain increase the signaling rate within the lateral spinothalamic pain pathway. Physiological changes occurring during chronic pain result in stimulation of tactile receptors (e.g., touch or vibration) activating lateral spinothalamic pathways, which results in the false interpretation by the brain that pain-sensitive nerve endings have been activated.

This model has been tested in humans with the use of preemptive analgesia, i.e., locally anesthetizing an area prior to pain exposure. Preemptive analgesia is intended to reduce persistent pain by blocking spinal input from an acute injury. Preemptive analgesia has been shown to effectively reduce postoperative pain and narcotic use in patients undergoing limb surgery or mastectomy *(10)*. In one study of individuals with lower extremity amputations, painful phantom limb pain developed in 64% of patients within 1 week after standard surgery *(11)*.

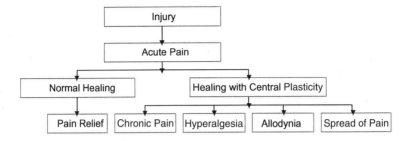

Fig. 3. Course of acute pain. The injury causing acute pain may heal and the pain may resolve. Alternatively, extensive neural changes may occur during the healing process, resulting in persistent pain and changes in neural physiology.

Table 1
Neurological Changes With Injury and Resultant Symptomatic Complaints

Physiological change	Medical symptom	Typical patient complaints	Typical exam finding
Lower pain threshold Increased action potentials Spontaneous firing	Hyperalgesia: increased sensitivity to painful stimuli	Increased sensitivity to scratches, pinches, or hot water	Exaggerated pain response to gentle pinprick
Touch mechanoreceptor neurons reconnect to pain pathways	Allodynia: nonpainful touch stimuli perceived as painful	Bedclothes touching bare feet is painful Wind blowing across or cool water touching a limb is painful	Limb withdrawal and grimacing from light touch Guarding painful area to prevent touching
Increase in receptive field size	Spread of pain to adjacent, noninjured areas	Pain spreads from originally injured ankle to affect entire foot	Tenderness to palpation in areas near site of original injury

Preemptive analgesia with epidural bupivacaine administered for 72 hours before surgery reduced the incidence of phantom limb pain to 27%. Preemptive analgesia studies have shown that the risk for the development of persistent pain is minimized by preventing the initial activation of spinal pain pathways.

2. EXPECTED COURSE OF CHRONIC PAIN

Pain persisting longer than 3 months is unlikely to resolve spontaneously *(12)*. Prospective studies of patients with a complaint of new low back pain who are

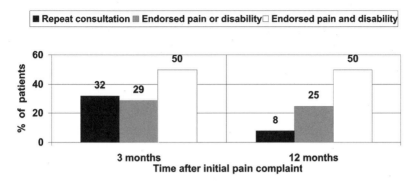

Fig. 4. Discrepancy between reconsultation rate and persistence of symptoms following acute back pain. Disability involves difficulty performing activities of daily living. (Based on data from ref. *13.*)

seen in a primary care setting have demonstrated symptoms persisting longer than 3 months in 48 to 79% of these patients and longer than 12 months in 42 to 75% of these patients *(13–15)*. Anecdotally, however, doctors often notice only a small minority of patients consult with them again following the initial assessment of acute pain. This suggests that most instances of acute pain resolve spontaneously. In a sample of 463 new consultations to a general practitioner for acute back pain, the percentage of patients returning with pain complaints was very low *(13)*. When patients were contacted and asked directly about persistent and troublesome symptoms, however, reports of chronic pain and disability were high (Fig. 4). These data suggest that significant pain complaints often do persist, despite a lack of reconsultation to the doctor. In addition, pain failing to resolve after 3 months is likely to persist for at least 12 months. Therefore, treatment should be initiated for pain that persists at least 3 months.

3. PREDICTORS OF CHRONIC PAIN

Medical science is unable to explain why two persons exposed to a seemingly similar injury will have different pain outcomes—one with only acute pain and the other with years of chronic pain. Several studies have identified physical, psychological, and social features that predict a greater likelihood of persistent pain *(14,16–21)* (Table 2). Interestingly, gender and premorbid psychological characteristics predict persistent pain for seemingly disparate pain conditions, such as myofascial masticatory pain and chronic low back pain. These features can be used to predict a greater likelihood of persistent pain when positive predictive features are present and indicate the need for a more aggressive type of therapy.

Table 2
Predictors of Chronic Pain

Pain indicators	Factors predicting chronic pain
Physical findings	Back pain associated with restricted lumbar flexion
	Abnormal neurological examination
Symptoms	Nonlocalized pain
	Insidious pain onset
	Back pain radiates to leg
Psychosocial factors	
Personal issues	Female sex
	History of chronic pain
	History of trauma
	Delay before consultation (>30 days)
	Dissatisfaction with consultant
	Depression or psychological distress
	Nicotine use
Family issues	Lack of social support
	Family delegitimizes pain
	Family history of chronic pain
Occupational issues	Dissatisfaction with work or work status
	Unemployment
	Previous job change related to pain

Certain types of chronic pain also occur more commonly in people with certain occupations. For example, professions strongly associated with high risk for developing chronic low back pain include those that require lifting, pushing, or pulling 25 lb or more; prolonged standing; or sustained postures *(22,23)*. Such high-risk occupations include some health care occupations (e.g., nurse's aides, nurses, dentists, and chiropractors), construction workers, automobile mechanics, housekeepers/janitors, and hairstylists *(24–27)*. A recent survey of nurses' aides, for example, revealed complaints of musculoskeletal pain during the previous 2 weeks in 89% of respondents, with 51% rating the pain as intense *(28)*. A work-related back injury is more likely to occur in individuals with these high-risk occupations than in sedentary workers. In addition, identifying a worker as being at high risk for chronic pain based on physical, psychological, or social characteristics may result in early and more aggressive treatment.

4. IDENTIFYING THE MALINGERER

To provide appropriate care for patients with chronic pain, the clinician must be able to trust the patient's self-reports of discomfort and pain experiences, because there are no objective measures of pain. The clinician must also con-

---

Box 1
Warning Signs for Malingering

- Uncooperative with providing historical data.
- Uncooperative with basic physical examination, including gait testing.
- Refuses additional testing or reports tests were completed and normal, although the doctor cannot access them because they are lost, destroyed, or at a facility whose name is unknown to the patient.
- Insists on one particular treatment and refuses all other options.
- Interview focuses exclusively on completion of disability forms or providing specific requested prescriptions rather than on improving patient symptoms.

---

sider the fact that the patient's descriptions and displays of pain are influenced by past pain experiences, gender, and cultural background. Different responses to pain can be readily noted in the labor suite, for example, where uterine contractions of the same magnitude result in quiet, deep breathing in one woman and loud cries from another. The stoic person may report pain as discomfort, with little display of pain mannerisms, whereas a more demonstrative person may use pain descriptors like "searing" or "crippling" and frequently change positions, grimace, or moan in pain during the interview. Health care providers may question the validity of reports from either type of patient and be reluctant to prescribe potentially habit-forming medications to patients with either seemingly minor or exaggerated pain complaints. It is important to remember, however, that the most reasonable patient can be frustrated by chronic pain and the resulting sleep deprivation, along with an apparent need to "prove" there's really something wrong when all test results are normal can result in seemingly exaggerated complaints. It is essential to treat all patients with respect and openness and let them see that you trust each patient as a treatment partner, not an adversary. When patients trust their health care provider in return, they are most likely to cooperate with evaluations.

Malingering patients are fortunately rare and are usually easy to spot (Box 1). Malingerers are consciously aware that they are reporting false symptoms. They typically believe that they can fool most doctors, but it is doubtful that they will be able to fool every doctor. Therefore, malingerers try to avoid providing information, either during the history or examination, that could identify the false character of their complaints. They will avoid providing any historical information and insist the doctor rely on available medical records or that the doctor provide descriptions to which they can agree. Later, if a discrepancy is identified, they will rightly remind the doctor that *they* didn't state the falsehood; either the chart or doctor did. These patients will also insist that they cannot complete a pain questionnaire or a physical examination because their pain is intolerable. Malingerers have learned to successfully make health care providers feel guilty about not treating them, even when the provider does not feel comfortable prescribing therapy. Malingerers will usually insist that they need medication first before undergoing any diagnostic evaluations and will threaten to go to the emergency department if the doctor fails to provide pain relief. In contrast to the malingerer, who will refuse additional testing, most patients with chronic pain are eager to have additional tests to identify their pathology.

Patients with "legitimate" pain typically want to get better and will, therefore, cooperate with examinations. Some patients will seem to exaggerate the severity of their symptoms, although this may be in anticipation of a painful examination or their perception that the doctor does not believe the pain is real. If a patient cannot be adequately cooperative during an examination to allow the clinician to establish a diagnosis, the clinician should explain that his or her ability to select an effective treatment is contingent on establishing a diagnosis; if necessary, a second appointment should be made at a time when the patient is more likely to be cooperative. The malingerer will take his or her business elsewhere, whereas the person who is truly interested in improvement is likely to cooperate during a repeat visit.

Signs of nonorganic pathology, symptom magnification, or malingering have been categorized by Waddell and colleagues (29). These categories were recently evaluated for their usefulness in identifying nonorganic symptoms in patients with pain (30). Waddell's signs include superficial skin tenderness, diffuse tenderness, pain with pressing on the top of the head or rotation of the thorax, change in straight leg-raise performance when distracted from testing, give-away weakness, nondermatomal sensory loss, and excessive expression of pain. As expected, patients with these signs tend to endorse higher pain levels and greater disability. Contrary to prediction, however, they do not correlate with psychological distress or secondary gain, nor do they discriminate between patients with organic and nonorganic pathology. For example, patients may produce a greater straight leg-raise test when distracted because they anticipate pain with testing and tense muscles before testing occurs. This does not mean that the patient is exaggerating the level of restriction, but rather that straight leg-raise testing should be performed during distraction to achieve optimal testing accuracy.

5. SUMMARY

Experimental rodent studies clearly demonstrate changes in neural connections and activity that persist despite the recovery of gross neural function. Documentation of neural abnormalities that result in symptoms of hyperalgesia, allodynia, and the spread of pain in rodent models adds credence to patient reports of similar symptoms after recovery from an acute injury is complete. Knowledge of these studies is beneficial for both the health care provider and patient, particularly because there are no objective measures of pain that can be identified with gross clinical, laboratory, or radiographic testing.

REFERENCES

1. Turk DC, Okifuji A, Starz TW, Sinclair JD. Effects of type of symptom onset on psychological distress in fibromyalgia syndrome patients. Pain 1996; 68:423–430.
2. Turk DC, Okifuji A. Perception of traumatic onset, compensation status, and physical findings: impact on pain severity, emotional distress, and disability in chronic pain patients. J Behav Med 1996; 19:435–453.
3. Marcus DA. Disability and chronic post-traumatic headache. Headache 2003; 43: 117–121.
4. Spertus IL, Burns J, Glenn B, Lofland K, McCracken L. Gender differences in associations between history and adjustment among chronic pain patients. Pain 1999; 82:97–102.
5. Decosterd I, Woolf CJ. Spared nerve injury: animal model of persistent peripheral neuropathic pain. Pain 2000; 87:149–158.
6. Bennett GJ, Xie YK. A peripheral mononeuropathy in rat that produces disorders of pain sensation like those seen in man. Pain 1988; 33:87–107.
7. Seltzer Z, Dubner R, Shir Y. A novel behavioral model of neuropathic pain disorders produced in rats by partial sciatic nerve injury. Pain 1990; 43:205–218.
8. Guilbaud G, Gautron M, Jazat F, et al. Time course of degeneration and regeneration of myelinated nerve fibers following chronic loose ligatures of the rat sciatic nerve: can nerve lesions be linked to the abnormal pain-related behaviours? Pain 1993; 53:147–158.
9. Behbehani MM, Dollberg-Stolik O. Partial sciatic nerve ligation results in an enlargement of the receptive field and enhancement of the response of dorsal horn neurons to noxious stimulation by an adenosine agonist. Pain 1994; 58: 421–428.
10. Aida S, Baba H, Yamakura T, et al. The effectiveness of preemptive analgesia varies according to the type of surgery: a randomized, double-blind study. Anesth Analg 1999; 89:711–716.
11. Bach S, Noreng MF, Tjellden NU. Phantom limb pain in amputees during the first 12 months following limb amputation after preoperative lumbar epidural blockade. Pain 1988; 33:156–161.
12. Carey TS, Garrett JM, Jackman A, Hadler N. Recurrence and care seeking after acute back pain: results of a long-term follow-up study. North Carolina Back Pain Project. Med Care 1999; 37:157–164.
13. Croft PR, Macfarlane GJ, Papageogiou AC, et al. Outcome of low back pain in general practice: a prospective study. BMJ 1998; 316:1356–1359.
14. Thomas E, Silman AJ, Croft PR, et al. Predicting who develops chronic low back pain in primary care: a prospective study. BMJ 1999; 318:1662–1667.
15. Schiotz-Christensen B, Nielsen GL, Hansen VK, et al. Long-term prognosis of acute back pain in patients seen in general practice: a 1-year prospective follow-up study. Fam Pract 1999; 16:223–232.

16. Macfarlane GJ, Thomas E, Croft PR, et al. Predictors of early improvement in low back pain amongst consulters to general practice: the influence of premorbid and episode-related factors. Pain 1999; 80:113–119.
17. Reis S, Hermoni D, Borkan JM. A new look at low back pain complaints in primary care: a RAMBAM Israeli Family Practice Research Network study. J Fam Pract 1999; 48:299–303.
18. Croft PR, Papageogiou AC, Ferry S, et al. Psychological distress and low back pain. Evidence from a prospective study in the general population. Spine 1995; 20:2731–2737.
19. Scott SC, Goldberg MS, Mayo NE, Stock SR, Poitras B. The association between cigarette smoking and back pain in adults. Spine 1999; 24:1090–1098.
20. Palmer KT, Syddall H, Cooper C, Coggon D. Smoking and musculoskeletal disorders: findings from a British national survey. Ann Rheum Dis 2003; 62:33–36.
21. Velly AM, Gornitsky M, Philippe P. Contributing factors to chronic myofascial pain: a case-control study. Pain 2003; 104:491–499.
22. Macfarlane GJ, Thomas E, Papageogiou AC, et al. Exercise and physical activities as predictors of future low back pain. Spine 1997; 22:1143–1149.
23. Smedley J, Egger P, Cooper C, Coggon D. Prospective cohort study of predictors of incident low back pain in nurses. BMJ 1997; 314:1225–1228.
24. Leighton DJ, Reilly T. Epidemiological aspects of back pain: the incidence and prevalence of back pain in nurses compared to the general population. Occup Med (Lond) 1995; 45:263–267.
25. Diakow PR, Cassidy JD. Back pain in dentists. J Manipulative Physiol Ther 1984; 7:85–88.
26. Mior S, Diakow PR. Prevalence of back pain in chiropractors. J Manipulative Ther 1987; 10:305–309.
27. Guo HR, Tanakas S, Cameron LL, et al. Back pain among workers in the United States: national estimates and workers at high risk. Am J Int Med 1995; 28:591–602.
28. Eriksen W. The prevalence of musculoskeletal pain in Norwegian nurses' aides. Int Arch Occup Environ Health 2003; 76:625–630.
29. Waddell G, McCulloch JA, Kummel E, et al. Nonorganic physical signs in low-back pain. Spine 1980; 5:117–125.
30. Fishbain DA, Cole B, Cutler RB, et al. A structured evidence-based review on the meaning of nonorganic physical signs: Waddell signs. Pain Medicine 2003; 4:141–181.

CME QUESTIONS—CHAPTER 3

1. Experimental nerve injuries can result in rewiring of the central nervous system that causes:
   a. Lowered pain threshold
   b. Increased sensitivity to pain
   c. Spread of pain to contiguous body regions
   d. All of the above

2. Choose the correct statement:
   a. Ninety percent of injuries causing acute pain will lead to chronic pain
   b. Pain persisting for 3 mo will likely persist if untreated
   c. Pain beginning after an automobile accident is usually a sign of malingering
   d. None of the above

3. Which of the following occupations is not associated with high risk for developing chronic back pain?
   a. Hairstylist
   b. Receptionist
   c. Carpenter
   d. Janitor
   e. Nurse

4. Which of the following patient characteristics is associated with high risk for chronic pain?
   a. Male gender
   b. No history of depression or anxiety
   c. No history of previous injury or chronic pain
   d. Supportive family
   e. Nicotine use

III

Common Chronic Pain Conditions

CASE HISTORY

Ms. Sharpe is a 38-year-old high school administrator. She describes incapacitating headaches associated with vomiting that take her to bed. She reports having troublesome headaches two to three times a week, although she rarely misses work for headache. She does report that her family becomes angry with her for wanting to spend Friday evenings in bed rather than going to the movies or some other family activity. She has never found relief from analgesics or triptans. Her primary care physician (PCP) prescribes a nighttime dose of amitriptyline and arranges a follow-up visit in 3 weeks. Three weeks later, she reports no headache improvement and her PCP subsequently prescribes trials with propranolol, verapamil, and valproate, all without relief. At this point, Ms. Sharpe is given a daily headache-recording diary, which she is asked to keep over the next month. When the diary is reviewed, her PCP notes that, in addition to the one or two severe migraine episodes each week, she also records a daily headache that fluctuates in severity between mild and moderate, lasting most of the day. She also records daily use of four to six tablets of Excedrin per day, four ibuprofen tablets 3 days a week, and Imitrex twice a week. In her history, she also notes drinking approximately six cups of coffee daily. Because excessive use of analgesics, caffeinated products, and other acute care medications (e.g., triptans) typically aggravates underlying headache disorders, Ms. Sharpe's PCP asks her to discontinue all acute therapies and limit coffee to two cups a day. She is also prescribed Relafen twice daily as treatment for rebound headache, and is allowed to take one additional Relafen dose on days with severe headache. One month later, she reports that she is no longer having daily headache, but still has a severe migraine once a week. This is easily managed with infrequent use of Imitrex, which had previously proven ineffective when taken in conjunction with daily analgesics.

* * *

This case demonstrates the importance of extracting an accurate history of headache pattern to correctly assign a headache diagnosis and prescribe effective therapy. Because headaches often begin in childhood or adolescence, a

From: *Chronic Pain: A Primary Care Guide to Practical Management*
Edited by: D. A. Marcus © Humana Press, Totowa, NJ

full headache history can become quite lengthy, especially because headache characteristics may change with age and reproductive status in women. This chapter provides tools to help focus patient questioning to accurately identify diagnosis(es). After identifying headache diagnosis(es), treatment is relatively straight forward, with treatments divided into first-, second-, and third-line therapies for most commonly recurring headaches.

KEY CHAPTER POINTS

- Chronic headache needs to be treated because of its association with significant disability.
- Migraine is the most common type of headache presenting to a PCP.
- Hallmarks of serious headache include change in headache pattern, posterior head pain, headache beginning after middle age, and neurological abnormalities.
- Regular, frequent use of analgesics and other acute headache medications aggravates underlying headaches and prevents efficacy of standard therapy.

1. EPIDEMIOLOGY AND IMPACT OF CHRONIC HEADACHE

Headache is a common chief complaint for the primary care physician (PCP), listed among the top 10 reasons for women to seek a PCP office visit in national surveys conducted in 1997 and 1998 *(1)*. In addition, most patients with headache are managed by their PCPs. The National Ambulatory Medical Care Survey showed that 72% of migraineurs were treated by PCPs compared with only 17% who saw neurologists *(2)*.

1.1. Chronic Headache Diagnoses Seen in Primary Care

A survey of European adults revealed a 93% lifetime prevalence of headache, with a 3-month prevalence of 70% *(3)*. The most common types of chronically recurring headaches are tension-type and migraine headaches. Tension-type headache affects approximately 88% of females and 69% of males over their lifetimes *(4)*. The American Migraine II survey of nearly 30,000 Americans identified migraine in 18% of females and 6.5% of males *(5)*. Although tension-type headache is more prevalent than migraine, migraineurs are more likely to seek care, with the number of family practitioner office visits for migraine surpassing that for tension-type headache *(6)*. An international survey of patients seeking treatment for headache from PCPs revealed a diagnosis of migraine in 94%, with tension-type headache in only 4% (Fig. 1) *(7)*.

Cluster headache is an uncommon, but important chronic headache, occurring in fewer than 1% of adults. Curiously, the male predominance of cluster has decreased in recent decades, with a 6:1 male predominance reported during the 1960s decreasing to a 2:1 predominance in the 1990s *(8)*. Changes in lifestyle, such as increased female use of tobacco and nicotine products, as well as increased role in the workforce, have been postulated to contribute to

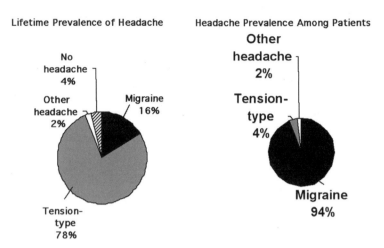

Fig. 1. Comparison of the prevalence of migraine and tension-type headache in the general population vs individuals who seek treatment from primary care physicians. Although migraine occurs in only 16% of the general population, 94% of patients who seek care for headache through a primary care physician have migraine. (Based on refs. *4* and *7*.)

this changing epidemiology. Patients with cluster headaches often engage in bizarre behavior during a cluster attack, such as hitting their heads against the wall or pounding the painful eye. Many patients and their families become concerned that this signifies serious psychiatric disease, rather than a reaction to intense pain. It is, therefore, useful to ask patients with cluster headaches about any of these behaviors to assure them that they represent typical cluster behaviors. Clearly, potentially harmful behaviors should be discouraged. As cluster pain is controlled, behaviors will remit.

Chronic headache may also begin as a consequence to head injury. A survey of college athletes who had sustained sport-related concussions revealed headache in 87% of football players and 50% of soccer players *(9)*. Posttrauma headache begins within 14 days of a head injury associated with concussion. In 60% of cases, headache will persist longer than 2 months *(10)*. Posttraumatic headache resolves for most patients within 6 to 12 months after injury, persisting longer than 1 year in 33% and longer than 3 years in 15 to 20% *(11)*. Type of injury may predict likelihood of persistent posttraumatic headache. A survey of victims of rear-end collisions revealed headache 7 years after the accident in 22% who reported associated whiplash vs 7% without whiplash *(12)*. Headache prevalence in a comparator, nonaccident group was 5%. Interestingly, the presence or resolution of litigation does not significantly impact posttraumatic headache *(11,13–15)*.

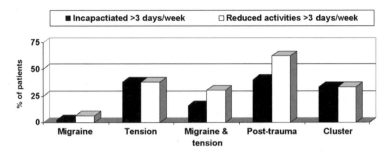

Fig. 2. Rate of disability owing to chronic headache. Non-migraine headaches are associated with significantly greater disability than migraine ($p < 0.001$). (Based on ref. *19*.)

1.2. Headache Impact and Disability

Societal impact from chronic headache is large because of the high prevalence of headache. In addition, individual impact is also significant. A recent study showed similar economic impact from headache-related disability in Europe, North America, and Central America *(16)*. Migraineurs reported an average of 19.6 lost workdays annually because of absenteeism and reduced productivity. Additional employer cost for each employed migraineur was estimated at more than $3000 annually. Significant disability may also be associated with non-migraine headache *(17)*. Schwartz and colleagues evaluated headache-related work disability in a community sample of more than 13,000 employed adults *(18)*. Work absenteeism or reduced productivity as a result of headache occurred in 9.4% of adults. Migraine was more likely to be associated with work absenteeism than tension-type headache (57 vs 43%), whereas tension-type headache was more likely to cause reduced work productivity (64 vs 36%). A recent survey of 289 treatment-seeking headache sufferers similarly identified greater overall disability for work and daily activities in patients with non-migraine headache (Fig. 2) *(19)*.

As noted by our patient, Ms. Sharpe, headache-related disability extends beyond work loss. The American Migraine II survey identified frequent disability for school or work activities, household chores, and social functions (Fig. 3) *(5)*. A similar survey of more than 8000 households in the United States and England identified significant impact of migraine on both headache sufferers and their household members *(20)*. For migraineurs who lived with a household partner, 85% reported significant reduction in ability to perform household chores, 45% missed family or social activities, and 32% avoided making plans because of fear of having a headache. In addition, parents with migraine

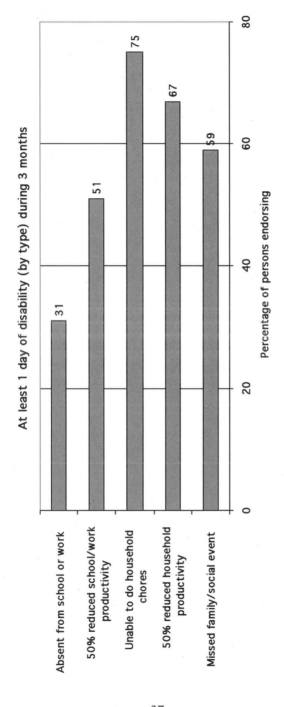

Fig. 3. Disability identified in migraineurs by American Migraine II survey. (Based on data from ref. 5.)

Box 1
Warning Signs and Symptoms Suggesting the Need for Additional Work-Up

- New headache or significant change in headache character within 2 years
- Posterior head or neck pain
- Patient ≥ 50 years old
- Abnormal neurological examination findings

Based on ref. *21.*

---

reported substantial impact on their children, including reduced ability to parent children and school absenteeism for the child because of the parent's headache. Like Ms. Sharpe, migraineurs are more likely to reduce productivity, household chores, and family or social commitments rather than miss work or school.

2. EVALUATION OF HEADACHE COMPLAINTS

Patients address headache complaints with their PCPs to ensure that the pain is not caused by serious pathology, such as a brain tumor, and to obtain symptomatic relief from benign headache. Several clinical characteristics have been associated with more serious headache (*see* Box 1) *(21)*. Patients with any warning signs of serious headache or associated additional medical or neurological symptoms should be evaluated to rule out serious causes of headache (*see* Box 2). Fortunately, most patients who seek treatment for headache have migraine, a benign and fairly easy-to-treat headache. Interestingly, although tension-type headache is a more prevalent headache than migraine, the vast majority of treatment-seekers are migraineurs *(7)*.

When asking diagnostic questions, it is essential to specify if a patient has one or more unique types of headache, for example, frequent, mild tension-type headache and infrequent, incapacitating migraine. If this is not clarified, patients may lump the symptoms from all different headaches together as they are described. In this case, a patient with both migraine and tension-type headache may report daily headache and being bedridden with headache episodes, leading to the false perception that the patient is exaggerating headache symptoms. Patients rarely have more than two unique types of headache. If patients report many headache "types," ask them to describe their most severe headache and their most frequent headache for diagnostic purposes.

A structured diagnostic interview can help focus patients to identify worrisome headache features, as well as patterns of common benign headaches (*see*

Box 2
Evaluation of New-Onset or Worrisome Headaches

- History and physical examination
  - Complete review of systems
  - Cervical spine examination
    - Resting posture
    - Active range of motion
    - Palpation
  - Neurological evaluation
    - Gait
    - Fundoscopy for papilledema
    - Assess symmetry of face and eye movements
    - Strength and reflex testing
    - Sensation to touch
    - Able to identify two of three numbers drawn in the palm without looking
- Laboratory
  - Radiological testing
    - Computed tomography or magnetic resonance imaging (MRI) of brain
    - X-ray of cervical spine for mechanical abnormalities [a]
    - MRI of cervical spine for radiculopathy [b]
  - Blood work
    - Autoimmune tests (antinuclear antibody)
    - Hematology (blood count)
      - Sedimentation rate and temporal arteritis workup for new headache in patients aged >50 years
    - Chemistries (electrolytes; liver and kidney function tests)
    - Endocrine (thyroid function tests)
    - Infectious (rapid plasma reagin for syphilis)

---

[a] Mechanical abnormalities include abnormal posture, restricted range of motion, or pain reproduced with neck motion.

[b] Radiculopathy should be considered if focal strength, reflex, or sensory loss in an arm is present.

Box 3). Stable headache patterns can often be distinguished by applying the information learned through the structured interview to a diagnostic algorithm (*see* Fig. 4).

3. HEADACHE DIAGNOSIS

Benign headaches are diagnosed by identifying common patterns. Recall of headache patterns can be difficult for many patients, particularly if they have

---

Box 3
Questions To Be Answered by New Headache Patients

---

1. How long have your headaches been the way they are now?
   If new or change in headache occurred within past 2 years, consider more extensive evaluation.
2. Do you have one type of headache or more?
   If > type, ask questions to identify each type of headache.
3. Does your headache occur intermittently, or do you always have head pain?
   Ask about daily prescription or over-the-counter analgesic use if daily.
4. How often do you get your headache?
5. How long does each headache episode usually last?
   Headaches lasting <2 hours may be indicate cluster headaches. Also, the time course of headache may dictate therapy: short-acting medications are best for headaches that reach maximum intensity quickly; long-acting medications are often needed for headaches lasting ≥12 hours.
6. What do you typically do when you have a headache?
   a. *Are usual activities reduced or curtailed?*
   b. *Do you go to bed?*
   c. *Do you need to turn off the television, radio, or lights in the room?*
7. Are you having a headache right now? If so, it this how severe your headaches usually get, or is this an especially "good" or "bad" day?
   Patient behavior in the clinic can be compared with historical reports if the patient is having a typical headache during the examination.
8. Where is the pain located? Is it always in the same location?
   Headache pain typically shifts among different areas on the head during different headache episodes. Pain that is always located in the same spot (with the exception of cluster headache, which usually involves the same eye with each episode) or is located in the back of the head or neck often requires additional work-up.
9. Any other new problems since the headache began?
   Identification of new medical or neurological symptoms will suggest the need for additional evaluations.

---

frequent headache or two types of headache. In this circumstance, daily headache diary recordings for 1 month can be a useful tool to help elucidate headache pattern and diagnosis (Fig. 5). (A sample diary is provided in Appendix E.)

Patients with frequent or daily headache often focus on their most troubling headache, neglecting to mention the additional frequent headache that is often associated with medication overuse. Diaries will also help identify if menstruation is a consistent headache trigger.

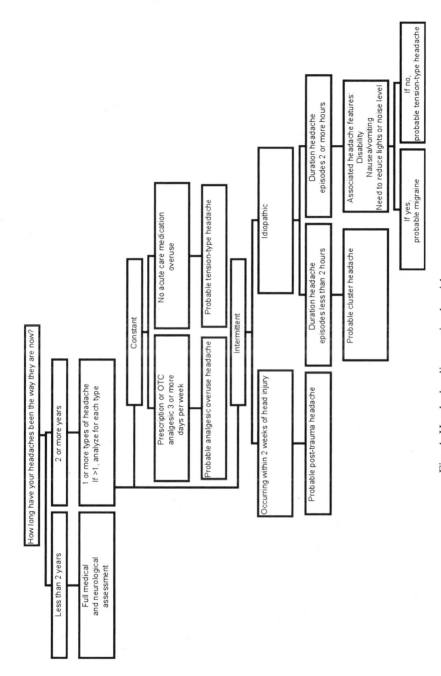

Fig. 4. Headache diagnostic algorithm.

Patient A. Intermittent, moderate-to-severe headache lasting >24 hours

Day 08 / 03 / 03	Severity (0-10)				Medication used (Prescription & OTC)	Menstrual days
Sunday	0	0	0	0		
Monday	0	0	0	0		
Tuesday	0	5	8	4	4 Excedrin	
Wednesday	3	0	0	0	1 Excedrin	
Thursday	0	0	0	0		
Friday	0	0	0	0		X
Saturday	0	0	0	0		X

Patient A diagnosis: Episodic migraine, nonmenstrual
Treatment recommendation: Acute therapy with long-acting triptan

Patient B. Intermittent, disabling headache occurring with menses

Day 12 / 14 / 01	Severity (0-10)				Medication used (Prescription & OTC)	Menstrual days
Sunday	0	0	0	0		
Monday	4	6	0	0	2 Excedrin	X
Tuesday	0	5	8	4	4 Excedrin	X
Wednesday	0	0	7	6	2 Aleve	X
Thursday	0	0	0	0		X
Friday	0	0	0	0		
Saturday	0	0	0	0		

Patient B diagnosis: Menstrual migraine
Treatment recommendation: 5-day course of treatment perimenstrually

Patient C. Daily headache

Day 06 / 20 / 02	Severity (0-10)				Medication used (Prescription & OTC)	Menstrual days
Sunday	2	4	3	2	4 Excedrin, 2 Tylenol	
Monday	1	3	0	0	2 Tylenol	
Tuesday	0	4	6	4	6 Excedrin, 2 Fiorinol	
Wednesday	1	3	2	2	3 Ibuprofen	
Thursday	4	2	1	0	2 Imitrex	
Friday	2	3	5	0	2 Imitrex, 1 Fiorinol	
Saturday	1	2	2	1	3 Ibuprofen	

Patient C diagnosis: Medication overuse headache
Treatment recommendation: Discontinue current therapy; use Aleve twice daily;
reassess diary in one month

Fig. 5. Diary samples compared with headache diagnoses and treatment recommendations.

Patient D. Daily mild headache, with occasional incapacitating headache lasting 8-12 hours

Day 06 / 20 / 02	Severity (0-10)				Medication used (Prescription & OTC)	Menstrual days
Sunday	2	1	3	2		
Monday	1	3	0	0		
Tuesday	0	6	8	7	6 Excedrin, 2 Fiorinol	
Wednesday	0	0	2	2		X
Thursday	0	2	1	0		X
Friday	2	3	0	0		X
Saturday	0	0	2	1		X

Patient D diagnosis: Combined migraine & tension-type headache
Treatment recommendation: Preventive therapy plus fast-acting triptan when headache severity exceeds 5/10

Patient E. Cycle of brief, excruciating nightly headaches lasting 90 minutes

Day 10 / 13 / 01	Severity (0-10)				Medication used (Prescription & OTC)	Menstrual days
Sunday	0	0	0	10		
Monday	0	0	0	10		
Tuesday	0	0	0	10		
Wednesday	0	0	0	9		Headache 24
Thursday	10	0	0	9		
Friday	0	0	0	10		
Saturday	0	0	0	10		

Patient E diagnosis: Cluster headache
Treatment recommendation: Verapamil daily plus O$_2$ with attacks

Fig. 5. *(Continued from previous page.)*

Contrasting features of different headache patterns help distinguish most common, chronically recurring headaches (Fig. 6). Migraine headaches are intermittent and result in patients needing to curtail work activities. Although migraine is disabling, it usually occurs infrequently, usually once or twice monthly. Some patients have frequent migraine, at most typically twice weekly. Migraine is not a daily headache. Each episode of migraine typically lasts approximately 6 to 12 hours. Tension-type headache, by contrast, is more frequent and long lasting, with milder episodes often lasting all day. Cluster headache is a very short-lasting, high intensity headache that often occurs at night, approximately 90 minutes after initiating sleep, when dream sleep occurs. Pain is typically unilateral orbital

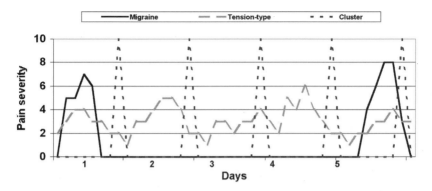

Fig. 6. Pattern of common recurring headaches. Some patients will have a combination of migraine and tension-type patterns, experiencing both patterns simultaneously. Posttraumatic headache may resemble migraine or tension-type headache. Medication overuse headache has a daily headache pattern similar to that for tension-type headache. Cluster headaches are characteristically very brief and very intense, and tend to recur predictably during a cluster period.

or periorbital. Although cluster headache is generally associated with autonomic features, like pupillary changes or discharge from the eye and nostril, few cluster headache patients will note these features in their history, possibly because of the extreme intensity of the head pain. By contrast, migraineurs often endorse eye tearing and nasal discharge, although these features are very mild in comparison to their occurrence with cluster headache. Therefore, using the presence of autonomic features to distinguish migraine from cluster headache is often counterproductive.

Medication overuse or rebound headache can be difficult to diagnosis unless a high index of suspicion is maintained. Medication overuse will not cause headache in a headache-free patient; however, the headache pattern of the chronic headache sufferer will be aggravated by medication overuse. Typically, patients experience a change from intermittent migraine to a daily tension-type headache. Another common scenario is the perpetuation of posttraumatic headache, with frequent headaches persisting longer than expected. Every patient reporting frequent headache should be repeatedly queried about medication overuse and required to complete a headache diary to log both headache and medication use. Any acute care medication (triptans, ergotamine, analgesic or analgesic combinations, opioids, and butalbital combinations) may contribute to medication overuse headache. Patients with benign headache taking any acute care medication or combination of acute care medications on a regular basis at least 3 days per week for at least 6 weeks should be diagnosed with probable medication overuse headache. Switching among different acute care agents on different days does not minimize risk of medication overuse headache. Patients should have at least 5 days per week during which they use no acute care medication.

Posttraumatic headaches occur within 2 weeks of a head injury. The head injury should be significant enough to have produced a concussion, which may be experienced as "feeling dazed," "seeing stars," having amnesia for events before or after the accident, or a brief loss of consciousness. Postconcussive syndrome features often accompany posttraumatic headaches: depressed or irritable mood, memory loss, dizziness or vertigo, and tinnitus. Posttraumatic headache should improve from constant and severe to milder and less frequent over the first 2 weeks. Headaches failing to improve, worsening, or associated with progressive postconcussive symptoms should be reevaluated with imaging studies to rule out subacute pathology, such as subdural hematoma or undiagnosed fracture. Headache features are often consistent with migraine in the early phases of posttraumatic headache, and become milder like tension-type headache when posttraumatic headache persists.

4. HEADACHE TREATMENT

The same types of treatment may be used to treat migraine, tension-type, and posttraumatic headache *(22)*. Most nonmedication and medication treatments work equally well for all three types of headache, with the exception of valproate, which is more effective for migraine. The first step in headache treatment is identifying the contribution to headache of analgesic overuse. Patients regularly using prescription or over-the-counter acute care or analgesic medications at least 3 days a week are at risk for medication overuse headache. Standard acute care and preventive therapies are ineffective in patients with concomitant analgesic overuse; therefore, discontinuation of analgesics or triptans and tapering of opioids and butalbital compounds must be completed before patients can expect headache improvement.

Monitoring the benefit from headache treatment is best accomplished using a daily headache diary. Patients should record headache severity three or four times daily. In this way, reduced headache duration can be identified, as well as reduced severity and frequency of headaches. Many patients initially experience reduction in only one of these three variables. If headache duration is not monitored, a potentially beneficial treatment may be prematurely discontinued if it initially impacts headache duration only. In addition, identifying the unique features of a patient's headache allows the clinician to individualize treatment recommendations. For example, patients with combined migraine and tension-type headache may be instructed to use acute-care medications only when the headache reaches the level of intensity that is typical of migraine in that patient; this restriction will avoid use of acute therapy excessively for mild, daily headaches.

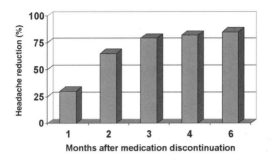

Fig. 7. Medication overuse headache: improvement following drug discontinuation. (Based on ref. *23.*)

4.1. Analgesic-Overuse Headache

Both patients and their doctors must be convinced that analgesic overuse can aggravate chronic headaches. Data clearly show that discontinuation of daily or near-daily acute-care medication with no additional treatment effectively reduces headaches for the majority of patients (Fig. 7) *(23)*. Regrettably, improvement typically takes approximately 6 to 8 weeks. During that time, patients may supplement acute care medications with such medications as non-ibuprofen nonsteroidal anti-inflammatory drugs (NSAIDs), COX-2 inhibitors, or tramadol with little chance of promoting analgesic overuse. These medications may reduce aggravation caused by headaches and the psychological anxiety associated with medication abstinence during the withdrawal period. After patients have successfully eliminated acute care medications for 1 month, standard preventive therapies may be initiated (*see* Box 4). Preventive therapies will not be effective if used concomitantly with daily acute care therapies; therefore, therapies that previously failed while the patient was also overusing acute therapy may be tried again.

4.2. Common Primary Recurring Headaches (Migraine, Tension-Type, Posttrauma)

The selection of therapy for common headaches requires an initial evaluation of headache severity and frequency (Fig. 8). Headaches occurring on no more than 2 days per week may be managed by acute therapy (Fig. 9), whereas those occurring more frequently will require preventive therapy (Fig. 10). Patients who are not overusing acute-care medication but have frequent mild headaches and infrequent severe headaches (e.g., combined migraine and tension-type headache) may benefit from both preventive and acute therapy. Triptans are particularly beneficial for patients with moderate to severe disabling attacks. The choice of triptan is based on slight differences in time course of action and formulation preference (*see* Box 5). Most patients will respond to at least one of three triptan

---

Box 4
Steps for Treating Medication Overuse Headache

---

1. Discontinue analgesics and triptans.
2. Taper opioids, butalbital combinations, and ergotamines by one-half to one pill per week.
3. Prescribe a low-dose non-ibuprofen nonsteroidal anti-inflammatory drug, COX-2 inhibitor, or tramadol twice daily, with an additional dose permitted once daily for severe pain during first month after discontinuing analgesics or throughout period of taper.
4. Reassess headache pattern 1 month after discontinuing analgesics and triptans or completing drug taper.
5. Treat frequent headache with standard preventive therapy (Fig. 10).
6. Allow acute-care medications for infrequent, severe headaches only; maximum: 2 days/week.
7. Maintain headache diary to ensure no return of excessive acute care medication.

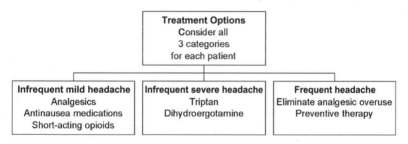

Fig. 8. Therapeutic options for migraine, tension-type, and posttrauma headaches.

trials *(24)*. Combining a triptan with an analgesic may increase the duration of headache relief *(25)*. The selection of preventive therapy is often based on concomitant treatment of comorbid conditions. For example, patients with migraine and hypertension may be treated with a β- or calcium channel blocker, whereas patients with migraine and depression or anxiety may be treated with a tricyclic or selective serotonin reuptake inhibitor antidepressant. Combining both medication and first-line nonmedication therapy (e.g., relaxation and biofeedback) maximizes headache reduction *(26)*.

4.3. Cluster Headache

The intensity of each individual cluster headache attack is so severe that therapy must focus on prevention (*see* Box 6). In addition, most acute therapies will not become effective during the course of these brief attacks. Episodic cluster headache is typically treated with preventive therapy for the ache

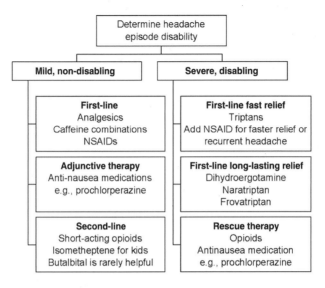

Fig. 9. Choosing acute care medication.

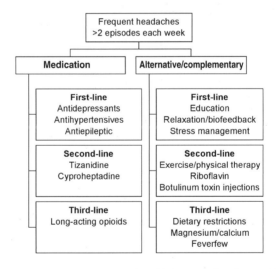

Fig. 10. Choosing preventive therapy. Combining medication and alternative therapies maximizes treatment outcome.

expected duration of the cluster cycle, usually approximately 6 weeks. Chronic cluster, which has no or only brief headache-free periods, is treated with daily, ongoing, preventive therapy. If patients are initially diagnosed when a cluster period has already reached peak severity, treatment with a short course of steroids is usually necessary. Plans should be made at that time, however, for initiation of preventive therapy at the start of the next cluster cycle.

Box 5
Choosing a Triptan

- Weigh needs for immediate relief against convenience/desirability of oral therapy
  - ○ Fastest relief from injectable or intranasal sumatriptan
  - ○ Patients typically prefer oral formulations
    - ▪ Fast-acting oral triptans include rizatriptan, eletriptan, zolmitriptan, and sumatriptan
- Need for sustained relief
  - ○ Add nonsteroidal anti-inflammatory drugs to fast-acting triptan *(25)*
  - ○ Choose slower acting triptan
    - ▪ Naratriptan and frovatriptan
- Desire for convenient formulation
  - ○ Orally disintegrating formulations (Maxalt MLT or Zomig ZMT)
- Sumatriptan nonresponders usually respond to alternative triptan.
  - ○ Only 19% of sumatriptan nonresponders fail zolmitriptan and rizatriptan *(24)*

Box 6
Treatment of Cluster Headache

- Episodic cluster (cluster duration ≥7 days, with pain-free period between clusters ≥1 month)
  - ○ Preventive therapy: onset of cluster
    - ▪ Discontinuation of nicotine and alcohol during cluster
    - ▪ 240–480 mg/day verapamil for 6 weeks
    - ▪ 2–8 mg/day methysergide for 6 weeks
  - ○ Preventive therapy: cluster at maximum intensity at time of treatment initiation
    - ▪ Prednisone 10–60 mg/day for 1 week
  - ○ Rescue therapy
    - ▪ 6 mg subcutaneous sumatriptan
    - ▪ 100% O_2 7 L/minute for 10 minutes by face mask
    - ▪ Intranasal butorphanol
- Chronic cluster (cluster duration >1 year, with any pain-free periods during that year lasting <1 month)
  - ○ Preventive therapy
    - ▪ Discontinuation of nicotine and alcohol
    - ▪ 240–480 mg/day verapamil
    - ▪ 250–1000mg/day valproic acid
    - ▪ 900–1800 mg/day gabapentin
  - ○ Rescue therapy
    - ▪ 100% O_2 7 L/minute for 10 minutes by face mask

Response to cluster therapy is typically different for patients with migraine or tension-type headache. Successful cluster therapy typically results in reduced frequency and duration of headaches. The intensity of each headache is often not reduced, however. For this reason, reduction in headache frequency is the main goal of cluster headache therapy.

4.4. Headache Patterns in Women

Headache patterns often change in a predictable fashion during the reproductive cycle in women. Estradiol is an important pain modulator, directly influencing neural function through a variety of neurotransmitters important for transmitting pain signals, including endorphins, serotonin, γ-aminobutyric acid (GABA), and dopamine *(27)*. Generally, estradiol protects against pain, reducing pain perception as estradiol levels rise. Therefore, the pain threshold increases and headache frequency decreases for the majority of women during pregnancy *(28,29)*. Conversely, when estradiol levels fluctuate or drop from high to low levels—as occurs with ovulation, menses, the placebo week of oral contraceptives, and after delivery—headache frequency increases. Because estradiol levels fluctuate during the perimenopausal period, headaches tend to worsen while other somatic symptoms of menopause—e.g., hot flashes—occur during early menopause. Headaches may also be aggravated during menopause by estrogen supplementation *(30)*.

Headache management in women should focus on either minimizing changes in estradiol levels with estrogen supplementation when a decline in estradiol levels is expected or by pharmaceutically manipulating other important neurochemicals, such as using antidepressants or triptans to modulate serotonin levels, valproate or gabapentin to modulate GABA, or antinausea medications to modulate dopamine *(see* Boxes 7 and 8) *(31)*. Consideration should also be given to the risk for adverse effects of medications on the developing fetus when treating headaches during pregnancy *(see* Box 9). Most medications that can be used safely during pregnancy can be continued when breastfeeding. Injectable sumatriptan, which is restricted during pregnancy, may be used when by a nursing mother if she pumps her milk and discards it for 4 hours after an injection and supplements the baby's feeding with stored milk.

5. SUMMARY

Managing chronic headache begins with a reliable headache history to aid the health care provider in identifying common headache patterns. Worrisome headaches are generally associated with new headache patterns, pain in the back of the head or neck, aging (>50 years old), or abnormal neurological examination findings *(21)*. A diary that is used to record both headache activity and medication use can be helpful to the clinician in correctly identifying head-

---

Box 7
Treating Menstrual Headache: Perimenstrual Prevention

- Hormone therapy
  - 7-day 100-mg estrogen patch
  - Eliminate placebo week from oral contraceptives for 2 or 3 months
- Acute-care medications
  - Nonsteroidal anti-inflammatory drugs (excluding aspirin or ibuprofen)
  - 2.5 mg naratriptan twice daily
  - 2.5 mg frovatriptan once or twice daily
- Preventive medications
  - β-blocker
  - Antidepressant (excluding fluoxetine)
  - Calcium channel blocker
  - Antiepilepsy drug (valproic acid or gabapentin)

All medications should be used at usual dose for 3 days before the expected menstrual period and during first 2–4 days of menses. Do not use unless diary confirms headache occurrence exclusively in association with menses.

Box 8
Treating Headache During Menopause

- Determine if there has been a change in headache pattern notable enough to warrant additional evaluation
- Adjust estrogen replacement therapy if it aggravates headache
  - Use noncycling, transdermal route
  - Reduce estrogen dose
  - Change estrogen-replacement product
- Add standard headache-preventive therapy in conjunction with estrogen replacement

---

patterns, the contribution of medication overuse to headache, and the relationship of headache to menstruation. Identification and elimination of medication overuse is the first step in successful headache management. Choice of headache therapy depends on headache frequency and disability. Combining medication and nonmedication therapies maximizes treatment outcome.

REFERENCES

1. Brett KM, Burt CW. Utilization of ambulatory medical care by women: United States, 1997–98. Vital Health Stat 2001; 13:1–46.
2. Gibbs TS, Fleischer AB, Feldman SR, Sam MC, O'Donovan CA. Health care utilization in patients with migraine: demographics and patterns of care in the ambulatory setting. Headache 2003; 43:330–335.

Box 9
Treating Headache During Pregnancy

- Eliminate excessive or daily analgesics
- Acute-care treatment (maximum: 2–3 days/week)
  ○ Acetaminophen
  ○ Short-acting opioids
  ○ Antiemetics
- Preventive treatment for frequent headache
  ○ Medications
    ▪ β-blocker
    ▪ Selective serotonin reuptake inhibitor antidepressant
    ▪ Bupropion
    ▪ Gabapentin (in early pregnancy; stop in third trimester)
  ○ Nonmedication therapy
    ▪ Relaxation and biofeedback
    ▪ Stress management
    ▪ Discontinuation of nicotine and caffeine
    ▪ Regular meals and sleep

---

3. Boardman HF, Thomas E, Croft PR, Millson DS. Epidemiology of headache in an English district. Cephalalgia 2003; 23:129–137.

4. Rasmussen BK, Jensen R, Schroll M, Olesen J. Epidemiology of headache in a general population: a prevalence study. J Clin Epidemiol 1991; 44:1147–1157.

5. Lipton RB, Stewart WF, Diamond S, Diamond ML, Reed M. Prevalence and burden of migraine in the United States: data from the American Migraine Study II. Headache 2001; 41:646–657.

6. Hasse LA, Ritchey N, Smith R. Predicting the number of headache visits by type of patient seen in family practice. Headache 2002; 42:738–746.

7. Tepper S, Newman L, Dowson A, et al. The prevalence and diagnosis of migraine in a primary care setting in the US: insights from the Landmark Study. Poster presented at 16th Annual Practicing Physician's Approach to the Difficult Headache Patient; February 11–15, 2003; Rancho Mirage, CA.

8. Manzoni GC. Gender ratio of cluster headache over the years: a possible role of changes in lifestyle. Cephalalgia 1998; 18:138–142.

9. Delaney JS, Lacroix VJ, Gagne C, Antoniou J. Concussions among university football and soccer players: a pilot study. Clin J Sport Med 2001; 11:234–240.

10. Lance JC, Arciniegas DB. Post-traumatic headache. Curr Treat Options Neurol 2002; 4:89–104.

11. Packard RC. Posttraumatic headache: permanency and relationship to legal settlement. Headache 1992; 32:496–500.

12. Berglund A, Alfredsson L, Jensen I, Cassidy JD, Nygren A. The association between exposure to a rear-end collision and future health complaints. J Clin Epidemiol 2001; 54:851–856.

13. Kolbinson DA, Epstein JB, Burgess JA, Senthilselvan A. Temporomandibular disorders, headaches, and neck pain after motor vehicle accidents: a pilot investigation of persistence and litigation effects. J Prosthet Dent 1997; 77:46–53.
14. Kolbinson DA, Epstein JB, Burgess JA. Temporomandibular disorders, headaches, and neck pain following motor vehicle accidents and the effect of litigation: review of the literature. J Orofac Pain 1996; 10:101–125.
15. Mureriwa J. Head injury and compensation: a preliminary investigation of the postconcussional syndrome in Harare. Cent Afr J Med 1990; 36:315–318.
16. Gerth WC, Carides GW, Dasbach EJ, Visser WH, Santanello NC. The multinational impact of migraine symptoms on healthcare utilisation and work loss. Pharmacoeconomics 2001; 19:197–206.
17. Marcus DA. Identification of headache subjects at risk for psychological distress. Headache 2000; 40:373–376.
18. Schwartz BS, Stewart WF, Lipton RB. Lost workdays and decreased work effectiveness associated with headache in the workplace. J Occup Environ Med 1997; 39:320–327.
19. Marcus DA. Headache disability and headache diagnosis. Headache & Pain 2003; 14:180–185.
20. Lipton RB, Bigal ME, Kolodner K, et al. The family impact of migraine: population-based studies in the USA and UK. Cephalalgia 2003; 23:429–440.
21. Ramirez-Lassepas M, Espinosa CE, Cicero JJ, et al. Predictors of intracranial pathological findings in patients who seek emergency care because of headache. Arch Neurol 1997; 54:1506–1509.
22. Marcus DA: Migraine and tension headache: the questionable validity of current classification systems. Clin J Pain 1992; 8:28–36.
23. Rapoport AM, Weeks RE, Sheftell FD, Baskin SM, Verdi J. The "analgesic washout period": a critical variable in the evaluation of treatment efficacy. Neurology 1986; 36(Suppl 1):100–101.
24. Mathew NT, Kailasam J, Gentry P, Chernyshev O. Treatment of nonresponders to oral sumatriptan with zolmitriptan and rizatriptan: a comparative open trial. Headache 2000; 40:464–465.
25. Krymchantowski AV, Barbosa JS. Rizatriptan combined with rofecoxib vs rizatriptan for the acute treatment of migraine: an open label pilot study. Cephalalgia 2002; 22:309–312.
26. Holroyd KA, France JL, Cordingley GE, et al. Enhancing the effectiveness of relaxation-thermal biofeedback training with propranolol hydrochloride. J Consult Clin Psychol 1995; 63:327–330.
27. Marcus, DA: Sex hormones and chronic headache. Exp Opin Pharmacother 2001; 2:1839–1848.
28. Gintzler AR, Bohan MC. Pain thresholds are elevated during pseudopregnancy. Brain Res 1990; 507:312–316.
29. Sances G, Granella F, Nappi RE, et al. Course of migraine during pregnancy and postpartum: a prospective study. Cephalalgia 2003; 23:197–205.
30. Facchinetti F, Nappi RE, Granella F, et al. Effects of hormone replacement treatment (HRT) in postmenopausal women with migraine. Cephalalgia 2001; 21:452.
31. Marcus DA: Focus on primary care: diagnosis and management of headache in women. Obstetrical & Gynecological Survey 1999; 54:395–402.

CME QUESTIONS—CHAPTER 4

1. Which of the following statements about medication overuse headache is true?
   a. Medication overuse headache is a sign of drug addiction.
   b. Medication overuse headache only occurs in patients overusing narcotics.
   c. Medication overuse headache does not occur in patients with true head pain.
   d. Medication overuse headache may occur in patients regularly using any acute care prescription or over-the-counter headache treatment 3 days or more per week.

2. Features associated with potentially serious headache that requires additional evaluation include:
   a. Posterior head or neck pain
   b. Pain beginning after the age of 50 years
   c. Change in headache pattern
   d. Abnormal neurological examination
   e. All of the above

3. The most common type of chronic headache seen in the primary care office is:
   a. Migraine
   b. Tension-type
   c. Posttraumatic
   d. Cluster

4. Which of the following headaches is experienced as short pain episodes, typically lasting <2 hours?
   a. Migraine
   b. Tension-type
   c. Posttraumatic
   d. Cluster
   e. Medication overuse

5

Cervical and Lumbar Pain

CASE HISTORY

Ms. Hoffmann is a 45-year-old registered nurse who works in the busy intensive care unit (ICU) of a city hospital. She has worked in this environment for the past 15 years, with two previous episodes of work-related neck pain during the last 5 years. In both cases, her primary symptom was severe muscle spasm, and she returned to regular duties after 1 week. Her current injury occurred when she pulled an obese, sedated patient into a bed. At that time, she developed a searing pain in her neck and upper left arm. Physical examination the next day revealed a reduced biceps reflex and numbness in her upper arm. Magnetic resonance imaging revealed a herniated disc at C5/C6. No improvement was reported after 1 week of rest and treatment with prednisone, valium, and hydrocodone. After an uncomplicated discectomy, the pain was reduced to moderate severity, although numbness and sensitivity to touch in the upper arm persisted. An attempt to return to regular duties was unsuccessful because of intense pain experienced when lifting supplies, reaching across patient beds, and repositioning patients. Ms. Hoffmann was concerned that she would not be able to adequately care for the patients under her charge and went on sick leave. Her physician treated her with daily ibuprofen, and her pain was diminished when she performed reduced activities. Ms. Hoffmann discontinued ibuprofen after 1 month because of gastric upset. Six months later, she was still not working and developed a tendency to hold her arm splinted to her torso to avoid moving it or having anything touch it. Her workers' compensation caseworker suspected symptom magnification because of her prolonged work absence with this injury and recommended a physical capacity evaluation.

* * *

Ms. Hoffmann's story is typical for many patients with neck pain. Episodes of acute neck pain are quite common, especially among individuals whose work involves heavy lifting (e.g., nurses). With her latest injury, Ms. Hoffmann's symptoms suggested more than simple muscle pain. Postoperatively, she continued to report symptoms of persistent neuropathic changes that delayed her

From: *Chronic Pain: A Primary Care Guide to Practical Management*
Edited by: D. A. Marcus © Humana Press, Totowa, NJ

recovery. Ms. Hoffmann's long employment history and strong work ethic suggested that she would likely return to work. However, it is difficult to return initially to such work. In Ms. Hoffmann's case, the occupational therapist performing the physical capacity evaluation appropriately noted the signs of neuropathic pain (e.g., hypersensitivity to touch) and physical limitations caused by her pain. A recommendation was given to the treating physician to address Ms. Hoffmann's neuropathic pain and recommend restricted duty on her return to work, along with a work-hardening program. Ms. Hoffmann returned to work on light duty, 3 hours daily, while participating in a work-hardening program. Treatment with gabapentin plus physical therapy, pacing skills, and body mechanics helped reduce pain and increase her work capabilities. At the conclusion of the work-hardening program, Ms. Hoffmann was able to resume her daily household routine, but could not perform the type of lifting necessary for working in the ICU. She was, however, successfully returned to a full-time modified nursing job within her hospital.

KEY CHAPTER POINTS

- Chronic neck and back pain are the two most common pain problems seen by primary care physicians.
- Evaluation of chronic neck and back pain focuses on the identification of a specific pathology and factors that predict persistent pain.
- The primary focus of chronic neck and back pain treatment is a return to normal functioning at home and at work.
- The most effective therapy for acute neck and back pain is a reduction in intensity of activities to a tolerable level; complete restriction from all work duties is generally neither necessary nor beneficial.
- The most effective therapy for chronic neck and back pain is physical therapy exercise with behavioral intervention (e.g., cognitive restructuring, development of pacing skills, and modification of body mechanics for physical activities).
- Most neck and back pain can be managed successfully by primary care physicians. Patients with significant risk factors for chronic pain or prolonged disability should be referred for more aggressive rehabilitative therapy.

1. EPIDEMIOLOGY

Back and neck pain are the two most common pain complaints that result in a primary care physician (PCP) consultation *(1)*. A random, general population survey of more than 2000 adults in the United States indicated that back or neck pain occurred during the last 12 months in 31% of adults (Fig. 1) *(2)*. The pre-valence of these problems is significantly higher among treatment-seeking patients. In two large surveys of adults enrolled in general medical care or in a health insurance plan in Canada and Great Britain, neck pain, back pain, or both lasting at least 1 week was reported to have occurred during the preceding month in 33% of adults and within the previous 6 months in 80% (Fig. 2) *(3,4)*,

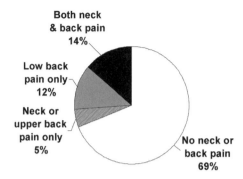

Fig. 1. Prevalence of neck and back pain during the preceding year in the general population. Almost one-third of adults in the general population reported experiencing neck or back pain during the preceding year. (Based on ref. 2.)

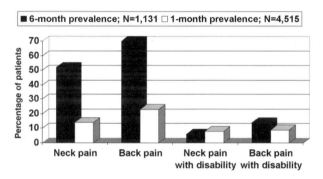

Fig. 2. Prevalence of neck and back pain in general medical patients. The Côté Canadian study reported the occurrence of neck or back pain during the previous 6 months. The Webb British study reported neck or back pain lasting at least 1 week during the previous 1 month. (Based on refs. 3,4.)

peaking at a younger age in women than in men (45–64 years vs 65–74 years, respectively) (4). Neck and back pain often occur in association with pain in other body regions. For example, 75% of people with back pain also report pain in other body areas (in order of frequency: the knee, shoulder, and neck); 89% of patients with neck pain report additional pain areas (in order of frequency: the shoulder, back, and knee) (4).

Although neck and back pain are highly prevalent, only a minority of affected individuals seek medical care. In a Canadian survey, neck or back pain symptoms were severe enough to completely prohibit participation in work, school, or household chores for 16% of the total population and to restrict work, school, or chores in another 21%, yet only 25% had consulted a health care provider within the previous month (3). Treatment seekers were more likely to have a

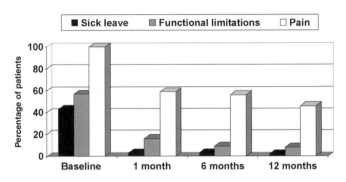

Fig. 3. Long-term prognosis for acute low back pain. (Based on ref. *10*.)

lower level of education and lower income, less likely to be employed full-time, and more likely to have comorbid illness. Similarly, a US survey showed that only 37% of people with neck or back pain sought conventional medical care during the preceding month, whereas 54% used alternative medicine (e.g., chiropracty, massage, relaxation therapy, and herbal remedies) *(2)*. The severity of both pain and disability correlate with the likelihood of seeking care *(5)*.

Chronic neck pain occurs less commonly than back pain. A survey of a sample of 6000 Swedish adults identified a history of neck pain in 43%, with women affected more frequently than men (48 vs 38%) *(5)*. The prevalence in women decreased after age 64 years. Neck pain persisting longer than 6 months was reported for 43% of women and 33% of men, with continuous, neck pain persisting longer than 6 months in 23% of women and 17% of men.

Low back pain is the most common chronic pain, affecting about 59% of adults at some point during their lives *(7)*. Low back pain is the fifth most common reason for PCP office visits *(1)*. Daily low back pain lasting longer than 1 week is experienced annually by 17.6% of workers and results in 150 million lost work days *(8)*. In one study, acute back pain resolved within 1.5 months in 61% of adults treated for acute back pain with the usual care of their primary practitioners or rheumatologists *(9)*. Back pain that does persist beyond the acute period, however, often persists long-term. A prospective survey of 503 Danish adults consulting a general practitioner for acute low back pain revealed that, despite returning to work, nearly half of these patients continued to report pain or functional limitations 1 year after the onset of their back pain (Fig. 3) *(10)*. Similarly, surveys conducted in Great Britain revealed a persistence of symptoms 12 months after first consultation to a primary care provider by 42 to 75% of patients *(12,13)*.

In several studies, patient, work, and psychological features have been identified that can be used to predict an increased risk for chronic neck or back pain

```
┌─────────────────────────────────────────────────┐
│                    Box 1                         │
│       Risk Factors for Chronic Neck or Back Pain │
├─────────────────────────────────────────────────┤
```

- General characteristics
  - Female
  - Increasing age
  - Living alone
  - History of pain
  - Poor general health
  - Nicotine use
  - Not a sports participant
- Work-related factors
  - Work dissatisfaction
  - Neck pain
    - Repetitive work
    - Prolonged neck flexion
  - Low back pain
    - Work duties require heavy lifting or pulling
    - Work duties require prolonged standing
    - Initial work absenteeism more than 8 days
- Pain variables
  - Widespread pain
  - Radiating pain
  - Difficulty standing or walking
- Physical factors
  - Obesity
  - Restricted spine movement
- Psychological factors
  - Depression
  - Anxiety
  - Stress
  - Poor coping strategies

Based on refs. *9,12,13,15,16*.

following an acute injury *(3,13–16; see* Box 1). Ms. Hoffmann has general work-related and pain variables associated with an increased risk for developing chronic neck pain. Occupations that put workers at highest risk for chronic neck or back pain include construction work and nurses aide *(8)*. Other workers at high risk for neck pain include carpenters, car mechanics, maids, janitors, and hairstylists, because these jobs require lifting or prolonged standing. It is important to remember that most patients who develop back pain will return to work, even if pain symptoms persist *(10)*. Successful return to work after absenteeism from low back pain can be predicted by a number of factors *(17,18; see* Box 2).

Box 2
Predictors of a Successful Return to Work Following Absence for Back Pain

- General characteristics
  - Age less than 30 years
  - Good general health
  - Medical evaluation occurs less than 30 days after pain begins
- Work-related factors
  - Steady employment for more than 2 years
  - Patient is main household breadwinner
  - High job satisfaction
  - Public job (rather than private)
  - Job duties allow unscheduled breaks
- Physical factors
  - Normal neurological examination
  - Good lumbar flexion for low back pain

Based on refs. *17,19*.

Van den Heuvel identified the ability to take frequent work breaks (with or without exercises during the break periods) as important to improved recovery from neck pain *(19)*. Although Ms. Hoffmann's solid work history is a good prognostic predictor, her general characteristics (age >30 years) and physical factors (abnormal neurological examination) predict a poor prognosis for returning to work and suggest the need for more aggressive occupational therapy interventions.

2. EVALUATION OF NECK AND BACK PAIN

Most patients seeking treatment from a PCP for neck or back pain do not have surgical pathology. The National Ambulatory Medical Care Survey showed nonspecific back pain to be the most common diagnosis for patients treating with a PCP (Fig. 4) *(1)*.

Patient evaluation for neck or back pain, therefore, needs to focus on identifying the minority of patients with identifiable pathology (e.g., radiculopathy from a herniated disc), and identifying patients at risk for persistent, chronic pain that will require more aggressive therapy.

Patient history should focus on factors that predict the chronic nature of symptoms (*see* Box 3). A history of back injury or pain, work duties satisfaction, and symptoms of depression and anxiety all need to be explored. Chronic pain or disability in other family or household members also influences the duration of pain and should be evaluated.

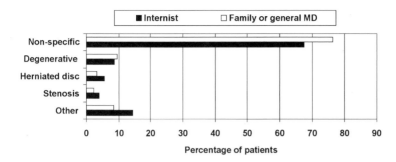

Fig. 4. Diagnoses for low back pain seen by the primary care physician. (Based on ref. *1*.)

Box 3
Historical Evaluation of Patient With Cervical or Lumbar Pain

Identify the following historical features that predict the chronicity of pain:

1. History of previous pain problems or prior injuries
2. Family history of chronic pain complaints
3. Occupational history
   a. Work duties: heavy work; prolonged posture or standing
   b. Poor work satisfaction
   c. Patient is not household breadwinner
4. Psychological history
   a. Anxiety
   b. Depression

The physical examination should include an evaluation of range of motion and neurological signs of strength, reflexes, and sensation (*see* Box 4). Identification of patterns of motor and sensory loss that suggest cervical or lumbar radiculopathy should be a major part of the neurological examination (*see* Tables 1 and 2). Figures 5 through 7 show motor tests for cervical radiculopathy and skin areas that will show signs of altered sensation caused by abnormal cervical and lumbar nerve function. Plain X-rays with flexion and extension views are helpful to rule out instability in patients with mechanical pain complaints (e.g., restricted movement or pain occurring during movement) or limited range of motion. Nerve conduction and electromyography testing may be useful to rule out acute radiculopathy in patients with a mixed pattern of motor and sensory loss (e.g., reflex loss suggests one nerve root, whereas sensory loss suggests another).

Box 4

Physical Examination of Patient With Cervical or Lumbar Pain

---

1. Musculoskeletal examination
   a. Muscle palpation for tenderness, spasm, and trigger points
   b. Skeletal assessment for posture and range of motion
2. Neurological examination
   a. Strength testing
   b. Reflexes
   c. Sensory examination to touch and pin
   d. Gait testing to assess casual movements and strength

Table 1

Evaluation of Common Cervical Radiculopathies

Nerve involved	Motor loss	Reflex loss	Sensory loss
C5	Biceps	Biceps	Lateral upper arm
C6	Brachioradialis	Biceps	Lateral lower arm
C7	Triceps	Triceps	Middle finger
C8	Finger flexors	None	Medial lower arm

Remember: A herniated cervical disc affects the nerve for the vertebra below. Thus, C5 radiculopathy occurs when the C4–C5 disc is herniated; C8 radiculopathy occurs with a C7–T1 herniated disc.

Table 2

Evaluation for Common Lumbar Radiculopathies

Nerve involved	Motor loss	Reflex loss	Sensory loss
L3	Knee extension	Knee reflex	Anterior medial thigh
L4	Knee extension	Knee reflex	Medial lower leg
L5	Foot dorsiflexion: walking on heels	None	Lateral lower leg and great toe
S1	Foot plantar flexion: walking on toes	Ankle jerk	Lateral foot and sole

Remember: A herniated lumbar disc usually affects the nerve for the vertebra below. Thus, an L4 radiculopathy usually occurs when the L3–L4 disc is herniated.

Magnetic resonance imaging (MRI) and computed tomography (CT) generally should be reserved for patients with clinical evidence for myelopathy (e.g., bilateral motor and sensory loss), radiculopathy, or spinal stenosis (e.g., pain with walking or a tendency to adopt forward lumbar flexion with walking). MRI scans of asymptomatic adult controls have shown radiographically signifi-

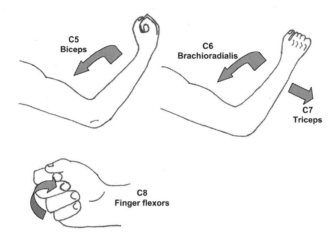

Fig. 5. Motor testing for cervical radiculopathy. Arrows denote direction of movement required to test specific muscles. Test biceps strength with palm facing up. Test brachioradialis strength with thumb pointed up.

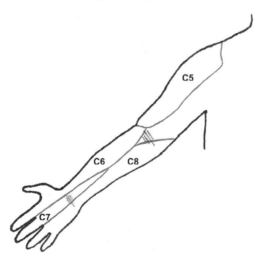

Fig. 6. Sensory testing for cervical radiculopathy. Arm viewed from the anterior aspect, with palm facing toward viewer. Skins areas served by specific cervical nerve roots are marked.

cant changes in both cervical and lumbar spines (Table 3) *(20–22)*. A study comparing cervical MRIs in young adults (ages 24–27) with recurrent and persistent neck and shoulder pain vs asymptomatic controls showed no difference in the prevalence of most MRI abnormalities, with the exception of disc protrusion (observed in 19% of symptomatic adults vs 32% of controls; $p < 0.05$) and disc herniation (4% of symptomatic adults vs 0% in controls; $p = 0.05$) *(22)*.

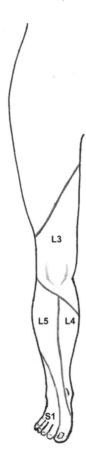

Fig. 7. Sensory testing for lumbar radioulopathy. Skin areas served by specific lumbar nerve roots are marked.

Table 3
Prevalence of Abnormal Magnetic Resonance
Imaging Findings in Asymptomatic Adults

Abnormality	Prevalence in normal adults (%)
Cervical spine	
Disc degeneration	73
Annular tear	67
Disc bulge	87
Lumbar spine	
Disc bulge	52
Disc herniation	24
Stenosis	4

Based on refs. *21* and *22*.

Although radiographically significant changes can be seen in young adults, the percentage of patients with such abnormalities increases with age. After the age of 60, 79% of asymptomatic controls will have bulging lumbar discs. In a study involving baseline and 12-month follow-up MRI evaluations in 89 men, 32% of men with no complaint of low back pain had an abnormality and 47% of men with a complaint of low back pain had a normal spine *(23)*. In addition, the development of low back pain during the study did not correlate with the change from baseline MRI. A 7-year prospective study similarly failed to link radiographic changes with a subsequent development of low back pain *(24)*. Nonspecific abnormalities are similar with CT scanning. In a group of 52 controls, 35% had abnormal lumbar studies; this rate increased to 50% after the age of 40 years *(25)*. In controls younger than 40 years, 20% had CT scans that revealed a herniated disc. The validity of discography remains controversial, however, and should not be used as a screening tool *(26)*.

3. TREATMENT

Treatments for acute and chronic neck and back pain are different, with acute pain therapy focused on symptomatic relief and chronic pain therapy focused on rehabilitation, with the goal of reducing pain, psychological distress, and disability to help the individual resume normal activity levels, including returning to work.

3.1. Acute Neck and Back Pain Treatment

Patients with acute neck or back pain require evaluation to distinguish pain-specific pathology from nonspecific pathology. For the vast majority of patients with nonspecific pathology, noninvasive symptomatic treatment is effective. Many episodes of acute back pain resolve on their own or improve significantly without specific medical intervention. Studies show that patients improve best after acute injury when they reduce activities to as tolerated and allow healing to occur, compared with patients who are treated with either complete bed rest or acute physical therapy *(27–29)*. A survey of 281 adults with acute back pain reported similar outcomes when treated with bed rest or activities as tolerated, which suggests that there is little need for most patients to restrict work activities *(30)*.

Malmivaara and colleagues selected 165 patients with acute back pain or a brief exacerbation of chronic back pain and randomized them to treatment with 2 days of bed rest, mobilizing exercises, or ordinary activities as tolerated *(31)*. Both the extent and speed of improvement were greatest for the ordinary activity group and worst in the bed-rest group. These findings suggest that neither brief bed-rest nor light exercise should be prescribed for acute back pain. Rather, it should be managed with medical evaluation and brief education to avoid even short-term bed rest and maintain activities as tolerated (Fig. 8).

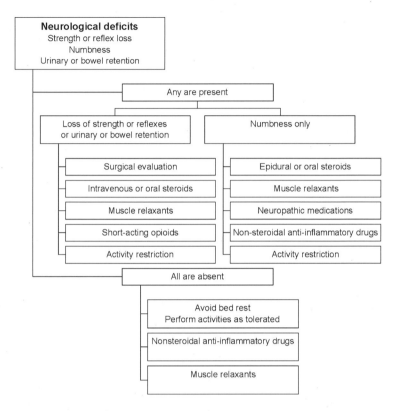

Fig. 8. Management of acute cervical or lumbar pain.

3.2. Chronic Neck and Back Pain Treatment

A 2-year follow-up of patients with chronic low back pain receiving no treatment revealed a slight reduction in pain severity during the first 3 months, but no improvement in either functional status or psychological distress *(32)*. Standard conservative therapy (physical therapy, injections, and/or medications) resulted in improvement in both pain and disability. A variety of physical and psychological treatments have been tested for chronic neck and back pain *(33–37)* (Table 4). Active physical therapy with behavioral interventions is the most effective method of achieving long-term pain relief and the ability to resume normal activities. The specific type of rehabilitative therapy to be offered to patients depends on the presence or absence of chronic radicular changes and neuropathic pain, which may benefit from targeted neuropathic therapy (Fig. 9). (Additional information about treatment for neuropathic symptoms can be found in Chapter 8.) Opioids may be used to manage severe, infrequent flares or in low doses for constant, disabling pain. (More complete coverage of recom-

Table 4
Effective Therapies for Patients With Chronic Neck and Low Back Pain

Treatment	Effective	Ineffective	Insufficient data
Chronic neck pain			
Exercise	X (long-term)		
Acupuncture	X (short-term)		
Traction		X	
Ultrasound		X	
Massage			X
Electrical stimulation			X
Multidisciplinary rehabilitation			X
EMG biofeedback			X
Behavioral interventions			X
Chronic low back pain			
Exercise	X		
TENS		X	
Acupuncture		X	
Traction		X	
Ultrasound		X	
Massage			X
Electrical stimulation			X
Multidisciplinary rehabilitation			X
EMG biofeedback		X	
Behavioral interventions	X		

EMG, electromyography; TENS, transcutaneous electrical nerve stimulation. (Based on refs. *33–37*.)

mendations for the use of opioids appears in Chapter 17.) Nerve blocks are reserved for adjunctive therapy in patients with clearly identified nerve root irritation, such as chronic radiculopathy or spinal stenosis *(38,39)*. Trigger-point injections generally result in only short-term, symptomatic relief *(38)*.

3.2.1. Work and Chronic Pain

Treatment for chronic pain focuses on helping the individual return to his or her previous functional level, including returning to or continuing work. The average cost per worker for work-related low back pain in 1989 was $8321 *(40)*. Interestingly, most of this cost was incurred from lost wage payments; only one-third of this amount reflects medical costs. Three recent studies reported similar data, with 75 to 93% of the cost of back pain attributed to indirect costs (e.g., work absenteeism and disability) and only 7 to 25% to medical expenses *(41–43)*. Therefore, reducing the cost of care should focus primarily on facilitating the return to work, rather than reducing medical treatment expenses. It should be more cost-effective to treat patients aggressively initially to achieve a speedy return to work. Suter demonstrated the benefits of working for back pain *(44)*.

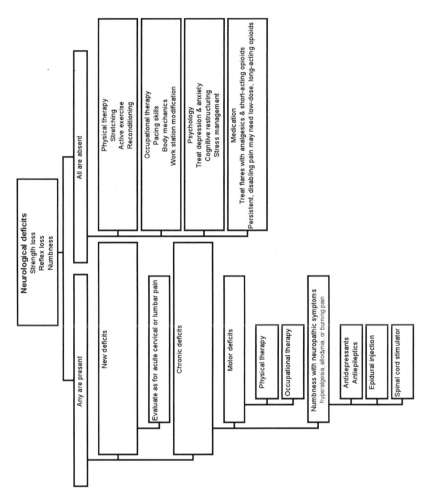

Fig. 9. Management of chronic cervical or lumbar pain.

Pain, depression, and disability measures were obtained from a sample of 200 patients with chronic back pain. Although litigation tended to increase patient perceptions of pain severity and disability, these effects were mitigated if the patients were working. Indeed, all measures of symptomatology were superior in working patients. Comparison of baseline demographics and injury variables between working and nonworking participants did not show a significant difference; in particular, injuries were not more severe in the nonworking group. These data suggest a need to minimize lost time from work for patients with either acute or chronic back pain.

3.2.2. Effective Chronic Neck and Back Pain Treatment

Therapy for chronic neck and back pain with the strongest data supporting good long-term efficacy are stretching, strengthening, and mobility exercises *(36,45)*. Intensive, active exercise and graded activity programs are effective for chronic pain, but ineffective for acute pain *(46–48)*. Exercise programs focusing on weight training, however, are not effective *(49)*. Acupuncture provides short-term relief for neck pain *(35,50)*, with no benefit over treatment with transcutaneous electrical nerve stimulation *(33)*. Acupuncture is, therefore, not recommended for most patients. There is no clear consensus on the effectiveness of chiropractic manipulation, and controlled studies are needed to provide efficacy data *(51)*. Opioids, either alone or as adjunctive therapy with other analgesics, help improve back pain by modest amounts *(52,53)*. The benefits of behavioral interventions for neck pain require additional testing *(37)*, although moderate benefit has been shown in patients with low back pain *(34)*. Occupational therapy or work conditioning programs can effectively help patients with neck or back pain return to work sooner than general treatment from a PCP. A review of 18 randomized, controlled clinical trials showed that intensive physical reconditioning for work tasks, in association with cognitive-behavioral treatment (e.g., work-hardening programs), reduced work absenteeism by an average of 45 days during a 12-month period *(54)*. Ms. Hoffmann's case illustrates how a focus on work disability by the occupational therapist can result in more rapid return to work. The strong influence that work factors (including duties, breaks, and job satisfaction) play in successful return to work (Box 2) also supports the need for intervention by an occupational therapist.

Intensive, multidisciplinary forms of therapy are typically reserved for recalcitrant or disabled patients. Hagen and colleagues randomized patients with low back pain who had missed work for 2 to 3 months to multidisciplinary rehabilitation (exercise and addressing activity restrictions and psychosocial issues) or standard medical care through a PCP *(55)*. One year later, 68% of the patients in rehabilitation had returned to full work duty compared with 56% in the standard care group. Studies investigating the effectiveness of multidisciplinary pain rehabilitation programs show improvement for compliant patients who complete treatment. However, noncompliance is a significant problem in this population. Intensive rehabilitation programs that combine active exercise and psychology treatment (coping skills, distraction techniques, and relaxation) with education are the most effective for improving function and reducing pain for recalcitrant, disabled patients with chronic pain *(56)*. This type of treatment, however, results in improvement and successful return to work in only about half of those patients treated *(57)*. In addition, the outcome is worse in patients who receive compensation for back pain *(58)*. Clearly, the focus in managing chronic pain must be on early intervention and the prevention of the development of chronic pain patterns.

4. SUMMARY

Neck and back pain are the two most common chronically painful conditions seen by PCPs. Evaluation of both conditions focuses on identifying the pain-specific pathology (e.g., radiculopathy) and factors associated with a poor prognosis (e.g., female gender, heavy work duties, history of depression/anxiety, and nicotine use). Although the treatment of acute neck and back pain emphasizes symptomatic pain relief and restriction of activities as tolerated, the treatment of chronic pain emphasizes facilitation of returning to regular household and work activities. Although work-duty restrictions may be needed for patients with physically demanding jobs, complete work restriction is generally not effective in reducing pain symptoms and can result in prolonged disability. Most patients with neck and back pain can be managed successfully by PCPs.

Patients with significant risk factors for chronic pain or prolonged disability should be referred for more aggressive rehabilitative therapy.

REFERENCES

1. Hart LG, Deyo RA, Cherkin DC. Physician office visits for low back pain. Frequency, clinical evaluation, and treatment patterns from a U.S. national survey. Spine 1995; 20:11–19.
2. Wolsko PM, Eisenberg DM, Davis R, Kessler R, Phillips R. Patterns and perceptions of care for treatment of back and neck pain: results of a national survey. Spine 2003; 28:292–297.
3. Côté P, Cassidy JD, Carroll L. The treatment of neck and low back pain. Who seeks care? Who goes where? Medical Care 2001; 39:956–967.
4. Webb R, Brammah T, Lunt M, et al. Prevalence and predictors of intense, chronic, and disabling neck and back pain in the UK general population. Spine 2003; 28:1195–1202.
5. Jacob T, Zeev A, Epstein L. Low back pain-a community-based study of care-seeking and therapeutic effectiveness. Disabil Rehabil 2003; 25:67–76.

6. Guez M, Hildingsson C, Nilsson M, Toolanen G. The prevalence of neck pain: a population-based study from northern Sweden. Acta Orthop Scand 2002; 73: 455–459.

7. Waxman R, Tennant A, Helliwell P. A prospective follow-up study of low back pain in the community. Spine 2000; 15:2085–2090.

8. Guo HR, Tanakas S, Cameron LL, et al. Back pain among workers in the United States: national estimates and workers at high risk. Am J Int Med 1995; 28: 591–602.

9. Valat J, Goulippe P, Rozenberg S, Urbinelli R, Allaert F. Acute low back pain: predictive index of chronicity from a cohort of 2487 subjects. Joint Bone Spine 2000; 67:456–461.

10. Schiøttz-Christensen B, Nielsen GL, Hansen VK, Sørensen HT, Olesen F. Long-term prognosis of acute low back pain in patients seen in general practice: a 1-year prospective follow-up study. Family Practice 1999; 16:223–232.

11. Croft PR, Macfarlane GJ, Papageogiou AC, et al. Outcome of low back pain in general practice: a prospective study. BMJ 1998; 316:1356–1359.

12. Thomas E, Silman AJ, Croft PR, et al. Predicting who develops chronic low back pain in primary care: a prospective study. BMJ 1999; 318:1662–1667.

13. Leboeuf-Yde C, Kyvik KO, Brun NH. Low back pain and lifestyle. Part I: Smoking. Information from a population-based sample of 29,424 twins. Spine 1998; 23:2207–2213.

14. Thomas E, Silman AJ, Croft PR, et al. Predicting who develops chronic low back pain in primary care: a prospective study. BMJ 1999; 318:1662–1667.

15. Linton SJ. A review of psychological risk factors in back and neck pain. Spine 2000; 25:1148–1156.

16. Andersen JH, Kaergaard A, Mikkelsen S, et al. Risk factors in the onset of neck/shoulder pain in a prospective study of workers in industrial and service companies. Occup Environ Med 2003; 60:649–654.

17. Infante-Rivard C, Lortie M. Prognostic factors for return to work after a first compensated episode of back pain. Occup Environ Med 1996; 53:488–494.

18. Van der Giezen A, Bouter LM, Nijhuis FJN. Prediction of return-to-work of low back pain patients sicklisted for 3–4 months. Pain 2000; 87:285–294.

19. Van den Heuvel SG, de Looze MP, Hildebrandt VH, The KH. Effects of software programs stimulating regular breaks and exercises on work-related neck and upper-limb disorders. Scand J Work Environ Health 2003; 29:106–116.

20. Jensen MC, Brant-Zavadzki MN, Obuchowski N, et al. Magnetic resonance imaging of the lumbar spine in people without back pain. NEJM 1994; 331: 69–73.

21. Boden SD, Davis DO, Dina TS, Patronas NJ, Wiesel SW. Abnormal magnetic resonance scans of the lumbar spine in asymptomatic subjects. A prospective investigation. J Bone Joint Surg 1990; 72:403–408.

22. Siivola SM, Levoska S, Ilkko E, Vanharanta H, Keinänen-Kiukaanniemi S. MRI changes of cervical spine in asymptomatic and symptomatic young adults. Eur Spine J 2002; 11:358–363.

23. Savage RA, Whitehouse GH, Roberts N. The relationship between the magnetic resonance imaging appearance of the lumbar spine and low back pain, age and occupation in males. Eur Spine J 1997; 6:106–114.

24. Borenstrein DG, O'Mara JW, Boden SD, et al. The value of magnetic resonance imaging of the lumbar spine to predict low-back pain in asymptomatic subjects: a seven-year follow-up study. J Bone Joint Surg Am 2001; 83-A:1306–1311.
25. Wiesel SW, Tsourmas N, Feffer HL, Citrin CM, Patronas N. A study of computer-assisted tomography. I. The incidence of positive CAT scans in an asymptomatic group of patients. Spine 1984; 9:549–551.
26. Carragee EJ. Is lumbar discography a determinate of discogenic low back pain: provocative discography reconsidered. Curr Rev Pain 2000; 4:301–308.
27. Malmivaara A, Hakkinen U, Aro T, et al. The treatment of acute low back pain-bed rest, exercises, or ordinary activity? NEJM 1995; 332:351–355.
28. Faas A, Chavannes AW, van Eijk JT, Gubbels JW. A randomized, placebo-controlled trial of exercise therapy inpatients with acute low back pain. Spine 1993; 18:1388–1395.
29. Faas A, van Eijk JT, Chavannes AW, Gubbels JW. A randomized trial of exercise therapy in patients with acute low back pain. Efficacy on sickness absence. Spine 1995; 20:941–947.
30. Rozenberg S, Delval C, Rezvani Y, et al. Bed rest or normal acitivty for patients with acute low back pain: a randomized controlled trial. Spine 2002; 27:1487–1493.
31. Malmivaara A, Hakkinen U, Aro T, et al. The treatment of acute low back pain-bed rest, exercises, or ordinary activity? NEJM 1995; 332:351–355.
32. Bendebba M, Torgerson WS, Boyd RJ, et al. Persistent low back pain and sciatica in the United States: treatment outcomes. J Spinal Disord Tech 2002; 15:2–15.
33. Van Tulder MW, Cherkin DC, Berman B, Lao L, Koes BU. The effectiveness of acupuncture in the management of acute and chronic low back pain. A systematic review with the framework of the Cochrane Collaboration Back Review Group. Spine 1999; 24:1113–1123.
34. Van Tulder MW, Ostelo R, Vlaeyen JW, et al. Behavioral treatment for chronic low back pain: a systematic review within the framework of the Cochrane Back Review Group. Spine 2001; 26:270–281.
35. Nabeta T, Kawakita K. Relief of chronic neck and shoulder pain by manual acupuncture to tender points: a sham-controlled randomized trial. Complement Ther Med 2002; 10:217–222.
36. Harris GR, Susman JL. Managing musculoskeletal complaints with rehabilitation therapy: summary of the Philadelphia Panel evidence-based clinical practice guidelines on musculoskeletal rehabilitation interventions. J Fam Pract 2002; 51:1042–1046.
37. Swenson RS. Therapeutic modalities in the management of nonspecific neck pain. Phys Med Rehabil Clin N Am 2003; 14:605–627.
38. Deyo RA. Drug therapy for back pain. Which drugs help which patients? Spine 1996; 21:2840–2849.
39. Stanton-Hicks M. Nerve blocks in chronic pain therapy - are there any indications left? Acta Anaesthesiol Scand 2001; 45:1100–1107.
40. Webster BS, Snook SH. The cost of 1989 workers' compensation low back pain claims. Spine 1994; 19:1111–1115.
41. Van Tulder MW, Koes Bw, Bouter LM. A cost-of-illness study of back pain in the Netherlands. Pain 1995; 62:233–240.

42. Maniadakis N, Gray A. The economic burden of back pain in the UK. Pain 2000; 84:95–103.
43. Seferlis T, Lindholm L, Nemeth G. Cost-minimisation analysis of three conservative treatment programmes in 180 patients sick-listed for low low-back. Scand J Prim Health Care 2000; 18:53–67.
44. Suter PB. Employment and litigation: improved by work, assisted by verdict. Pain 2002; 1000:249–257.
45. Ylinen J, Takala E, Nykänen M, et al. Active neck muscle training in the treatment of chronic neck pain in women: a randomized controlled trial. JAMA 2003; 289:2509–02516.
46. Snook SH, Webster BS, McGory RW, et al. The reduction of chronic nonspecific low back pain through the control of early morning lumbar flexion. A randomized controlled trial. Spine 1998; 23:2601–2607.
47. Frost H, Klaber Moffett JA, Moser JS, Fairbak JL. Randomised controlled trial for evaluation of fitness programme for patients with chronic low back pain. BMJ 1995; 310:151–154.
48. Faas A. Exercises: which ones are worth trying, for which patients, and when? Spine 1996; 21:2877–2878.
49. Viljanen M, Malmivaara A, Uitti J, et al. Effectiveness of dynamic muscle training, relaxation training, or ordinary activity for chronic neck pain: randomized controlled trial. BMJ 2003; 327:475.
50. Irnich D, Behrens N, Gleditsch JM, et al. Immediate effects of dry needling and acupuncture at distant points in chronic neck pain: results of a randomized, double-blind, sham-controlled crossover trial. Pain 2002; 99:83–89.
51. Ernst E, Assendelft WJ. Chiropractic for low back pain. BMJ 1998; 317:160.
52. Jamison RN, Slawsby EA, Nedeljkovic SS, Katz ND. Opioid therapy for chronic noncancer back pain. A randomized prospective study. Spine 1998; 23:2591–6000.
53. Schofferman J. Long-term opioid analgesic therapy for severe refractory lumbar spine pain. Clin J Pain 1999; 15:136–140.
54. Schonstein E, Kenny DT, Keating J, Koes BW. Work conditioning, work hardening and functional restoration for workers with back and neck pain. Cochrane Database Syst Rev 2003; CD001822.
55. Hagen EM, Eriksen HR, Ursin H. Does early intervention with a light mobilization program reduce long-term sick leave for low back pain? Spine 2000; 25:1973–1976.
56. Bendix AF, Bendix T, Lund C, Kirkbak S, Ostenfeld S. Comparison of three intensive programs for chronic low back pain patients: a prospective, randomized, observer-blinded study with one-year follow-up. Scand J Rehabil Med 1997; 29:81–89.
57. Lanes TC, Gauron EF, Spratt KF, et al. Long-term follow-up of patients with chronic back pain treated in a multidisciplinary rehabilitation program. Spine 1995; 20:801–806.
58. Rainville J, Sobel JB, Hartigan C, Wright A. The effect of compensation involvement on the reporting of pain and disability by patients referred for rehabilitation of chronic low back pain. Spine 1997; 22:2016–2024.

CME QUESTIONS—CHAPTER 5

1. Which occupations are associated with a high risk for chronic neck or back pain?

   a. Nurses
   b. Hairstylists
   c. Janitors/custodians/housekeepers
   d. Secretaries
   e. A and B
   f. A, B, and C

2. Which characteristic(s) predict a higher likelihood of developing chronic neck or back pain?

   a. Female gender
   b. Smoking
   c. Widespread pain
   d. Obesity
   e. A and C
   f. All of the above

3. Which feature(s) predict successful return to work after absence for back pain?

   a. Age less than 30 years
   b. Previous steady employment
   c. Normal lumbar flexion
   d. All of the above
   e. None of the above

4. Chose the correct statement(s):

   a. Acute back pain should be treated with physical therapy.
   b. Chronic back pain should be treated with physical therapy.
   c. Return to work should not be attempted by patients with chronic neck or back pain until their pain symptoms have resolved.
   d. A and B
   e. All of the above

CASE HISTORY

Ms. Stewart is an attractive, slender, 30-year-old professional who complains of recurrent bouts of abdominal pain, bloating, and diarrhea occurring over the last 6 years. The abdominal pain improves after bowel movements; however, despite having diarrhea, she always feels like her bowel movements are incomplete. She describes painful, loose, watery stools occurring approximately four to five times a day about twice a week. She has never had bowel accidents at night. She has never noticed blood in her stools, although they sometimes contain mucus. She was previously diagnosed with lactose intolerance because of some bloating episodes after drinking milk. Although she avoids milk and cheese, she eats ice cream without problems. She has no other medical symptoms and her weight is stable. She is currently not using any medications for her digestive symptoms. She has never seen a psychiatrist for depression or anxiety. When her primary care physician asks if she was ever the victim of sexual abuse, her lip begins to quiver and tears fill her eyes, but she won't provide any specific information. Physical examination shows mild, diffuse belly tenderness with no masses or enlarged organs. Laboratory testing shows a normal blood count and electrolytes and is negative for stool guaiac or stool ova and parasites. A previous sigmoidoscopy revealed only small external hemorrhoids. Ms. Stewart is treated with a low-fat diet and is referred for a psychological evaluation to rule out depression.

* * *

Ms. Stewart provides a typical history of irritable bowel syndrome (IBS), a common cause of chronic abdominal pain, especially in women. Although the literature describes a link between psychological distress and abuse history with IBS, most gastroenterologists agree that the gastrointestinal (GI) symptoms are not a manifestation of psychopathology. Indeed, psychological distress and abuse history occur commonly in all patients with chronic pain (*see* Chapter 15). In Ms. Stewart's case, the treating physician appropriately ensured the absence of identifiable organic disease. The absence of testing abnormalities,

From: *Chronic Pain: A Primary Care Guide to Practical Management*
Edited by: D. A. Marcus © Humana Press, Totowa, NJ

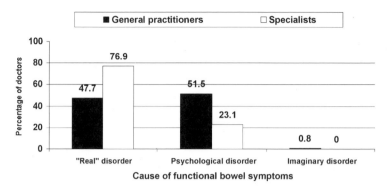

Fig. 1. Attitudes of physicians toward functional bowel disorders. (Based on ref. *1*.)

however, is not synonymous with the absence of pathology or a psychologically based disorder.

KEY CHAPTER POINTS

- Abdominal pain may be caused by a readily identified pathology or may occur as a chronic condition without correctable pathology. Chronic abdominal pain is typically diagnosed in patients with a stable pain history for at least 3 months who lack symptoms and signs of other types of pathology (e.g., fever, significant weight loss, or anemia).
- Functional abdominal pain disorders, such as IBS, are not part of a psychological syndrome.
- Although psychological distress is more common in patients with functional abdominal pain disorders, it does not occur at an elevated rate in individuals with the same disorders who are not seeking medical care. Therefore, psychological distress is a marker of treatment-seeking behavior rather than abdominal pain.
- Historical reports of symptoms and physical examination signs can help distinguish causes of chronic abdominal pain.
- Chronic abdominal pain is generally managed with both medication and non-medication pain management strategies.

Abdominal pain is often caused by readily identified pathology, such as gastritis or ulcer disease, gallbladder disease, or inflammatory bowel disease. Abdominal pain, especially in the absence of an identified structural pathology, is often equated with psychological or somatization disorders. A recent survey of perceptions of general practitioners and specialists demonstrated that general practitioners are significantly more likely to believe that functional bowel disorders were the result of psychological disorders, whereas specialists are more likely to assume that patients with this condition have a real but yet unidentified etiology ($p < 0.001$) (Fig. 1) *(1)*.

This chapter addresses some of the common syndromes of chronic abdominal pain. It is essential to remember that a diagnosis of chronic abdominal pain is only made in patients with a stable pain history for at least 3 months who lack symptoms and signs of other types of pathology, including fever, significant weight loss, and anemia. This important point was recently highlighted in a letter describing a woman with fever, diarrhea, and progressive abdominal pain over approximately 1 week *(2)*. Her condition was labeled "chronic abdominal pain," and she subsequently died with undiagnosed mesenteric ischemia. The author postulated that the chronic pain diagnosis restricted the ordering of tests that typically would have been completed in a patient with progressive, subacute abdominal pain.

1. EPIDEMIOLOGY

Persistent abdominal pain occurs in a significant minority of patients. A population-based community survey in the United Kingdom identified persistent abdominal pain (pain episodes during the preceding month lasting at least 24 hours) in 7.7% of adults, with a greater prevalence in women compared with men (9.3 vs 5.6%; $p < 0.01$) *(3)*. A total of 1501 adults without abdominal pain were followed prospectively for 12 months. New abdominal pain developed in 69 people (4.6%), with no gender differences noted in development of new pain.

Abdominal pain is among the most common pain complaints seen by primary care practitioners. The 2000 National Ambulatory Medical Care Survey identified abdominal pain as the one of the top reasons for seeking an outpatient physician visit, ranking as the 12th most common complaint *(4)*. Abdominal pain accounts for 5% of all pain complaints made to general practitioners *(5)*.

1.1. Irritable Bowel Syndrome

IBS describes the combination of recurrent lower abdominal pain, change in bowel habits, and bloating or rectal urgency in patients without identified structural or biochemical pathology. The diagnosis of IBS has been standardized with the development of the Rome criteria, which were revised in 1999 (*see* Box 1). Ms. Stewart meets Rome II criteria, reporting a chronic history of abdominal pain associated with diarrhea and relieved by bowel movements. She also reports feelings of incomplete evacuation, mucus in stool, and bloating.

An international, community-based survey of more than 40,000 individuals identified 11.5% with IBS, with a female to male ratio of 1.7:1 *(6)*. In this sample, IBS symptoms occurred on an average of 7 days/month with an average of two episodes daily, each lasting approximately 1 hour (Fig. 2). The majority of patients with IBS reported a variety of gastrointestinal (GI) symptoms (Table 1).

Box 1
Rome II Criteria for Diagnosis of Irritable Bowel Syndrome

- Abdominal pain for at least 12 weeks of the preceding year, with two of the following:
  - ○ Relief with bowel movement (BM)
  - ○ Onset associated with change in BM frequency
  - ○ Onset associated with change in stool appearance
- Additional symptoms often include:
  - ○ BMs more than three times daily or less than three times weekly
  - ○ Abnormally loose or hard stools
  - ○ Straining, urgency, or feeling of incomplete bowel evacuation
  - ○ Mucus in stool
  - ○ Bloating or abdominal distention

Based on ref. *5a*.

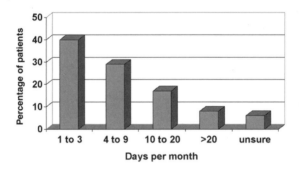

Fig. 2. Frequency of symptoms in irritable bowel syndrome. (Based on ref. *6*.)

In addition to pain and GI symptoms, individuals with IBS have significant disability, including reduced productivity and increased frequency of medical visits (Fig. 3).

1.2. Myofascial Abdominal Wall Pain

Myofascial pain, which is related to tight muscle bands and muscular trigger points, may also affect abdominal muscles. (*See* Chapter 9 for a full discussion of this syndrome and its treatment.) Chronic abdominal pain caused by tight and tender abdominal muscles (e.g., rectus abdominis, pyramidalis, obliques, and transversus abdominus) occurs in a significant minority of patients with chronic abdominal pain and is commonly overlooked. Myofascial pain was determined to be the cause of pain in 26% of patients diagnosed with chronic abdominal pain that is not related to an underlying visceral pathology *(7)*.

Table 1
Common Symptoms of Irritable Bowel Syndrome

Symptom	Prevalence (%)
Abdominal pain	88
Bloating	80
Trapped wind	66
Tiredness	60
Diarrhea	59
Tightness of clothing	58
Constipation	53
Heartburn	47

Based on ref. 6.

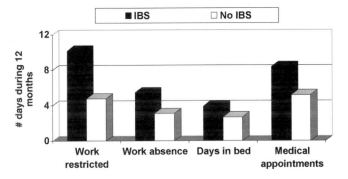

Fig. 3. Impact of irritable bowel syndrome (IBS). Comparison of disability in a community survey of individuals with IBS and without IBS (no IBS). (Based on ref. 6.)

1.3. Chronic Pancreatitis

Studies conducted in the United States, Europe, Central America, and Asia indicate that chronic pancreatitis affects approximately 4 out of every 100,000 people annually *(8)*. Alcoholism accounts for more than 50% of all cases of chronic pancreatitis, with the risk for chronic pancreatitis increasing linearly in relation to the amount of alcohol consumed. It is important to remember, however, that approximately 20 to 30% of all cases are idiopathic, with the remainder caused by biliary and other diseases.

2. EVALUATION

As with all types of chronic pain, the physician needs to ensure the absence of correctable, organic pathology during the initial history taking and physical examination in patients with abdominal pain. Patients with subacute symptoms,

---

Box 2
Symptoms and History That Suggest Irritable Bowel
Syndrome and Warrant a More Detailed Evaluation

- At least a 10-lb weight loss (unintentional)
- Bloody stools
- Fever; recent use of antibiotics
- Nocturnal diarrhea
- Family history of colon cancer

Based on ref. *3*.

---

symptoms related to eating, associated medical symptoms or signs (e.g., change in skin or stool color, bloody stools, organomegaly, or abdominal masses), constitutional symptoms (e.g., weight loss, fatigue, or fever), or a family history of GI cancer warrant a more detailed evaluation.

In addition to a general abdominal examination, patients with abdominal pain require a digital rectal examination and female patients require a thorough pelvic examination. Patients reporting abdominal pain should also receive a neurological examination to identify bands of sensory loss or dysethesia in the abdomen (to rule out local nerve entrapment syndromes, thoracic spine disease, or postherpetic neuralgia) and changes in strength, reflexes, and sensation in the lower extremities (to rule out spinal disease). A neurological examination is particularly important because the midthoracic spine is a vascular watershed area, with a predilection for metastatic disease. Patients suspected of having a thoracic pathology that is not well localized may be evaluated using sagittal magnetic resonance imaging, which demonstrates multiple thoracic levels.

2.1. Irritable Bowel Syndrome

Young patients with IBS symptoms without associated symptoms (*see* Box 2), such as Ms. Stewart, require a minimal amount of testing (*see* Box 3) *(9,10)*. Screening for thyroid disease and lactose intolerance is best reserved for patients with specific symptoms of these conditions, such as fatigue and weight change (thyroid disease) and intolerance to milk products, including ice cream (lactose intolerance). Patients aged 50 years and older warrant additional screening with a colonoscopy and thyroid function testing. Abdominal ultrasound is generally not helpful.

2.2. Myofascial Pain

Evaluation of myofascial pain is covered elsewhere in this book (*see* Chapter 9). Several questions are useful to differentiate patients with musculoskeletal causes of abdominal pain from those with nonmusculoskeletal pain (*see*

Box 3
Diagnostic Evaluation of Patients
With Symptoms of Irritable Bowel Syndrome

- Stools: Test for
  - Blood
  - Ova and parasites
- Laboratory testing
  - Complete blood count
  - Chemistry panel
  - Erythrocyte sedimentation rate
  - Add thyroid function testing for patients aged 50 years or older
- Gastrointestinal procedures
  - Aged younger than 50 years: flexible sigmoidoscopy
    - Include biopsy to rule out inflammatory disease or microscopic colitis if diarrhea is a symptom
  - Aged at least 50 years: colonoscopy to screen for cancer

Based on ref. *3*.

Box 4
Questions That Can Be Used to Distinguish Musculoskeletal
Etiologies From Other Causes of Chronic Abdominal Pain

Patients responding positively to the first set of questions and negatively to the second set are likely to have a musculoskeletal cause for their chronic abdominal pain.

- If patients give a positive response to the following questions, the pain is probably musculoskeletal:
  - Is pain worsened by coughing, sneezing, or taking a deep breath?
  - Is pain aggravated by change in posture, such as getting out of bed or a chair, bending, turning over in bed, or lifting?
- If patients give a negative response to the following questions, their pain is probably musculoskeletal:
  - Has there been a recent change in your bowel habits?
  - Does eating aggravate your pain?
  - Have you lost weight unintentionally since your pain started?

Based on ref. *11*.

Box 4) *(11)*. On examination, tender, tight muscle bands causing myofascial pain are best identified in the activated muscle. Patients with abdominal pain that is not associated with bowel symptoms or eating should be examined while lying flat. They should be asked to elevate the head and shoulders a few inches off of the examination table to induce abdominal muscle tensing.

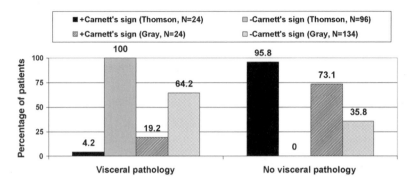

Fig. 4. Diagnostic function of Carnett's sign. A positive Carnett's sign was used to distinguish visceral and nonvisceral (functional) causes of abdominal pain in 120 emergency department patients with acute abdominal pain *(12)* and 158 hospital admissions for abdominal pain *(13)*.

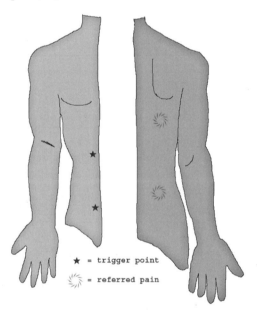

Fig. 5. Myofascial abdominal wall pain: rectus abdominis trigger points and referral pattern.

Aggravation of pain and abdominal tenderness with this maneuver is typical in patients with muscular pain (positive Carnett's sign). Carnett's sign is useful for distinguishing myofascial and visceral pain (Fig. 4) *(12,13)*. Examining the tensed belly while the patient maintains this position can reveal tender muscles and trigger points in the abdominal muscles, such as the rectus abdominis muscles (Fig. 5), as well as painful abdominal hernias.

Box 5
Diagnostic Testing for Patients With Suspected Chronic Pancreatitis

- Serum trypsinogen (in patients with diarrhea and steatorrhea)
- Secretin hormone stimulation test
- Endoscopic retrograde cholangiopancreatography
- Abdominal X-ray or computed tomography

2.3. Chronic Pancreatitis

The pain of chronic pancreatitis is constant and severe, and may radiate to the back. The pain is often aggravated by food or alcohol and is associated with malabsorption and weight loss. Chronic pancreatitis is diagnosed by clinical examination and a finding of abnormalities on tests for pancreatic enzymes and secretin stimulation (if available) or endoscopic retrograde cholangiopancreatography, and radiographic evidence of pancreatic calcifications (*see* Box 5). Patients with chronic pancreatitis should be evaluated for signs of poor pancreatic function, including weight loss, steatorrhea, and glucose intolerance, in addition to abdominal pain.

2.4. Psychological Factors

A large, prospective survey of individuals with abdominal pain identified psychological distress as an important predictor of new abdominal pain *(3)*. Patients without abdominal pain who had the highest levels of psychological distress were three times more likely to develop abdominal pain within the following 12 months compared with individuals without psychological distress. Anxiety doubled the risk for abdominal pain. This study suggests that patients with abdominal pain will be more likely to have comorbid psychological distress compared with patients without pain. This relationship, however, does not confirm that abdominal pain is a manifestation of psychological distress.

Childhood abuse has also been linked with the development of chronic abdominal pain in adulthood, especially pain related to functional GI disorders, such as IBS. A survey of 226 consecutive GI outpatients identified a history of physical or sexual abuse in approximately one-third of patients with either functional or organic GI disease *(14)*. A similar study of 206 female gastroenterology clinic patients identified a greater prevalence of both sexual and physical abuse in patients with functional disorders (53 and 13%, respectively) vs patients with organic disorders (37 and 2%, respectively) *(15)*. Interestingly, the treating physician was aware of abuse in only 17% of patients. Hobbis and colleagues questioned adults with IBS, Crohn's disease, or non-GI disease about the incidence of abuse during childhood and adulthood *(16)* and found that the prevalence of childhood and adult experiences of sexual abuse (17–28%) or physical abuse (49–61%) was similar in all groups. Although a history of abuse itself does not necessarily predict the occurrence or type of abdominal pain, symptom severity and comorbid somatic complaints are higher in GI patients with more significant abuse histories *(17,18)*. For this reason, gentle questioning about abuse is appropriate for patients with abdominal pain.

It is important to remember that, as with all types of chronic pain, patients seeking treatment for chronic abdominal pain have a higher prevalence of psychological distress. This does not, however, confirm a suspicion that the pain symptoms are a sign of or caused by psychological distress. Drossman and colleagues compared psychological tests for patients with IBS, individuals with IBS who had not sought medical treatment (non-patients with IBS), and pain-free controls *(19)*. Although psychological distress was significantly higher in patients with IBS, it was not greater in non-patients with IBS compared with pain-free controls. A similar study revealed an increased rate of psychological abnormalities in patients with fibromyalgia compared with individuals with fibromyalgia who had not sought medical care *(20)*. These studies suggest that psychological distress influences treatment-seeking behaviors, driving patients to initiate self-care. The data refute the hypothesis that these chronic pain complaints are themselves symptoms of psychological distress. In the case of Ms. Stewart and similar patients, a history of abuse, depression, and anxiety are important to determine. Although these factors are not likely to cause chronic abdominal pain, they are linked to more severe symptoms and suggest the need for more aggressive therapy.

3. TREATMENT

The same principles used to manage other types of nonmalignant chronic pain apply to chronic abdominal pain. As with chronic pain in general, patients with chronic abdominal pain typically benefit from both medication- and nonmedication-based pain management therapies. In a large, multicenter trial in which patients with functional bowel disorders were randomized to nonpharmacological (cognitive-behavioral therapy [CBT] vs education) and pharmacological (desipramine 150 mg/day vs placebo) therapy or placebo (Fig. 6) *(21)*, the responses to CBT and desipramine were similar.

3.1. Irritable Bowel Syndrome

Therapy for IBS targets individual symptoms. A variety of effective medications are available, although most treat diarrhea or constipation rather than global IBS symptoms (Table 2) *(10,22)*. Effective alternative therapy includes traditional Chinese medicine, relaxation training, CBT, and peppermint oil

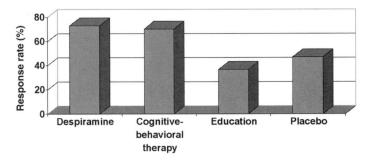

Fig. 6. Treatment of functional bowel disorders. (Based on ref. *21.*)

Table 2
Medication Therapy for Irritable Bowel Syndrome (IBS)

Medication	Condition improved	Significant side effects
5HT receptor agents		
5HT$_3$ antagonist alosetron	Global IBS symptoms in women with diarrhea	Constipation
5HT$_4$ agonist tegaserod	Global IBS symptoms in women with constipation	Diarrhea
Antidepressants		
Tricyclic	Abdominal pain	Constipation
SSRI	Abdominal pain	Better tolerated than tricyclics
Gastrointestinal		
Loperamide	Diarrhea	Constipation
Fiber/bulking agents	Constipation	Bloating
Oral cromolyn sodium	Diarrhea	Constipation

5HT, serotonin; SSRI, selective serotonin reuptake inhibitor.
(Based on refs. *10* and *22.*)

(10,22). Elimination diets and the use of probiotics (such as lactobacillus or yogurt) are generally not beneficial.

3.2. Myofascial Abdominal Wall Pain

Patients with myofascial abdominal wall pain should be treated using modalities similar to those used in patients with other myofascial pain syndromes. Abdominal stretching exercises, physical therapy, and trigger-point injections may all be beneficial. (For a complete review of myofascial pain treatment, *see* Chapter 9.)

Table 3
Treatment of Chronic Pancreatitis

Condition to treat	Treatment
All chronic pancreatitis symptoms	Abstinence from alcohol
Pain	Non-enteric-coated pancreatic enzymes
	(including a bedtime dose)
	Analgesics
	Somatostatin analog (e.g., octreotide)
	Cholecytokinin antagonist (e.g., loxiglumide[a])
Steatorrhea	Pancreatic enzymes
Glucose intolerance	Insulin

[a] Currently not available in the United States.

3.3. Chronic Pancreatitis

Treatment for patients with chronic pancreatitis focuses on minimizing future pancreatic damage (e.g., by avoiding alcohol) and symptoms of pain and abnormal exocrine and endocrine function (Table 3). Chronic pancreatitis pain tends to be severe and typically requires opioid analgesics. The use of opioids may be particularly challenging in patients with alcohol-related chronic pancreatitis because of the risk for medication misuse and abuse (*see* Chapter 17). Pancreatic enzymes and other agents may also improve pain severity. In a recent large, randomized study, investigators found an improvement rate of more than 50% in patients with chronic pancreatitis treated with the cholecystokinin A-receptor antagonist loxiglumide 600 mg/day (currently not available in the United States) *(23)*. Pancreatic surgery and celiac plexus blocks or neurolysis are not recommended for most patients with chronic pancreatitis.

Patients with poor exocrine function, manifested by steatorrhea and weight loss, should be treated with a low-fat diet and pancreatic enzyme supplementation. Patients with poor endocrine function and glucose intolerance typically require insulin therapy.

4. SUMMARY

Abdominal pain may be caused by a readily identified pathology (e.g., gastritis, ulcer disease, or inflammation) or present as a chronic pain complaint without a correctable pathology. Chronic abdominal pain is typically diagnosed in patients with a stable pain history for at least 3 months who lack symptoms and signs of other pathology (e.g., fever, significant weight loss, or anemia). Although blood tests and radiographs often fail to identify obvious abnormalities in patients with chronic abdominal pain, functional abdominal pain disorders (e.g., IBS) are not psychological syndromes. Measures of psychological distress are indeed higher in patients with functional abdominal pain disorders; however, the rate of psychological distress is not elevated in individuals with these disorders who are not seeking medical care. Therefore, psychological distress is a marker of treatment-seeking behavior rather than abdominal pain.

Historical reports of symptoms (changes in bowel habits, occurrence of bloating, and pain with lifting or change in posture) and physical examination signs (e.g., Carnett's sign of myofascial pain) can help the clinician distinguish the causes of chronic abdominal pain. In general, most types of chronic abdominal pain can be managed with a both medication- and nonmedication-based pain management strategies. Treatment strategies, however, are often specific to individual pain diagnostic categories (e.g., serotonin receptor agents or antidepressants for IBS, trigger-point injection for myofascial pain, and enzyme supplementation and analgesics for chronic pancreatitis).

REFERENCES

1. Gladman LM, Gorard DA. General practitioner and hospital specialist attitudes to functional gastrointestinal disorders. Aliment Pharmacol Ther 2003; 17:651–654.
2. Jones MP. Death by diagnosis. Ann Intern Med 2001; 135:307.
3. Halder SS, McBeth J, Silman AJ, Thompson DG, MacFarlane GJ. Psychosocial risk factors for the onset of abdominal pain: results from a large prospective population-based study. Int J Epidemiol 2002; 31:1219–1225.
4. Cherry DW, Woodwell DA. National Ambulatory Medical Care Survey: 2000 summary. Adv Data 2002; 5:1–32.
5. Hasselström J, Liu-Palmgren J, Rasjö-Wrååk G. Prevalence of pain in general practice. Eur J Pain 2002; 6:375–385.
5a. Thompson WG, Longstreth GF, Drossman DA, et al. Functional bowel disorders and functional abdominal pain. Gut 1999; 45(suppl 2):1143–1147.
6. Hungin AS, Whorwell PJ, Tack J, Mearin F. The prevalence, patterns and impact of irritable bowel syndrome: an international survey of 40,000 subjects. Aliment Pharmacol Ther 2003; 17:643–650.
7. McGarrity TJ, Peters DJ, Thompson C, McGarrity SJ. Outcome of patients with chronic abdominal pain referred to chronic pain clinic. Am J Gastroenterol 2000; 95:1812–1816.
8. Otsuki M. Chronic pancreatitis in Japan: epidemiology, prognosis, diagnostic criteria, and future problems. J Gastroenterol 2003; 38:315–326.
9. Olden KW. The challenge of diagnosing irritable bowel syndrome. Rev Gastroenterol Dis 2003; 3(Suppl 3):S3–S11.
10. Holten KB. Irritable bowel syndrome: minimize testing, let symptoms guide treatment. J Fam Pract 2003; 52:942–949.
11. Sparkes V, Prevost AT, Hunter JO. Derivation and identification of questions that act as predictors of abdominal pain of musculoskeletal origin. Eur J Gastroenterol Hepatol 2003; 15:1021–1027.
12. Thomson H, Francis DM. Abdominal-wall tenderness: a useful sign in the acute abdomen. Lancet 1977; 2:1053–1054.

13. Gray DW, Dixon JM, Seabrook G, Collin J. Is abdominal wall tenderness a useful sign in the diagnosis of non-specific abdominal pain? Ann R Coll Surg Engl 1988; 70:233–234.
14. Baccini F, Pallotta N, Calabrese E, Pezzotti P, Corazziari E. Prevalence of sexual an physical abuse and its relationship with symptom manifestations in patients with chronic organic and functional gastrointestinal disorders. Dig Liver Dis 2003; 35:256–261.
15. Drossman DA. Sexual and physical abuse and gastrointestinal illness. Scand J Gastroenterol Suppl 1995; 208:90–96.
16. Hobbis IA, Turpin G, Read NW. A re-examination of the relationship between abuse experience and functional bowel disorders. Scand J Gastroenterol 2002; 4: 423–430.
17. Leserman J, Li Z, Drossman DA, Hu YJ. Selected symptoms associated with sexual and physical abuse history among female patients with gastrointestinal disorders: the impact on subsequent health care visits. Psychol Med 1998; 28:417–425.
18. Drossman DA. Do psychosocial factors define symptom severity and patient status in irritable bowel syndrome? Am J Med 1999; 107(Suppl 5A):41S–50S.
19. Drossman DA, McKee DC, Sandler RS, et al. Psychosocial factors in the irritable bowel syndrome: a multivariate study of patients and nonpatients with irritable bowel syndrome. Gastroenterology 1998; 95:701–708.
20. Aaron LA, Bradley LA, Alarcon GS, et al. Psychiatric diagnoses in patients with fibromyalgia are related to health care-seeking behavior rather than to illness. Arthritis Rheum 1996; 39:436–445.
21. Drossman DA, Toner BB, Whitehead WE, et al. Cognitive-behavioral therapy versus education and desipramine versus placebo for moderate to severe functional bowel disorders. Gastroenterology 2003; 125:19–31.
22. Spanier JA, Howden CW, Jones MP. A systematic review of alternative therapies in the irritable bowel syndrome. Arch Intern Med 2003; 163:265–274.
23. Shiratori K, Takeuchi T, Satake K, Matsuno S. Clinical evaluation of oral administration of a cholecystokinin: a receptor antagonist (loxiglumide) to patients with acute, painful attacks of chronic pancreatitis: a multicenter dose-response study in Japan. Pancreas 2002; 25:E1–E5.

CME QUESTIONS—CHAPTER 6

1. Which of the following symptoms are common in patients with musculoskeletal abdominal pain?
   a. Pain aggravated by lifting
   b. Pain aggravated by eating
   c. Pain coughing or deep breaths
   d. A and C
   e. All of the above

2. Rome II diagnostic criteria for irritable bowel syndrome include:
   a. Pain occurring in 12 or more weeks during the preceding year
   b. Pain relieved by bowel movements
   c. Change in bowel frequency when pain began
   d. Change in stool appearance when pain began
   e. All of the above

3. Medications used to treat diarrhea in patients with irritable bowel syndrome include:
   a. Alosetron
   b. Loperamide
   c. Oral cromolyn sodium
   d. All of the above

4. Which of the following is not a routine therapy for chronic pancreatitis?
   a. Abstinence from alcohol
   b. Pancreatic enzymes
   c. Opioid analgesics
   d. Celiac plexus neurolysis

CASE HISTORY

Mr. Harris is a 68-year-old retired construction worker. He has had a very active life, playing football through high school and college and continuing to play in amateur leagues during his early work years. He comes to his doctor with a chief complaint of right knee pain, which has been increasing progressively over the last 8 years. An earlier evaluation revealed positive rheumatoid factor (RF), and he was diagnosed with rheumatoid arthritis (RA). This was managed with nonsteroidal anti-inflammatory drugs (NSAIDs) and steroids. Although he experienced pain reduction with the anti-inflammatory analgesics, he developed severe gastritis and needed to discontinue therapy. He was referred to a rheumatologist for more aggressive therapy, but was fearful of the side effects of methotrexate, which he had read about on the Internet. He decided to discontinue all exercise programs and began sedentary activities. During this time, he sprained his ankle twice after stepping off curbs and had recurrent attacks of low back sprain after carrying small loads, such as groceries or laundry. Mr. Harris subsequently tried to resume his previous jogging program without success. At this new consultation, Mr. Harris reports that his knee is most bothersome after prolonged sitting or after jogging for about 15 minutes. He also reports stiffness in both hands and in his left hip, and right knee when he first gets up in the morning, although this goes away after he "works it out" with range-of-motion exercises and a few minutes of walking. On examination, Mr. Harris is slow to get out of his chair and reports feeling "stiff" after sitting in the waiting room for 1 hour. Examination of the knee shows slight bony deformity with no inflammation of the joint. Passive range of motion is slightly reduced with joint crepitus. No joint instability is identified. Radiographs of the knee show narrowing of the joint space and the presence of osteophytes. His primary care physician (PCP) makes a diagnosis of osteoarthritis and treats him with acetaminophen. He also enrolls Mr. Harris in an arthritis pool therapy program at the local YMCA and recommends a bicycling program as well. Two months later, Mr. Harris reports improvement in both pain and activity tolerance.

* * *

From: *Chronic Pain: A Primary Care Guide to Practical Management*
Edited by: D. A. Marcus © Humana Press, Totowa, NJ

Mr. Harris shows characteristic features of osteoarthritis (OA), the most common form of arthritis in adults. OA typically affects the large, weight-bearing joints in a nonsymmetrical fashion, with the knee frequently affected. Interestingly, RF is not specific for RA; in fact, it may be positive in patients with OA and negative in RA, particularly during the early stages of the disease. Mr. Harris' PCP treated him appropriately with a well-tolerated analgesic. Anti-inflammatory medications are not the first choice for patients with OA because it is not an inflammatory condition.

Distinguishing between degenerative and inflammatory arthritis is essential in patients with chronic joint complaints. Disease pathology, pattern of joint involvement, and recommended treatments are dissimilar for degenerative and inflammatory arthritis. In addition, maintaining good condition of supportive tissues around joints is essential for minimizing new pain complaints and maintaining good function. Although the OA identified in Mr. Harris is likely the result of years of joint overuse, too much rest for the joints will not improve symptoms. As he discovered, too much rest increases the risk for injury from minor trauma because of a lack of the normal protection of the joint that is provided by strong and flexible muscles, tendons, and ligaments.

KEY CHAPTER POINTS

- Arthritis is a common cause of chronic joint pain, with the prevalence increasing with age.
- The most common type of chronic arthritis is degenerative OA.
- Patients with OA are treated with symptomatic therapy and rehabilitation.
- RA therapy requires specific disease-modifying drugs that are often prescribed after consultation with a rheumatologist.
- Aerobic exercise is important for reducing pain and maintaining function in both OA and RA.

1. EPIDEMIOLOGY AND IMPACT

Arthritis is one of the most common chronic pain disorders and is diagnosed in 8 to 16% of the population in Europe and the United States *(1)*. Because the incidence of arthritis increases with age, it has been predicted that its prevalence will increase substantially over the next decade because of aging populations in both Europe and the United States. The 2002 revision of the United Nations' population survey predicts a substantial increase in age over the next several decades *(2)*. People aged over 60 years currently comprise 19% of the population in developed countries and 8% in less developed countries. It is believed that by 2050 the percentage of individuals in this age group will increase to an estimated 32% in developed countries and 20% in less developed countries. In addition, the elderly currently outnumber children in developed countries. By 2050, there will be two elderly adults for every child.

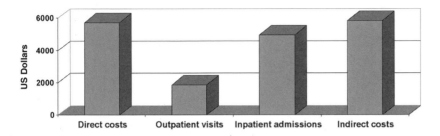

Fig. 1. Mean annual per-patient costs associated with rheumatoid arthritis, in US dollars. (Based on ref. *8*.)

The most common arthritic conditions are degenerative (e.g., osteoarthritis [OA]), and inflammatory (e.g., rheumatoid arthritis [RA]). A Dutch population survey reported OA in 28% of men and women, with RA in 2% of men and 5% of women *(3)*. In the United States, OA affects 68% of adults aged 55 and older, with RA diagnosed in 2% of Americans aged 60 or older *(4,5)*. An estimated 7.1 million ambulatory visits in the United States in 1997 were for OA, with an additional 3.9 million for RA *(6)*. The economic impact of arthritis is high. Arthritis sufferers lose an average of 5.2 hours of work productivity weekly *(7)*. In a meta-analysis of 14 studies addressing costs associated with RA, the mean annual cost per patient (including both direct and indirect costs) was estimated at more than $11,500 (Fig. 1) *(8)*. Costs are high even early in the disease. Söderlin and colleagues evaluated the direct and indirect costs of arthritis in Sweden from the onset of disease through 6 months of follow-up *(9)* and determined that the median cost per patient cost was $3362 ($4385 for RA). In a similar study conducted in the United States in patients with RA during the first year of their disease, investigators reported an average $200 per month in the cost of direct care and $281 per month for indirect costs *(10)*. The average number of days of activity lost each month because of RA symptoms was 3.8 ± 7.7.

2. ARTHRITIS EVALUATION

The evaluation of chronic arthritis focuses on distinguishing degenerative and inflammatory arthritis. This distinction relies primarily on historical data. For example, OA generally affects weight-bearing joints in an asymmetric fashion, whereas RA affects small joints symmetrically (Fig. 2). Radiographs can also be used to help distinguish OA from RA. OA is associated with the development of osteophytes and cartilage erosion (Fig. 3A,B). RA is associated with inflammatory changes and reduced cartilage; bony erosion may also be present, especially with disease progression (Fig. 3A,C).

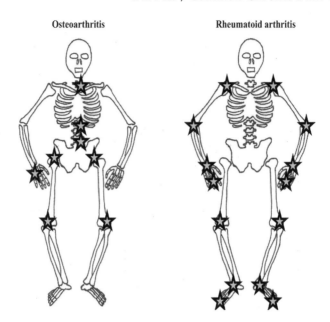

Fig. 2. Typical patterns of joint involvement. Star denotes joints typically involved in each type of arthritis. Osteoarthritis typically affects overused and large weight-bearing joints. Joint involvement is often asymmetrical. Rheumatoid arthritis typically produces symmetrical inflammatory changes in small joints.

Degenerative arthritis is typically evaluated and managed by PCPs, whereas patients with inflammatory arthritis are often referred for consultation with a rheumatologist. Because of the relatively low prevalence of RA compared with OA, many PCPs have limited experience in evaluating and managing RA. A comparative survey of PCPs and rheumatologists to determine the relative rate of diagnosis of rheumatic disease showed poor agreement for both OA (Cohen's $\kappa = 0.51$; positive predictive value [PPV] of PCP diagnosis = 51%) and RA (Cohen's $\kappa = 0.53$; PPV = 46%) *(11)*. Physician education can improve diagnostic accuracy.

In a recent study, Gormley and colleagues developed specific criteria to distinguish inflammatory joint disease from noninflammatory arthritis (*see* Box 1) *(12)*. These criteria were provided to PCPs and nurses to serve as diagnostic guidelines for identifying inflammatory joint disease. Patients identified by non-rheumatologists with any of the criteria in Box 1 were referred to a rheumatologist to confirm early inflammatory disease. Utilization of these screening criteria by general practitioners or rheumatology nurses resulted in excellent agreement between non-rheumatologists and rheumatologists for the diagnosis of inflammatory disease (Cohen's $\kappa = 0.77$ for general practitioners and 0.79 for nurses).

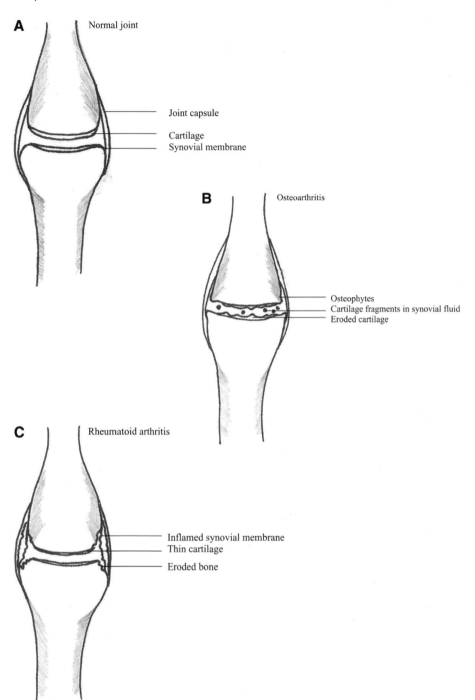

Fig. 3. Joint changes with arthritis.

Box 1
Clinical Features Suggesting Inflammatory Arthritis

- Historical features
  - Pain and/or swelling in several joints
  - Significant joint stiffness in the morning or after rest
  - Progressive loss of joint function
  - Symmetrical joint involvement
  - Good response to nonsteroidal anti-inflammatory drugs
- Physical examination features
  - Joint inflammation (swelling, warmth, tenderness)
  - Restricted joint range of motion

Based on ref. *12*.

Of the features used in the guidelines, historical reports of significant joint stiffness in the morning or after rest and identification of joint swelling on examination most significantly discriminated between inflammatory from non-inflammatory joint disease.

The American College of Rheumatology recommends referrals to a rheumatologist or other physicians familiar with the diagnosis and treatment of arthritis in all patients with newly diagnosed or suspected RA or when it is difficult to distinguish a diagnosis of degenerative vs inflammatory arthritis *(13)*. This recommendation is supported by data showing that RA care directed by a specialist results in superior functional status and pain reduction *(14)*. This is particularly important in the early stages of RA, because joint erosion is already evident in 13% of patients with RA at their initial assessment and subsequent erosion can be minimized by aggressive, disease-modifying RA treatment *(15)*. RA may also be associated with significant systemic complications—including cardiac, renal, ocular, and pulmonary complications—as well as vasculitis. Rheumatologist consultation will also include an evaluation for systemic features of RA.

Figure 4 can be used in the clinic in patients reporting chronic joint pain to help establish symptom chronicity, pain location, and the presence of historical symptoms of degenerative versus inflammatory arthritis. Some symptoms, such as joint pain and morning stiffness, are reported in both OA and RA, although morning stiffness tends to be prolonged in RA. RA patients with multisystem complaints should be evaluated by a rheumatologist. Figure 5 provides completed joint assessment sheets and diagnoses for three typical arthritis patients.

Please complete the following questions:
1. Mark all areas on the figure where you typically experience pain with an X.

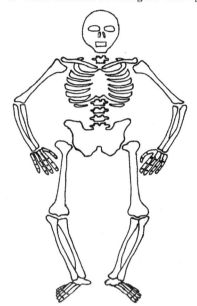

2. How long have you had these pain complaints? _____

3. Circle the best description for your pain:
   NEW PROBLEM   PROGRESSIVELY WORSENING   STABLE   IMPROVING

4. Check any problems you experience with your pain
   ❏ **JOINT SWELLING**
   ❏ **PROLONGED MORNING STIFFNESS**
   ❏ **PROLONGED STIFFNESS AFTER REST**
   ❏ **REDUCED JOINT MOVEMENT**
   ❏ **PAIN IN THE SAME JOINTS ON BOTH SIDES OF THE BODY**
   ❏ **GOOD PAIN RELIEF WITH IBUPROFEN OR NAPROXEN**

5. Check any other body areas that are causing problems:
   ❏ **Heart or chest pain**
   ❏ **Lungs or shortness of breath**
   ❏ **Kidneys**
   ❏ **Swollen legs (other than at the joints)**
   ❏ **Eye**
   ❏ **Skin**

Fig. 4. Assessment sheet for patients reporting joint pain. Patients with chronic or worsening pain may have degenerative or inflammatory arthritis. Placement of marks on drawing will help determine the location of affected joints to distinguish the asymmetrical large (weight-bearing) joint involvement of degenerative arthritis from the symmetrical small-joint involvement of inflammatory arthritis. Patients reporting symptoms described in Question 4 should be examined for the possibility of inflammatory arthritis.

A Diagnosis: acute arthritis – gout

Please complete the following questions:
 1. Mark all areas on the figure where you typically experience pain with an 'X.'

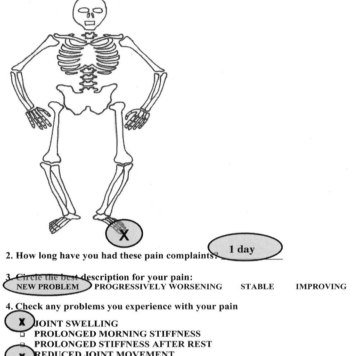

2. How long have you had these pain complaints?   1 day

3. Circle the best description for your pain:
 NEW PROBLEM   PROGRESSIVELY WORSENING   STABLE   IMPROVING

4. Check any problems you experience with your pain
 X JOINT SWELLING
 ❏ PROLONGED MORNING STIFFNESS
 ❏ PROLONGED STIFFNESS AFTER REST
 X REDUCED JOINT MOVEMENT
 ❏ PAIN IN THE SAME JOINTS ON BOTH SIDES OF THE BODY
 ❏ GOOD PAIN RELIEF WITH IBUPROFEN OR NAPROXEN

5. Check any other body areas that are causing problems:
 ❏ Heart or chest pain
 ❏ Lungs or shortness of breath
 ❏ Kidneys
 ❏ Swollen legs (other than at the joints)
 ❏ Eye
 ❏ Skin

Fig. 5. Completed patient assessment sheets. *(Continued on next page.)*

3. ARTHRITIS DIAGNOSIS

A diagnosis in patients with symptoms suggesting arthritis begins with a determination of whether the symptoms are acute or chronic before considering a diagnosis of OA vs RA.

3.1. Osteoarthritis

OA is a noninflammatory joint condition. Pain typically worsens with activity or weight bearing and improves with rest. Morning stiffness is often

B Diagnosis: chronic arthritis – OA

Please complete the following questions:
  1. Mark all areas on the figure where you typically experience pain with an 'X.

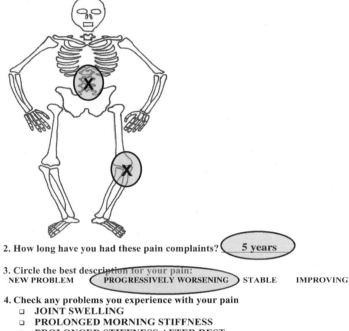

2. How long have you had these pain complaints? **5 years**

3. Circle the best description for your pain:
  NEW PROBLEM   **PROGRESSIVELY WORSENING**   STABLE   IMPROVING

4. Check any problems you experience with your pain
  ❑ JOINT SWELLING
  ❑ PROLONGED MORNING STIFFNESS
  ❑ PROLONGED STIFFNESS AFTER REST
  ❑ REDUCED JOINT MOVEMENT
  ❑ PAIN IN THE SAME JOINTS ON BOTH SIDES OF THE BODY
  ❑ GOOD PAIN RELIEF WITH IBUPROFEN OR NAPROXEN

5. Check any other body areas that are causing problems:
  ❑ Heart or chest pain
  ❑ Lungs or shortness of breath
  ❑ Kidneys
  ❑ Swollen legs (other than at the joints)
  ❑ Eye
  ❑ Skin

Fig. 5. *(Continued from previous page.)*

reported. The physical examination typically reveals joint tenderness, bony enlargement, crepitus on motion, and a restricted range of motion. Diagnostic criteria are shown in Box 2.

OA must be distinguished from both inflammatory arthritis and nonarthritic conditions (e.g., bursitis). Patients with a questionable diagnosis or normal radiograph findings should be referred to a rheumatologist for a definitive diagnosis.

C Diagnosis: chronic arthritis – RA

Please complete the following questions:
  1. Mark all areas on the figure where you typically experience pain with an 'X.'

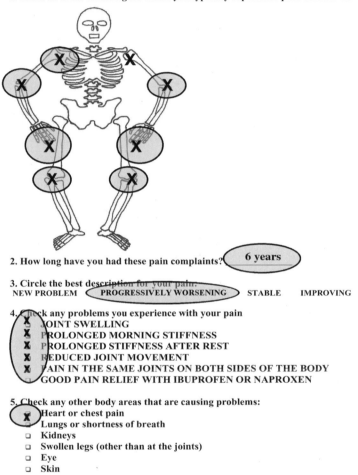

2. How long have you had these pain complaints? **6 years**

3. Circle the best description for your pain:
  NEW PROBLEM   **PROGRESSIVELY WORSENING**   STABLE   IMPROVING

4. Check any problems you experience with your pain
  X JOINT SWELLING
  X PROLONGED MORNING STIFFNESS
  X PROLONGED STIFFNESS AFTER REST
  X REDUCED JOINT MOVEMENT
  X PAIN IN THE SAME JOINTS ON BOTH SIDES OF THE BODY
  ☐ GOOD PAIN RELIEF WITH IBUPROFEN OR NAPROXEN

5. Check any other body areas that are causing problems:
  X Heart or chest pain
  ☐ Lungs or shortness of breath
  ☐ Kidneys
  ☐ Swollen legs (other than at the joints)
  ☐ Eye
  ☐ Skin

Fig. 5. *(Continued from previous page.)*

3.2. Rheumatoid Arthritis

RA is a symmetric, inflammatory arthritis of the small joints. Because RA affects joints, as well as other organ systems, a multisystem evaluation is required (*see* Box 3). Additionally, the severity of symptoms must be recorded initially and at each subsequent visit to identify and document the efficacy of disease-modifying agents.

```
┌─────────────────────────────────────────────┐
│                   Box 2                       │
│      Diagnostic Features of Osteoarthritis    │
│                                               │
│      • Joint pain                             │
│      • Morning stiffness                      │
│      • Joint changes on radiographs           │
│      • Crepitus with joint movement           │
└─────────────────────────────────────────────┘
```

Box 3
Evaluation of Rheumatoid Arthritis

Step 1. Evaluate and diagnose.

1. Establish a diagnosis.
2. Consider making a referral to a rheumatologist if diagnosis questionable
3. Document disease severity
   a. Record severity of pain, morning stiffness, fatigue, and disability
   b. Count number of swollen and tender joints
   c. Record joint deformity or restricted motion
   d. Record systemic symptoms
4. Perform baseline laboratory tests
   a. Erythrocyte sedimentation rate or C-reactive protein
   b. Rheumatoid factor
   c. Complete blood count
   d. Electrolytes, creatinine, and liver function tests
   e. Urinalysis
   f. Stool guaiac
   g. Synovial fluid analysis to rule out other conditions
   h. Radiographs of affected joints, as well as hands and feet

Step 2. Initiate treatment.

1. Patient education
2. Begin disease-modifying antirheumatic drug within 3 months
3. Consider nonsteroidal anti-inflammatory drugs
4. Consider local or low-dose systemic steroids
5. Refer to physical/occupational therapy

Step 3. Assess benefit of therapy. Prolonged morning stiffness or fatigue or signs of
inflammation suggest ineffective treatment and need for treatment modification.

1. Record severity of pain, morning stiffness, fatigue, and disability
2. Count number of swollen and tender joints
3. Record joint deformity or restricted motion
4. Periodically reassess laboratory inflammatory markers and radiographs

Step 4. Inadequate response after 3 months of maximal therapy necessitates
rheumatology referral.

1. Change disease-modifying antirheumatic drug
2. Consider addition of methotrexate or other therapies

Based on ref. *13*.

The rheumatoid factor (RF) auto-antibody can be detected in about 60 to 80% of patients with RA *(16)*. Disease specificity for RA is low (66%), with positive titers present in a variety of autoimmune diseases (e.g., Sjögren's syndrome) and nonautoimmune conditions (e.g., OA). RF, therefore, should not be used as a general screening tool in all patients with arthritis, but should be reserved for those with a clinical diagnosis of probable RA. In addition, RF titers may be low in early RA.

4. ARTHRITIS TREATMENT

Arthritis therapy involves the use of both pharmacologic and nonpharmacologic approaches. The pharmacological approach uses medications designed to reduce symptoms in patients with OA and to modify disease-specific entities in patients with RA. Nonpharmacological therapy includes both pain management and active exercise. Exercise is essential for improving joint flexibility and the strength of surrounding muscles. Good conditioning of surrounding tendons, ligaments, and muscles offers important protection of at-risk joints. Additionally, aerobic exercise with a minimal impact on weight-bearing joints, such as swimming and bicycling, reduces arthritis pain and improves joint function. Efforts to severely restrict normal activities and rehabilitative exercise actually increase the risk for subsequent injury.

4.1. Medications

In arthritis therapy, medications are used to complement, but not replace, nonpharmacologic therapy. Nonsteroidal anti-inflammatory drugs (NSAIDs) have been the mainstay of arthritis therapy. However, a meta-analysis of studies of the use of anti-inflammatory agents documented significant risks associated with the use of NSAIDs *(17)*. The relative risk for an upper gastrointestinal (GI) bleed was 3.8 in NSAID users, and the risk correlated with the drug dose, age of the patient, and history of peptic ulcer disease. The significance of adverse GI events with NSAIDs was also highlighted in a survey of the members of the Norwegian Rheumatism Association *(18)*, 68% of whom reported experiencing adverse GI events. In addition, 35% reported concomitant use of over-the-counter (OTC) gastroprotective agents and 30% reported using prescription gastroprotective agents. Almost half of these individuals used a gastroprotective agent at least every other day. Similar efficacy, with a substantial reduction in the risk for adverse GI events, can be achieved with cyclooxygenase-2 (COX-2) inhibitors *(19)*.

4.1.1. Osteoarthritis

OA is typically treated symptomatically with acetaminophen, NSAIDs, or COX-2 inhibitors. Because of gastric toxicity associated with long-term NSAID use, acetaminophen is considered first-line therapy for patients with OA. Topical analgesics, such as OTC capcaisin cream, may also be helpful.

Table 1
Disease-Modifying Anti-Rheumatic Drugs

Drug	Typical maintenance dosage
Adalimumab	40 mg SQ every other week
Anakinra	100 mg/day SQ
Azathioprine	25 mg/day
Cyclosporin	3 mg/kg/day
D-penicillamine	250–750 mg/day
Etanercept	25 mg SQ twice weekly
Gold (oral)	3 mg BID–TID
Hydroxychloroquine	200–400 mg/day
Infliximab	3 mg IV every 8 weeks
Leflunomide	20 mg/day
Methotrexate	7.5–30 mg/week
Minocycline	100 mg BID
Sulfasalazine	1000 mg BID

BID, twice daily; IV, intravenous; TID, three times a day; SQ, subcutaneous.

4.1.2. Rheumatoid Arthritis

Treatment recommendations for patients with RA are shown in Box 3. NSAIDs provide good symptomatic relief, reducing joint pain and swelling while facilitating motion. However, they do not retard joint destruction. Disease-modifying antirheumatic drugs (DMARDs) are considered the first-line treatment for patients with RA (Table 1). DMARDs significantly improve the quality of life *(20)*, with function preserved in patients treated early in the course of their disease *(21)*. Comparative studies of DMARDs show similar efficacy among various drug classes *(22)*. Hydroxychloroquine or sulfasalazine are often selected as initial therapy in the early stages of RA, whereas methotrexate is reserved for patients with more advanced disease. Sulfasalazine works faster than hydroxychloroquine and is better at retarding bony destruction. Patients who fail to achieve any benefit from traditional DMARDs may benefit from changing to tumor necrosis factor (TNF)-α inhibitors (e.g., adalimumab, etanercept, and infliximib) or interleukin-1 receptor antagonists (anakinra), or combining these agents with a traditional DMARD. Both drug categories effectively reduce joint erosions, but the onset of response is faster with TNF-α inhibitors.

4.2. Nonpharmacological Therapy

Patient education for arthritis patients typically involves information about the disease and specific self-management strategies (i.e., changing activities or activity scheduling, pain management skills, and physical exercises). Comprehensive programs addressing a wide variety of techniques *(23)* and focused

---
Box 4
Online Resources for Arthritis Exercise

Find local facilities trained to administer Arthritis Foundation Aquatic Program
 (AFAP) and People with Arthritis Can Exercise (PACE) classes
  ○ http://www.arthritis.org/events/getinvolved/ProgramsServices/default.asp
Exercise instruction sheet from the National Arthritis Foundation
  ○ http://www.arthritis.org.sg/101/treat/exercise.html
Free exercise and arthritis brochure
  ○ http://www.arthritis.org/AFStore/StartRead.asp?idProduct=3359

---

skills training (e.g., cognitive-behavioral therapy [CBT]) *(24,25)* both provide
significant short- and long-term reducing in pain and psychological distress
and improvement in functional ability. A brief educational intervention (a
single 30- to 60-minute educational session with a nurse, followed by two telephone calls) resulted in significant improvement in pain and disability for 1
year after the intervention *(26)*. Benefits did decrease over time, suggesting the
need for repeated or ongoing education in patients with arthritis. Additionally,
pharmacological compliance is enhanced by arthritis disease education. In one
study, brief educational sessions that focused on disease information and self-
management skills and were delivered by a nurse practitioner increased pharmacological compliance from 55 to 85% *(27)*.

4.2.1. Weight Reduction

Obesity increases mechanical load on joints, particularly in the lower extremities *(28)*, and increases the availability of proinflammatory cytokines that promote joint destruction *(29,30)*. Not surprisingly, increased body weight has been
linked with the development of OA, particularly in the hand, hip, and knee *(31)*.
Odds ratios for obese women compared with normal weight women for developing OA in these joints ranges from 3.0 to 10.5. Increased body mass index has
also been linked to knee and hand OA in men *(32,33)*. Fortunately, weight loss
significantly reduces stress on joints. The risk for knee OA decreased over a 10-
year period by more than 50% in women who lost 5.1 kg *(34)*.

4.2.2. Exercise

Physical therapy should focus on range-of-motion and strengthening exercises, as well as the implementation of devices to assist in ambulation and
activities of daily living. An occupational therapy referral should be made for
patients with significant disability or activity restriction. Aerobic exercises and
aquatic therapy tailored for arthritic patients are also recommended. A variety
of exercise resources are available online through the Arthritis Foundation (*see*

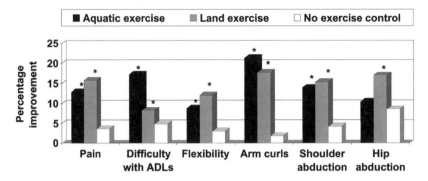

Fig. 6. Benefit from aquatic or land Arthritis Foundation exercise . * denotes significant improvement from study initiation to end ($p < 0.05$). Arm curls and shoulder and hip abduction tests are reported for right side of body. (Based on ref. *35.*)

Box 4). Both aquatic and land exercise programs are recommended for patients with arthritis. A comparative study evaluated the benefits of an exercise program versus no exercise in non-exercising patients with RA aged older than 60 yr *(35)*. Arthritis Foundation exercise programs were conducted in two 45-minute sessions each week for 8 weeks. Controls were asked to refrain from beginning any new exercise program. Both exercise programs resulted in a significant reduction in pain and disability and a significant improvement in flexibility and strength (Fig. 6).

Investigators involved in the Rheumatoid Arthritis Patients in Training trial compared long-term symptoms in patients participating in an intensive exercise program twice weekly with symptoms in those receiving usual care *(36)*. The exercise consisted of a warm-up period; 20 minutes each of bicycling, exercises, and a game (e.g., badminton, indoor soccer, volleyball, basketball, or relay games); and a cool-down period. Exercise program compliance was very good, with 81% of patients continuing to participate after 2 years *(37)*. Improvement in disability was significantly better in the exercise group compared with usual care after both 1 and 2 years of treatment ($p < 0.05$). Improvement in muscle strength and reduction in emotional distress were also significantly better in the exercise group ($p < 0.01$). In addition, although aerobic fitness increased in the exercise group, it diminished in those receiving usual care. Treatment safety was assessed using radiographs of the large joints, with no significant difference noted between usual care and aggressive exercise groups.

4.2.3. Psychological Treatments

Treatment with psychological pain management techniques, such as stress management and CBT, results in improved physical and psychological symp-

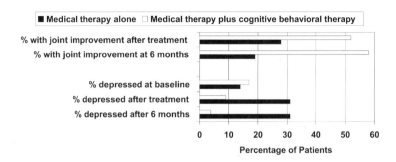

Fig. 7. Benefits of adding psychological treatment to usual medical care. (Based on ref. *38*.)

toms in patients with arthritis *(25)*. Although psychological treatments are not recommended as monotherapy, they are important adjunctive therapy. Sharpe and colleagues compared both psychological and physical benefits in patients with RA who were randomized to either medical therapy alone or medical therapy plus CBT *(38)*. Those who participated in CBT experienced superior short- and long-term improvement in measures of both physical and emotional health (Fig. 7).

As with all types of chronic pain, patients with comorbid psychological distress need additional therapy targeted to their emotional symptoms. Targeted depression therapy in patients with arthritis resulted in significantly superior improvement in depressive symptoms, as well as pain and pain interference in activities of daily living compared with usual care *(39)*.

4.2.4. Alternative/Complementary Medicine

The American College of Rheumatology does not recommend complementary or alternative therapies for rheumatologic disease. A 1-year, longitudinal study of effects of complementary therapies in rheumatology patients (15% with OA, 39% RA, and 19% with fibromyalgia) failed to find any benefit from a wide variety of treatments, including acupuncture, chiropracty, nutritional and herbal supplements, or copper bracelets and magnets *(40)*. Patients should alternatively focus on therapies with proven efficacy in arthritis, such as weight reduction, exercise, and psychological pain management.

5. SUMMARY

Arthritis is one of the most common chronic pain complaints, with the prevalence in most populations increasing with age. Most cases of chronic arthritis are caused by a degenerative or inflammatory pathology. Degenerative OA typically affects large, weight-bearing joints in a nonsymmetrical fashion. Inflammatory RA, conversely, usually causes symmetric symptoms in the small joints. The knee is a common site for either OA or RA.Treatment for arthritis includes both pharmacologic and rehabilitative therapy. Acetaminophen is considered first-line therapy for OA, whereas RA disease-modifying agents are used in inflammatory arthritis. Patients with either OA or RA should be treated with weight reduction, exercise, and pain management techniques. Although patients are often concerned that aerobic exercise will add further stress to painful joints and aggravate both pain and joint deformity, studies have shown that exercise improves the strength and flexibility of surrounding structures to provide support and protection to arthritic joints. Indeed, aerobic exercise improves both pain and function in patients with arthritis.

REFERENCES

1. Reginster JY. The prevalence and burden of arthritis. Rheumatology 2002; 41 (Suppl 1):3–6.
2. United Nations Population Information Network. World population prospects: the 2002 revision. (Available at Website: http://www.un.org/popin; accessed December 13, 2003).
3. Picavet HJ, Hazes JW. Prevalence of self reported musculoskeletal diseases is high. Ann Rheum Dis 2003; 62:644–650.
4. Elders MJ. The increasing impact of arthritis on public health. J Rheumatol Suppl 2000; 60:6–8.
5. Rasch EK, Hirsch R, Paulose-Ram R, Hochberg MC. Prevalence of rheumatoid arthritis in persons 60 years of age and older in the United States: effect of different methods of case classification. Arthritis Rheum 2003; 48:917–926.
6. Hootman JM, Helmick CG, Schappert SM. Magnitude and characteristics of arthritis and other rheumatic conditions on ambulatory medical care visits: United States 1997. Arthritis Rheum 2002; 47:571–581.
7. Stewart WF, Ricci JA, Chee E, Morganstein D, Lipton R. Lost productive time and cost due to common pain conditions in the US workforce. JAMA 2003; 290: 2443–2454.
8. Cooper NJ. Economic burden of rheumatoid arthritis: a systemic review. Rheumatology 2000; 39:28–33.
9. Söderlin MK, Kautiainen H, Jonsson D, Skogh T, Leirisalo-Repo M. The costs of early inflammatory joint disease: a population-based study in southern Sweden. Scand J Rheumatol 2003; 32:216–224.
10. Newhall-Perry K, Law NJ, Ramos B, et al. Direct and indirect costs associated with the onset of seropositive rheumatoid arthritis. Western Consortium of Practicing Rheumatologists. J Rheumatol 2000; 27:1156–1163.
11. Gamez-Nava JI, Gonzalez-Lopez L, Davis P, Suarez-Almazor ME. Referral and diagnosis of common rheumatic diseases by primary care physicians. Br J Rheumatol 1998; 37:1215–1219.
12. Gormley GJ, Steele WK, Gilliland A, et al. Can diagnostic triage by general practitioners or rheumatology nurses improve the positive predictive value of referrals to early arthritis clinics? Rheumatology 2003; 42:763–768.

13. American College of Rheumatology Subcommittee on Rheumatoid Arthritis Guidelines. Guidelines for the management of rheumatoid arthritis: 2002 update. Arthritis Rheum 2002; 46:328–346.
14. Yelin EH, Such CL, Criswell LA, Epstein WV. Outcomes for persons with rheumatoid arthritis with a rheumatologist versus a non-rheumatologist as the main physician for this condition. Med Care 1998; 36:513–522.
15. Machold KP, Stamm TA, Eberl GJ, et al. Very recent onset arthritis: clinical, laboratory, and radiological findings during the first year of disease. J Rheumatol 2002; 29:2278–2287.
16. Steiner G, Smolen J. Autoantibodies in rheumatoid arthritis and their clinical significance. Arthritis Res 2002; 4(Suppl 2):S1–S5.
17. Hernández-Díaz S, Rodríguez LG. Association between nonsteroidal anti-inflammatory drugs and upper gastrointestinal tract bleeding/perforation. Arch Int Med 2000; 160:2093–2099.
18. Steinfeld S, Björke PA. Results from a patient survey to assess gastrointestinal burden of non-steroidal anti-inflammatory drug therapy contrasted with a review of data from EVA to determine satisfaction with rofecoxib. Rheumatology 2002; 41(Suppl 1):23–27.
19. Lanas A. Clinical experience with cyclooxygenase-2 inhibitors. Rheumatology 2002; 41(Suppl 1):16-22.
20. Blumenauer B, Cranney A, Clinch J, Tugwell P. Quality of life in patients with rheumatoid arthritis: which drugs make a difference? Pharmacoeconomics 2003; 21:927–940.
21. Sokka T, Möttönen T, Hannonen P. Disease-modifying anti-rheumatic drug use according to the "sawtooth" treatment strategy improves the functional outcome in rheumatoid arthritis: results of a long-term follow-up study with review of the literature. Rheumatology 2000; 39:34–42.
22. Osiri M, Shea B, Robinson V, et al. Leflunomide for treating rheumatoid arthritis. Cochrane Database Syst Rev 2003; 1:CD002047.
23. Barlow JH, Turner AP, Wright CC. Long-term outcomes of an arthritis self-management programme. Br J Rheumatol 1998; 37:1315–1319.
24. Sharpe L, Snesky T, Timberlake N, Ryan B, Allard S. Long-term efficacy of a cognitive behavioural treatment from a randomized controlled trial for patients recently diagnosed with rheumatoid arthritis. Rheumatology 2003; 42:435–441.
25. Evers AW, Kraaimaat FW, van Riel PL, de Jong AJ. Tailored cognitive-behavioral therapy in early rheumatoid arthritis for patients at risk: a randomized controlled trial. Pain 2002; 100:141–153.
26. Mazzuca SA, Brandt KD, Katz BP, Chambers M, Byrd D, Hanna M. Effects of self-care education on the health status of inner-city patients with osteoarthritis of the knee. Arthritis Rheum 1997; 40:1466–1474.
27. Hill J, Bird H, Johnson S. Effect of patient education on adherence to drug treatment for rheumatoid arthritis: a randomized controlled trial. Ann Rheum Dis 2001; 60:869–875.
28. Sharma L, Lou C, Cahue S, Dunlop DD. The mechanism of the effect of obesity in knee osteoarthritis: the mediating role of malalignment. Arthritis Rheum 2000; 43:568–575.

29. Bastard JP, Jardel C, Bruckett E, et al. Elevated levels of interleukin 6 are reduced in serum and subcutaneous adipose tissue of obese women after weight loss. J Clin Endocrinol Metab 2000; 85:3338–3342.

30. Winkler G, Salamon F, Harmos G, et al. Elevated serum tumor necrosis factor-alpha concentrations and bioactivity in Type 2 diabetes and patients with android type obesity. Diabetes Res Clin Pract 1998; 42:169–174.

31. Oliveria SA, Felson DT, Cirillo PA, Reed JI, Walker AM. Body weight, body mass index, and incident symptomatic osteoarthritis of the hand, hip, and knee. Epidemiology 1999; 10:161–166.

32. Gelber AC, Hochberg MC, Mead LA, Wang NY, Wigley FM, Klag MJ. Body mass index in young men and the risk of subsequent knee and hip osteoarthritis. Am J Med 1999; 107:542–548.

33. Sayer AA, Poole J, Cox V, et al. Weight from birth to 53 years: a longitudinal study of the influence on clinical hand osteoarthritis. Arthritis Rheum 2003; 48:1030–1033.

34. Felson DT, Zhang Y, Anthony JM, Naimark A, Anderson JJ. Weight loss reduces the risk for symptomatic knee osteoarthritis in women: the Framingham Study. Ann Intern Med 1992; 116:535–539.

35. Suomi R, Collier D. Effects of arthritis exercise programs on functional fitness and perceived activities of daily living measures in older adults with arthritis. Arch Phys Med Rehab 2003; 84:1589–1594.

36. De Jong Z, Munneke M, Zwinderman AH, et al. Is a long-term high-intensity exercise program effective and safe in patients with rheumatoid arthritis? Arthritis Rheum 2003; 48:2415–2424.

37. Munneke M, de Jong Z, Zwinderman AH, et al. Adherence and satisfaction of rheumatoid arthritis patients with a long-term intensive dynamic exercise program (RAPIT Program). Arthritis Care Res 2003; 49:665–672.

38. Sharpe L, Sensky T, Timberlake N, Ryan B, Brewin CR, Allard S. A blind, randomized, controlled trial of cognitive-behavioral intervention for patients with recent onset rheumatoid arthritis: preventing psychological and physical morbidity. Pain 2001; 89:275–283.

39. Lin EB, Katon W, Von Korff M, et al. Effect of improving depression care on pain and functional outcomes among older adults with arthritis: a randomized controlled trial. JAMA 2003; 290:2428–2434.

40. Rao JK, Kroenke K, Mihaliak KA, Grambow SG, Weinberger M. Rheumatology patients' use of complementary therapies: results from a one-year longitudinal study. Arthritis Care Res 2003; 49:619–625.

CME QUESTIONS—CHAPTER 7

1. Which of the following feature(s) is typical of osteoarthritis?

    a. Symmetrical joint involvement
    b. Pain mainly in the small joints
    c. Pain in weight-bearing joints
    d. Joint inflammation
    e. All of the above

2. Select the correct first-line therapy or therapies for osteoarthritis

    a. Acetaminophen
    b. Nonsteroidal anti-inflammatory drugs
    c. Aerobic exercise
    d. A and B
    e. All of the above

3. Select the correct first-line therapy or therapies for rheumatoid arthritis

    a. Methotrexate
    b. Sulfasalazine
    c. Hydroxychloroquine
    d. Leflunomide
    e. All of the above

4. Which of the following nonpharmacological therapies should be prescribed for patients with rheumatoid arthritis?

    a. Acupuncture
    b. Aqua therapy
    c. Copper bracelets
    d. Magnets
    e. Bed rest

8

Neuropathic Pain

CASE HISTORY

Mrs. Showalter is a 60-year-old woman with well-controlled diabetes, which was diagnosed at age 45. She complains of cold, numb feet, noting pain primarily when water hits her feet after stepping into the shower or when the bedclothes brush against the feet after going to bed. She says that her feet often feel "dead" or "wooden" during the day. A physical examination reveals that she is wearing thick woolen socks, which she reports is necessary to keep her feet warm. Both feet appear normal, with good coloring, temperature, and pulses. Despite her complaints of "numbness," she is able to identify light touch throughout both feet. When approached with an open safety pin for pinprick testing, Mrs. Showalter reacts with dramatic withdrawal, complaining that the pin produces an intolerable, searing "fire" whenever it touches her feet. Her doctor orders Doppler studies and nerve conduction tests, both of which show relatively normal results. Because of the normal testing and lack of confirmatory examination evidence to support the claims of either coldness or numbness, Mrs. Showalter is advised to limit activities that may stress the foot and aggravate her pain. No other therapy is prescribed.

* * *

Mrs. Showalter's history is very typical of early neuropathic pain. Reports of pain symptoms often exceed any findings on examination. In addition, patients with neuropathic pain often guard the painful area, covering it with clothing to avoid access to air currents or incidental light touch, or refuse a sensory examination because of extreme pain with touch or pinprick. The excessive drawing away from pinprick is usually involuntary and may be very embarrassing for the patient who believes that she is being perceived as someone who is exaggerating pain severity. Neuropathic pain, however, changes the body's perception of touch and pain, heightening pain perception from even minor sensations, such as the sensation of air rushing across a bare arm, water beating onto a bare leg, or the gentlest prick from the examiner's pin.

From: *Chronic Pain: A Primary Care Guide to Practical Management*
Edited by: D. A. Marcus © Humana Press, Totowa, NJ

KEY CHAPTER POINTS

- Hallmarks of neuropathic pain include burning sensation, hyperalgesia, and allodynia.
- Peripheral neuropathy occurs in a variety of chronic medical conditions, including diabetes, thyroid disease, rheumatoid arthritis (RA), cancer, and human immunodeficiency virus infection.
- Postherpetic neuralgia occurs in approximately 30% of patients with herpes zoster. The incidence may be minimized by early treatment with antiviral agents and amitriptyline.
- Complex regional pain syndrome (formerly called reflex sympathetic dystrophy causalgia or sympathetically maintained pain) is recognized by excessive guarding of the painful extremity.
- First-line therapy for neuropathic pain includes gabapentin and tricyclic antidepressants.

Neuropathic pain is the 14th most common pain complaint seen in general practice *(1)*. Despite the availability of many well-tolerated therapies, patients like Mrs. Showalter often receive inadequate care. A recent survey of patients with neuropathic pain showed that the majority was undertreated *(2)*. In this survey, 73% of respondents reported inadequate pain control. In addition, 25% had never been treated with standard therapy, including antiepileptic drugs (AEDs), antidepressants, or opioids. Despite the widespread acceptance of AEDs and antidepressants as effective, first-line therapy, 72% of patients with neuropathic pain had never been treated with an AED and 60% had never been treated with a tricyclic antidepressant.

Neuropathy frequently accompanies a variety of general medical conditions, including diabetes, RA, and thyroid disease (*see* Box 1). Neuropathy may also occur as a consequence of peripheral nerve injury. Historical identification of conditions with frequent neuropathic comorbidity raises the index of suspicion of neuropathy as the cause of chronic pain, especially extremity pain.

1. DEFINITION

Neuropathic pain is characterized by altered, unpleasant sensations. Several adjectives used to describe pain are more commonly used by patients with neuropathic pain (Table 1) *(3)*. Textbook descriptions of neuropathy often focus on numbness. Patients, however, are generally less disturbed by the absence of normal sensation (or numbness) and are more concerned with new abnormal sensations perceived in the numb area, including burning, prickling, heat, cold, or a perception of swelling *(4)*. Patients may also refer to the affected area as feeling "wooden" or "dead." Although the painful area may become insensible to normal touch stimuli, patients will often describe the presence of intense sensations over the neuropathic area. Generally, these perceptions are greatest when the damaged area is stimulated (e.g., by wearing clothing, using bed-

```
┌─────────────────────────────────────────┐
│                  Box 1                   │
│   Common Neuropathic Pain Syndromes      │
│ ─────────────────────────────────────── │
│                                          │
│  • Peripheral neuropathy                 │
│     ○ Systemic disease                   │
│        ▪ Diabetes                        │
│        ▪ Thyroid disease                 │
│        ▪ Renal disease                   │
│        ▪ Rheumatoid arthritis            │
│     ○ Nutritional/toxicity               │
│        ▪ Alcoholism                      │
│        ▪ Pernicious anemia               │
│        ▪ Chemotherapy                    │
│     ○ Infectious                         │
│        ▪ HIV                             │
│  • Postherpetic neuralgia                │
│  • Complex regional pain syndrome        │
│                                          │
└─────────────────────────────────────────┘
```

Table 1
Percentage of Patients Endorsing Pain Descriptors:
Neuropathic vs Non-Neuropathic Pain

Pain descriptor	Neuropathic pain	Non-neuropathic pain
Electric shock	53	21
Burning	54	29
Cold	22	10
Pricking	37	18
Tingling	48	25
Itching	33	9

These seven pain descriptors are more commonly used by patients with neuropathic pain ($p < 0.05$). (Based on ref. *3*.)

clothes, or being exposed to the wind). Patients may occasionally report that the neuropathic area feels misshapen, deformed, or alien, although the external appearance may be quite normal.

The presence of hyperalgesia and allodynia effectively discriminate neuropathic from non-neuropathic pain *(5)*. Occasionally, the examiner may notice that the painful area is cool to the touch. Rarely, the same area may be warm and red.

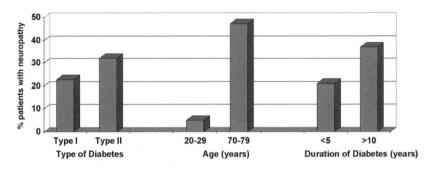

Fig. 1. Risk factors for diabetic neuropathy pain. (Based on refs. *6,7.*)

2. EPIDEMIOLOGY OF COMMON NEUROPATHIC PAIN SYNDROMES

Neuropathy is a common accompaniment of a variety of common medical conditions. The etiology of the neuropathy is usually identified based on a history of comorbid medical illnesses or previous nerve injury. Patients with evidence of peripheral neuropathy should be screened for these common medical conditions.

2.1. Diabetic Neuropathy

Neuropathy occurs in approximately 23 to 28% of patients with diabetes *(5,7)*. The risk of developing neuropathy increases with type 2 diabetes, aging, duration of diabetes, and medical consequences of diabetes (e.g., renal and cardiovascular disease) (Fig. 1) *(7)*. Peripheral neuropathy is common in older patients with diabetes, even when the blood sugar is well controlled. Peripheral neuropathy occurs in more than 50% of patients with type 2 diabetes who are older than 60 years *(6)*.

2.2. Postherpetic Neuralgia

Postherpetic neuralgia is defined as pain that persists for more than 1 month after the onset of herpes zoster. Postherpetic neuralgia occurs in approximately 30% of patients following acute zoster and lasts 1 year in approximately 10% of patients (Fig. 2) *(8)*. Persistence of postherpetic neuralgia increases with aging and pain severity. Interestingly, despite the focal nature of postherpetic neuralgia pain complaints, patients with these conditions report significant impairment in both physical and emotional quality of life *(9)*. Interestingly, quality of life for all eight domains of the Medical Outcome Health Survey (SF-36) is lower in patients with postherpetic neuralgia versus patients with acute herpes zoster.

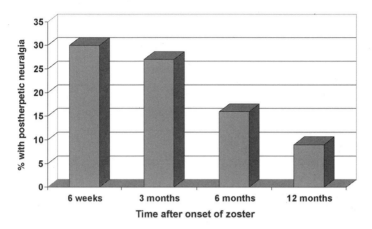

Fig. 2. Prevalence of postherpetic neuralgia in patients with herpes zoster. (Based on ref. *8*.)

2.3. Complex Regional Pain Syndromes

Complex regional pain syndrome (CRPS) develops following an identified injury or period of limb immobilization (e.g., casting). CRPS may be categorized as type 1 (occurring in the absence of a nerve injury; formerly called reflex sympathetic dystrophy) or type 2 (occurring after injury to a specific large nerve; formerly called causalgia). The terms "sympathetically maintained pain" and "sympathetically mediated pain" were also formerly used to describe this syndrome. Failure to achieve relief using sympathetic blocks, particularly in patients with long-standing complaints, led to the discontinuation of these terms.

CRPS patients are readily identified in the clinic by seemingly exaggerated guarding of the painful extremity, often holding the arm in a splinted posture and avoiding movement. They may also shroud the extremity with a cover to limit sensory exposure or, alternatively, hold the extremity away from the body as though trying to continually demonstrate the painful area to onlookers. Some patients will place an affected arm across the doctor's desk for history taking, often to the surprise of the examiner. These behaviors serve to reduce normal movement of or contact with the painful limb. The patient history reveals a persistently painful extremity with pain severity that is disproportionately in excess of that caused by any preceding injury *(10)*. Patients typically report changes in temperature in the painful limb, as well as intermittent redness and swelling. These findings may or may not be evident at the time of evaluation because they are generally transient *(see* Box 2). Interestingly, subjective patient reports of

---

Box 2
Diagnostic Criteria for Complex Regional Pain Syndrome

- Identification of inciting event or history of immobilization
- Persistent pain, allodynia, or hyperalgesia with severity in excess of expectations from inciting event
- History of changes in swelling, temperature, color, or sweating in the painful area

---

Based on ref. *10.*

CRPS changes (allodynia, edema, and sweating/color/temperature abnormality) have greater diagnostic sensitivity and specificity than objective clinical examination findings for the same conditions *(11)*. On examination, patients with CRPS excessively guard the painful limb, often splinting it and restraining an examiner from touching it. "Motor neglect" has also been described in some patients with CRPS, who have reported an inability to move the extremity, to move an extremity without mentally focusing on the extremity, or a perception that the extremity is no longer part of the person's body *(12)*.

Objective motor findings are rarely present in CRPS, but may include restricted range of motion, weakness, or tremor. Motor findings typically are seen with very long-standing, untreated CRPS. Ten or 20 years ago, it was common to see patients with end-stage CRPS, with contracted joints, as well as abnormal skin, hair, and nail growth. Better identification of this syndrome and an emphasis on rehabilitation and maintaining function in the painful limb has resulted in current patients typically displaying evidence of only early, more reversible disease stages, such as color and temperature changes and avoidance of movement by voluntary splinting.

A Mayo Clinic survey identified the prevalence of CRPS types I and II, respectively, as 0.02 and 0.004% *(13)*. Patients with CRPS type I were predominantly female (female:male ratio = 4:1). Pain typically affected an upper extremity in patients with either type I and II. The most common precipitating events for CRPS type I were fracture (46%) and sprain (12%). CRPS type I symptoms resolved in 74% of cases, with a mean time to resolution of 1 year. In this sample, clinical signs and symptoms were similar (Fig. 3). In clinical practice, however, symptoms reported by patients are usually not observed during the initial visit or visits but may be noted over time when multiple opportunities to observe the extremity have occurred.

2.4. Cancer-Related Neuropathy

Cancer-related neuropathy may occur as a consequence of compressive neuropathy, direct injury from surgery, chemotherapy, or nutritional deficits. Man-

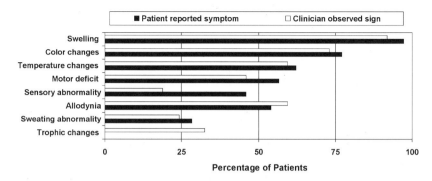

Fig. 3. Clinical symptoms and signs in patients with complex regional pain syndrome type I. (Based on ref. *13*.)

agement of cancer-related neuropathy with standard analgesics and neuropathic medications is effective in most patients. A survey of 213 cancer patients with neuropathy showed satisfactory to good efficacy with standard neuropathic treatment in 79 to 91% of patients *(14)*.

2.5. HIV-Related Neuropathy

Distal sensory polyneuropathy (with complaints of painful feet) is the most common neuropathy seen in human immunodeficiency virus (HIV)-infected patients and may be caused by immunological dysfunction related to the infection itself, as well as the toxicity of antiretroviral drugs *(15)*. Sensory neuropathy does occur in HIV-infected patients prior to treatment with antiretroviral medications. A recent survey of HIV patients who had never been treated with antiretroviral drugs showed symptomatic neuropathy in 35%, with a 1-year incidence rate for symptomatic distal sensory neuropathy of 36% *(16)*. The risk for neuropathy increases with antiretroviral therapy, with combination dideoxynucleoside therapy having synergistic effects on neurotoxicity and symptomatic neuropathy *(17)*.

3. EVALUATION OF NEUROPATHIC PAIN

Peripheral neuropathy is best recognized by the identification of symmetrical, distal dysesthesia, and sensory loss, such as a stocking or sock distribution of numbness or burning pain. Historical reports of hyperalgesia and allodynia, along with a history of predisposing medical conditions, establish a probable diagnosis for peripheral neuropathy. Diagnosis becomes more obvious as neuropathy severity increases and sensory loss becomes more dense. Other types of chronic neuropathic pain, such as postherpetic neuralgia and CRPS, are identified by eliciting a history of inciting events.

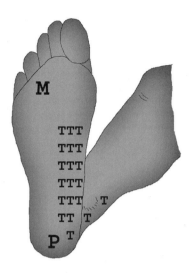

Fig. 4. Location of typical painful foot syndromes. M, Morton's neuroma, P, plantar fasciitis, T, tarsal tunnel syndrome.

In patients with painful feet, other common causes of chronic foot pain need to be ruled out. Unique pain locations and symptoms with nonneuropathic syndromes can help the clinician distinguish them from peripheral neuropathy (*see* Table 2 and Fig. 4). Morton's neuroma produces a unilateral pain that is located in the ball of the foot with weight bearing. Plantar fasciitis is an excruciating pain in the heel of one or both feet that occurs after taking the first steps on rising from bed or a prolonged sitting position. Tarsal tunnel syndrome produces a diffuse pain over the medial ankle and sole, caused by compression of the tibial nerve. The tibial nerve travels behind the medial malleolus, immediately posterior to the tibial artery. Both travel into the foot beneath the flexor retinaculum, a fibrous band between the medial malleolus and the calcaneous. Nerve impingement in the tarsal tunnel is similar to but less common than compression of the median nerve in the carpal tunnel of the wrist.

Loss of vibratory and joint position sensations is a good marker of early peripheral neuropathy. Except in cases of severe nerve impairment, when vibratory testing is no longer necessary because of marked loss of tactile sense, most patients with neuropathy will still perceive vibration from a tuning fork that has been struck hard enough to produce audible sound. Detection of early neuropathy requires a comparison of the level of tuning fork vibration that is perceived in the toe of the healthy examiner. Elderly patients and patients with diabetes who lack significant neuropathy should be able to sense the level of vibration that is just perceived in the healthy examiner's great toe when the tuning fork is immediately placed on the patient's lateral malleolus (Fig. 5).

Table 2
Common Causes of Painful Feet

Condition	Pain location	Response to walking	Typical symptoms	Treatment
Peripheral neuropathy	Bilateral, burning pain located over areas covered by socks. Early symptoms are more distal.	Aggravated by touch. Walking may worsen or relieve.	Symmetrical sensory loss and/or dysesthesia in a stocking distribution.	Antidepressants or antiepileptic drugs.
Plantar fasciitis	Excruciating heel pain.	Maximum severity with first morning step or after prolonged sitting. Improves with walking.	Painful heel and posterior sole, especially on waking and first walking on foot. Pain is relieved by "walking it off." Pain occurs with foot dorsiflexion.	Stretching exercise program with frequent foot dorsiflexion.
Tarsal tunnel syndrome	Vague pain and numbness over the medial ankle, heel, sole, and arch.	Aggravated by walking.	Diffuse ankle and foot pain, worsened with activity. Electric shock pain with percussing the flexor retinaculum posterior to the medial malleolus.	Orthotics. NSAIDs. Stretching exercises for calf muscles. Steroid injections into the flexor retinaculum. Surgical nerve release.
Morton's neuroma	Ball of the foot.	Pain with each weight-bearing step	Tingling and electric shock around the 2nd–4th metatarsals and toes during weight bearing. Feeling like you're "walking on a marble." Pain in the ball of the foot is worsened with walking.	Change to comfortable, roomy shoes. Orthotics. NSAIDs. Local steroid injections.
Peripheral vascular disease	Diffuse coldness in feet at rest. Diffuse pain with exercise.	Exercise produces ache, cramp, or muscle fatigue.	Cold, discolored feet at rest. Pain with walking.	Reduce vascular risk factors (smoking, high cholesterol, hypertension). Antiplatelet agents. Cilostazol (50–100 mg twice daily). Revascularization surgery.

NSAIDs, nonsteroidal anti-inflammatory drugs.

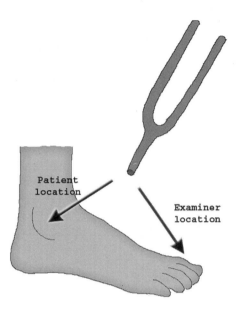

Fig. 5. Vibratory sense testing for early neuropathy. Tuning-fork vibration barely perceptible for the examiner at the great toe should be perceived at the lateral malleolus in normal elderly patients and patients with diabetes.

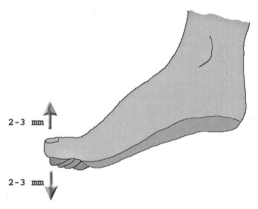

Fig. 6. Joint position sense testing for early neuropathy. Normal individuals perceive movement of the tip of the great toe that is 2–3 mm above or below resting position.

Few patients, even those with severe disease, will fail to perceive vibration at the knee, so testing above the ankle is not helpful. Reduction in joint position sense also occurs in early peripheral neuropathy. Normal patients should be able to detect a very small change in joint position (movement of as little as 2 to 3 mm) at the end of the great toe (Fig. 6). Movement of the joint to the extreme end of its range of motion elicits pain and does not test joint position sense.

Electromyographic (EMG) and nerve conduction velocity (NCV) studies are very helpful to identify mononeuropathies, such as radiculopathy and compressive neuropathies (e.g., carpal tunnel syndrome). Often abnormalities are also seen in peripheral neuropathy. Unfortunately, abnormal EMG/NCV findings indicating peripheral neuropathy do not necessarily correspond with clinical symptoms. Therefore, electrical testing should be used to rule out alternative causes of pain in the extremities of patients with atypical symptoms, such as unilateral neuropathic symptoms, rather than as a routine test for patients with symmetrical bilateral sensory neuropathy.

Quantitative sensory testing and the quantitative sudomotor axon reflex test (sweat test) are frequently used research tools. The sensitivity and specificity of these tests for different types of painful neuropathies are low. Therefore, these tools are not recommended for routine clinical practice.

4. TREATMENT OF NEUROPATHIC PAIN

In patients with neuropathy caused by a treatable medical condition, improvement in pain symptoms may occur during the management of the primary disease. For example, studies suggest that tight glucose control minimizes peripheral neuropathy in patients with diabetes *(18)*. Symptomatic treatment of neuropathic pain involves the use of both first- and second-line medications (Table 3).

4.1. First-Line Therapy

Neuropathic pain is most likely to be reduced when patients are treated with an AED (e.g., gabapentin) or a tricyclic antidepressant. For this reason, these agents are considered first-line choices for neuropathic pain. Excellent efficacy and superior tolerability make gabapentin the first choice among neuropathic medications.

4.1.1. Antiepileptic Drugs

Newer AEDs enhance the activity of neurochemicals that inhibit pain messages, such as γ-aminobutyric acid. Animal studies show that AEDs effectively reduce both hyperalgesia and allodynia associated with neuropathic pain *(19)*.

Gabapentin should be considered first-line therapy for painful neuropathy because of its good efficacy and tolerability. Gabapentin effectively relieves dysesthesia, hyperalgesia, and allodynia *(20)*. It is important to remind patients that gabapentin is not expected to restore normal sensation; rather, it decreases the annoying abnormal sensations that occur in numb areas. A comparative study of gabapentin (mean dose: 1800 mg/day) and amitriptyline (mean dose: 50 mg/day) in patients with diabetic neuropathy showed significant pain reduction with both treatments *(21)*. Pain relief, however, was superior with gabapentin (65% decrease) compared with amitriptyline (46% decrease; $p <$ 0.05). Paresthesias also were reduced to a significantly greater extent with

Table 3
Medication for Neuropathic Pain

First-line therapy	Dosage
Antiepileptics	
• Gabapentin	Start at 300 mg/day. Increase to 300 mg three times a day over 2 weeks. Failure to achieve effective control calls for further titration to 1800 mg/day in divided doses for most patients; a few patients will require up to 3600 mg/day in divided doses.
Antidepressants	
• Tricyclic	Nortriptyline, imipramine, or desipramine: 25–150 mg administered 2 hours before bed. Amitriptyline is too sedating for many patients.
• SSRI	Paroxetine or citalopram: 40 mg/day.
Second-line therapy	
Topical	Topical agents are applied directly over the area of pain.
• Capsaicin cream	Start with 0.025% cream. Apply a small drop—the size of a small pea or half a chocolate chip—to the painful area three to four times daily. After completing one tube, if burning from capsaicin is not too intense, switch to 0.075% cream, applied in the same fashion. Wash hands *thoroughly* with soap and water and avoid putting hands into eyes or mouth. Do not use over open skin or mucous membranes. Use for 6 weeks before assessing efficacy.
• Lidocaine patch	5% patch: one to three patches daily, worn for 12 hours on, then 12 hours off. Number of patches is determined by size of painful area. Patches ideally cover painful area (if area is not too large). Patches may be cut to smaller sizes. Do not use over open skin. Use for 2 weeks before assessing efficacy.
• Long-acting opioids	Methadone 10 mg twice a day. Sustained-release oxycodone (10 mg three times a day or 20 mg twice a day).

gabapentin compared with amitriptyline. In addition, tolerability was better with gabapentin. In another study, gabapentin therapy resulted in reduced reliance on opioid therapy in patients with postherpetic neuralgia *(22)*. The percentage of patients who continued to use opioids decreased when gabapentin was used adjunc-tively (from 89% to 71%) and the total number of opioid prescriptions was reduced by 23% in those who continued to use opioids.

Other AEDs—such as carbamazepine, topiramate, and lamotrigine—are also effective for neuropathic pain. The superior tolerability of gabapentin, however, makes the other AEDs second choices for patients who fail trials with gabapentin.

4.1.2. Antidepressants

Antidepressants have significant analgesic properties in addition to their mood-altering effects. Analgesic effects are not a reflection of mood enhancement. For example, in a study comparing the analgesic benefits derived from transdermal antidepressants vs anesthetics in rodents, investigators found that the anesthetic blockade produced by amitriptyline lasted longer than that produced by lidocaine *(23)*. Newer antidepressants, such as venlafaxine, have also demonstrated an ability to inhibit neuropathic hyperalgesia in experimental animal pain models *(24)*.

TCAs are more effective in reducing peripheral neuropathy pain than are other antidepressants. In randomized, double-blind, controlled clinical trials, investigators observed efficacy with TCAs and, to a lesser extent, the selective serotonin reuptake inhibitors paroxetine and citalopram *(25)*. Newer antidepressants—including nefazodone, venlafaxine, and mirtazapine—also show promise in reducing neuropathic pain, but should be considered second-line therapy.

4.2. Second-Line Therapy

Patients who fail to achieve adequate symptomatic relief or who experience intolerable side effects from a first-line therapy may be offered a second-line therapy. Second-line therapy should not be used before first-line therapy, however, unless the patient has a medical condition that precludes the use of a first-line therapy.

4.2.1. Topical Agents

Topical therapies are typically well tolerated, although they are generally less effective than antidepressants and AEDs. In a controlled study of neuropathic pain patients, investigators found that lidocaine patches reduced both pain severity and allodynia by approximately 30% *(26)*. In a double-blind comparison of topical capsaicin (0.075% four times a day) and oral amitriptyline (titrated to 125 mg/day, as tolerated), investigators found a similar reduction in pain (approximately 40%) and improved function in both treatment groups *(27)*. This level of improvement with capsaicin is superior to what is typically seen in clinical practice.

4.2.2. Opioids

Although traditional teachings suggest that opioids are ineffective for neuropathic pain, low doses of long-acting opioids can be beneficial in patients who have failed other types of therapy. For example, in controlled trials, investigators have found that low-dose methadone (10 mg twice a day) or sustained-release oxycodone (20 mg twice a day) effectively reduced chronic neuropathic pain symptoms *(28,29)*. *(See* Chapter 17 for additional treatment recommendations.)

4.3. Treatment of Individual Pain Syndromes

Postherpetic neuralgia and CRPS typically require supplemental treatment modalities. Early treatment of each condition with general neuropathic medication and condition-targeted therapy may help reduce the risk for more prolonged and recalcitrant pain.

Table 4
Antiviral Therapy for Early Herpes Zoster

Drug	Dosage
Acyclovir	800 mg five times a day for 7–10 days
Famciclovir	500 mg three times a day for 7 days
Valacyclovir	1 g three times a day for 7 days
Brivudin [a]	125 mg once a day for 7 days

[a] Not available in the United States.

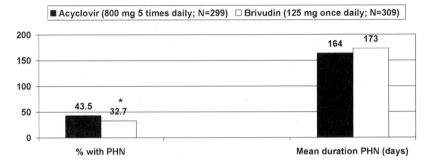

Fig. 7. Comparison of rate of development of postherpetic neuralgia after antiviral treatment. Brivudin was superior to acyclovir ($p = 0.006$). PHN, postherpetic neuralgia. (Based on ref. *30*.)

4.3.1. Postherpetic Neuralgia

Early and aggressive treatment of herpes zoster reduces the risk for postherpetic neuralgia. Early antiviral therapy of herpes zoster (within 72 h of symptom onset) can effectively minimize symptoms of postherpetic neuralgia (Table 4). In a large, prospective, double-blind study comparing the rate of postherpetic neuralgia in patients treated with acyclovir or brivudin (a new antiviral agent that is not yet available in the United States), investigators found that the incidence of postherpetic neuralgia was significantly lower with brivudin, although mean duration of postherpetic neuralgia pain was similar in both groups (Fig. 7). Neuropathic therapy administered during the early stages of zoster may also reduce the incidence of postherpetic neuralgia. Low-dose amitriptyline (25 mg/day) administered within 48 hours of the onset of zoster rash significantly reduced the rate of postherpetic neuralgia in elderly patients (mean age: 68 years) (Fig. 8) *(31)*.

Inflammation and increased prostaglandin activity occur in early postherpetic neuralgia *(32)*. In one study, treatment with topical aspirin (750–1500 mg plus 20–30 mL diethyl ether), but not other nonsteroidal anti-inflam-

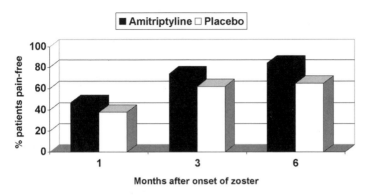

Fig. 8. Reduction in persistent pain in patients aged >60 years with acute zoster treated within 48 hours of rash onset with amitriptyline 25 mg/day vs placebo. Difference between amitriptyline and placebo is significant ($p < 0.05$). (Based on ref. *31*.)

matory drugs, reduced pain more than placebo (–66% with aspirin vs –34% with placebo) *(33)*. The onset of pain relief was rapid (approximately 4 minutes), with relief lasting a mean of 3.6 hours.

Patients with established postherpetic neuralgia are treated with the neuropathic medications listed previously. Both first- and second-line therapies are effective for postherpetic neuralgia.

4.3.2. Complex Regional Pain Syndrome

Complex regional pain syndrome is treated with a combination of medications to achieve symptomatic relief and physical rehabilitation to prevent progression to motor changes, such as reduced range of motion, joint contracture, and motor loss. CRPS occurring during the first few weeks of therapy is often managed with oral corticosteroids (30 mg/day for 2 weeks, followed by a tapering schedule) and sympathetic blocks, including sympathetic ganglion blocks (i.e., stellate, thoracic, or lumbar ganglion blockade) or intravenous regional sympathetic blocks (i.e., Bier blocks) *(34)*. These therapies are combined with vigorous physical therapy. The goal of early intervention with steroids, blocks, or both is to provide temporary symptomatic reduction to allow optimal participation in rehabilitative therapy. Both early and late treatment of CRPS focus on physical and occupational therapy designed to maintain or improve range of motion and maximize active use of the painful extremity. The goal of such therapy is to help the patient resume normal use of the extremity for both functional and casual use, including a return to a normal arm posture when sitting and arm swing during walking. Gait training is essential for patients with lower extremity CRPS to help them regain a normal, unrestricted walking pattern. Although physical and occupational therapy are often contrary to the desires of the patient with CRPS, who often wishes to minimize movement and stimulation of the painful extremity, the clinician must insist on aggressive therapy and resumption of more normal extremity postures and use at all times. Psychological interventions may serve as invaluable adjunctive pain management for patients with CRPS. Antidepressants, AEDs, and long-acting opioids may also help the patient participate in rehabilitative therapy activities.

5. SUMMARY

Neuropathic pain is seen in general practice, typically in conjunction with systemic medical illness; nutritional deficiency, toxicity, or both; cancer; and infection. Pain reports that include a description of pain and aggravating factors, as well as a clinical examination will help the clinician distinguish neuropathic pain from other common pain conditions, including plantar fasciitis, Morton's neuroma, and entrapment syndromes. Hallmarks of neuropathic pain include a burning sensation, hyperalgesia, and allodynia. Laboratory testing may be needed to identify systemic medical illness but is rarely helpful for diagnosing neuropathic pain.

A variety of effective, symptomatic therapies are available for neuropathic pain. These therapies will not reduce numbness, but can decrease dysethesia, hyperalgesia, and allodynia. Treatment of underlying medical conditions— such as glucose control in diabetes and antiviral therapy in herpes zoster— reduces the severity of neuropathic pain. First-line therapy for neuropathic pain includes gabapentin and a tricyclic antidepressent. Neuropathic pain syndromes that result in restricted use of the painful area should be treated with physical therapy and occupational therapy to normalize the active use of the painful extremity.

REFERENCES

1. Hasselström J, Liu-Palmgren J, Rasjö-Wrååk G. Prevalence of pain in general practice. Eur J Pain 2002; 6:375–385.
2. Gilron I, Bailey J, Weaver DF, Houlden RL. Patients' attitudes and prior treatments in neuropathic pain: a pilot study. Pain Res Manag 2002; 7:199–203.
3. Boreau F, Doubrére, Luu. Study of verbal description in neuropathic pain. Pain 1990; 42:145–152.
4. Dworkin RH. An overview of neuropathic pain: syndromes, symptoms, signs, and several mechanisms. Clin J Pain 2002; 18:343–349.
5. Bennett M. The LANSS pain scale: the Leeds assessment of neuropathic symptoms and signs. Pain 2001; 92:147–157.
6. Young MJ, Boulton AJ, MacLeod AF, Williams DR, Sonksen PH. A multicentre study of the prevalence of diabetic peripheral neuropathy in the United Kingdom hospital clinic population. Diabetologia 1993; 36:150–154.

7. O'Hare JA, Abuaisha F, Geoghegan M. Prevalence and forms of neuropathic morbidity in 800 diabetics. Ir J Med Sci 1994; 163:132–135.
8. Scott FT, Leedhan-Green ME, Barrett-Muir WY, et al. A study of shingles and the development of postherpetic neuralgia in East London. J Med Virol 2003; 70 (Suppl 1):S24–S30.
9. Chidiac C, Bruxelle J, Daures JP, et al. Characteristics of patients with herpes zoster on presentation to practitioners in France. Clin Infect Dis 2001; 33:62–69.
10. Merskey H, Bogduk N. Classification of chronic pain. Seattle, WA: IASP Press, 1994.
11. Galer BS, Bruehl S, Harden RN. Diagnostic clinical criteria for CRPS and painful diabetic neuropathy. Clin J Pain 1998; 14:48–54.
12. Galer BS, Butler S, Jensen M. Case reports and hypothesis: a neglect like syndrome may be responsible for the motor disturbance in reflex sympathetic dystrophy. J Pain Symptom Mange 1995; 10:385–392.
13. Sandroni P, Benrud-Larson LM, McClelland RL, Low PA. Complex regional pain syndrome type I: incidence and prevalence in Olmstead county, a population-based study. Pain 2003; 103:199–207.
14. Stute P, Soukup J, Menzel M, Sabatowski R, Grond S. Analysis and treatment of different types of neuropathic cancer pain. J Pain Symptom Manage 2003; 26: 1123–1131.
15. Luciano CA, Pardo CA, McArthur JC. Recent developments in the HIV neuropathies. Curr Opin Neurol 2003; 16:403–409.
16. Schifitto G, McDermott MP, McArthur J, et al. Incidence of and risk factors for HIV-associated distal sensory polyneuropathy. Neurology 2002; 58:1764–1768.
17. Moore R, Wong WM, Keruly J, McArthur J. Incidence of neuropathy in HIV-infected patients on monotherapy versus those on combination therapy with didanosine, stavudine and hydroxyurea. AIDS 2000; 14:273–278.
18. Krishnan AM, Rayman G. New treatment for diabetic-neuropathy: symptomatic treatments. Curr Diabet Rep 2003; 3:459–467.
19. Fox A, Gentry C, Patel S, Kesingland A, Bevan S. Comparative activity of the anti-convulsants oxcarbazepine, carbamazepine, lamotrigine and gabapentin in a model of neuropathic pain in the rat and guinea-pig. Pain 2003; 105:355–362.
20. Backonja M, Glanzman RL. Gabapentin dosing for neuropathic pain: evidence from randomized, placebo-controlled clinical trials. Clin Ther 2003; 25:81–104.
21. Dallocchio C, Buffa C, Mazzarello P, Chiroli S. Gabapentin vs. amitriptyline in painful diabetic neuropathy: an open-label pilot study. J Pain Symptom Manage 2000; 20:280–285.
22. Berger A, Dukes E, McCarberg B, Liss M, Oster G. Change in opioid use after the initiation of gabapentin therapy in patients with postherpetic neuralgia. Clin Ther 2003; 25:2809–2821.
23. Haderer A, Gerner P, Kao G, Srinivasa V, Wang GK. Cutaneous analgesia after transdermal application of amitriptyline versus lidocaine in rats. Anesth Analg 2003; 96:1707–1710.
24. Marchand F, Alloui A, Pelissier T, et al. Evidence for an antihyperalgesic effect of venlafaxine in vincristine-induced neuropathy in rat. Brain Res 2003; 980:117–120.
25. Mattia C, Coluzzi F. Antidepressants in chronic neuropathic pain. Min Rev Med Chem 2003; 3:773–784.

26. Meier T, Wasner G, Faust M, et al. Efficacy of lidocaine patch 5% in the treatment of focal peripheral neuropathic pain syndromes: a randomized, double-blind, placebo-controlled study. Pain 2003; 106:151–158.
27. Biesbroeck R, Bril V, Hollander P, et al. A double-blind comparison of topical capsaicin and oral amitriptyline in painful diabetic neuropathy. Adv Ther 1995; 12:111–120.
28. Morley JS, Bridson J, Nash TP, Miles JB, White S, Makin MK. Low-dose methadone has an analgesic effect in neuropathic pain: a double-blind randomized controlled crossover trial. Palliat Med 2003; 17:576–587.
29. Watson CP, Moulin D, Watt-Watson J, Gordon A, Eisenhoffer J. Controlled-release oxycodone relieves neuropathic pain: a randomized controlled trial in painful diabetic neuropathy. Pain 2003; 105:71–78.
30. Wassilew SW, Wutzler P, Wutzler P. Oral brivudin in comparison with acyclovir for herpes zoster: a survey study on postherpetic neuralgia. Antiviral Res 2003; 59:57–60.
31. Bowsher D. The effects of pre-emptive treatment of postherpetic neuralgia with amitriptyline: a randomized, double-blind, placebo-controlled trial. J Pain Symptom Manage 1997; 13:327–331.
32. Pappagallo M, Haldey EJ. Pharmacological management of postherpetic neuralgia. CNS Drugs 2003; 17:771–780.
33. DeBeneditis G, Lorenzetti A. Topical aspirin/diethyl ether mixture versus indomethacin and diclofenac/diethyl ether mixture for acute herpetic neuralgia and postherpetic neuralgia: a double-blind, cross-over placebo controlled study. Pain 1996; 65:45–51.
34. Chung OY, Bruehl SP. Complex regional pain syndrome. Curr Treatment Options Neurol 2003; 5:499–511.

CME QUESTIONS

1. Diabetic neuropathy occurs more commonly with:
   a. Type 2 diabetes
   b. Increased age
   c. Increased duration of diabetes
   d. All of the above

2. Common features of complex regional pain syndrome include:
   a. Excessive extremity guarding
   b. Decreased hair growth
   c. Tremor
   d. Nail deformities
   e. All of the above

3. Postherpetic neuralgia can be reduced by treating herpes zoster early with:
   a. Antiviral agents
   b. Amitriptyline
   c. Opioids
   d. A and B
   e. All of the above

4. First-line therapy for neuropathic pain includes:
   a. 5% lidocaine patches
   b. Venlafaxine
   c. Gabapentin
   d. Low-dose opioids
   e. All of the above

9

Myofascial Pain

CASE HISTORY

Mr. Duffy is a 50-year-old electrical engineer whose work and hobbies cause him to be sedentary. One day, a shipment of new computers arrived at his job and he helped to carry the computer crates during his lunch break. At the end of the day, he complained of soreness over the left side of his back above his hip bone. The pain was aggravated by bending forward or to the side. Pain did not radiate into his leg, and he reported there was no numbness. Over the next 3 months, Mr. Duffy had persistent low back pain. After work, he would lie on the sofa to rest his back; pain was most severe when he arose from lying down and walked to the kitchen or bathroom. Although initial walking or bending forward was painful, the pain actually improved after walking for approximately 10 minutes or bending several times. On examination, there was no discomfort to palpation over the hip, spine, or ribs. Mr. Duffy yelled and jumped when the doctor pressed an area of muscle spasm between the top of his hip and the bottom of his ribs, telling the doctor that pressing his back in that spot created a severe pain in his lower left buttock. Mr. Duffy also complained of severe pain when asked to bend forward or to the side, although his response to a straight-leg-raise testing was normal. An X-ray revealed only mild arthritis in the lumbar spine. Because of his lack of physical findings (absence of pain over joints or an abnormal neurological examination) and dramatic response to palpation with a non-neurological pain referral pattern, Mr. Duffy's treating physician wondered if he was seeking workers' compensation benefits.

* * *

Mr. Duffy's story is typical for one of the most common causes of low back pain—quadratus lumborum syndrome—which is caused by muscle tightness and shortening in the lower back. This is the spot on the sides of the back above the waistband that one typically massages after stooping too long while gardening or doing too much housecleaning. Myofascial pain is a common cause of localized chronic pain. Like other myofascial or muscle-based chronic pain conditions, quadratus lumborum syndrome lacks the characteristics features of radicular pain (such as radiating extremity pain, numbness, or weakness).

From: *Chronic Pain: A Primary Care Guide to Practical Management*
Edited by: D. A. Marcus © Humana Press, Totowa, NJ

Mr. Duffy's examination is characterized by one of the hallmarks of myofascial pain—an active trigger point, that is, a focal area of exquisitely tender muscle spasm which, when palpated, causes pain vocalization and referral of pain to areas of the body that are characteristic for that muscle—in this case, the hip and buttock. Mr. Duffy's pain is characteristically located over a muscle bulk and affected by muscle stretching. Because muscles in myofascial pain syndrome are contracted, initial stretch is often painful. Once the muscle is stretched, however, pain is improved. For this reason, treatment focuses on returning contracted muscles to normal length through stretching techniques.

KEY CHAPTER POINTS

- Myofascial pain should be considered in patients with localized pain complaints without arthritic or neuropathic features.
- Myofascial pain syndrome should not be diagnosed in patients with no physical findings. Myofascial pain requires the presence of a taut band and muscular trigger points.
- Active trigger points refer pain in predictable patterns.
- Treatment of myofascial pain focuses on active stretching and range-of-motion exercises. Physical therapy modalities, injections, and medications may be used adjunctively.

1. DEFINITION

Myofascial pain is often diagnosed in patients with chronic, nonmalignant pain who lack clinical or laboratory evidence of radiculopathy, neuropathy, or joint disease. Under these circumstances, persistent pain is believed to be caused by chronic changes in muscles and surrounding soft tissues, or myofascial pain. The diagnosis of myofascial pain, however, is not a diagnosis of exclusion, but requires the presence of specific abnormalities.

Myofascial pain is characterized by localized shortened (contracted), tender muscles. The hallmark of myofascial pain is the trigger point—a tender area within contracted muscle bands that produces an involuntary contraction with stimulation (*see* Box 1) *(1)*. These taut bands have been shown to have spontaneous electrical activity on electromyographic testing *(2)*. Taut bands are important to identify for diagnosis and also because they may restrict normal muscle stretch, resulting in reduced active range of motion and muscle weakness related to muscle shortening. Taut bands are produced involuntarily and serve as an objective sign of myofascial pain. *Trigger points* are distinguished from *tender points*, which merely represent areas of increased sensitivity to stimulation.

Many doctors use the terms *myofascial pain* (with trigger points) and *fibromyalgia* (with tender points) interchangeably, often denoting chronic pain in patients without demonstrable pathology. Both myofascial pain and fibromyalgia, however, have specific diagnostic criteria (Table 1). (For addi-

---

Box 1
Diagnostic Criteria for Trigger Points

- Taut band
  - ○ Palpable contracted cord-like group of muscle fibers
  - ○ Point tenderness over taut band
- Local twitch response
  - ○ Involuntary contraction of taut band after physically plucking or inserting a needle into it
- Trigger points
  - ○ Active if palpation results in pain referred to chronic pain area
  - ○ Latent if locally tender, but without referred pain

Based on ref. *1*.

---

tional information about fibromyalgia, *see* Chapter 10.) Perhaps the most important distinction is that myofascial pain represents a localized pain complaint (e.g., low-back or shoulder-girdle pain), whereas fibromyalgia produces widespread pain, covering most regions of the body. Because fibromyalgia may result in modification of posture, gait, and activity, patients wtih fibromyalgia may develop additional myofascial pain complaints (localized areas of muscle spasm, trigger points, and contracted muscles on the background of widespread fibromyalgia pain).

2. EPIDEMIOLOGY

Myofascial pain occurred in approximately 30% of patients in a general medical clinic and is usually the most common diagnosis in specialty pain clinics *(3)*. Common myofascial syndromes include lateral epicondylitis (tennis elbow), quadratus lumborum syndrome (a common cause of nonradicular low back pain), and piriformis syndrome (a common cause of buttock and hip pain). Quadratus lumborum syndrome is one of the most common causes of low back pain. The quadratus lumborum muscle connects at the 12th rib, iliac crest, and lumbar vertebrae (Fig. 1). It is responsible for lateral bending of the lumbar spine. Patients with quadratus lumborum syndrome often have unilateral hip elevation because of muscle shortening. Active quadratus lumborum trigger points refer pain to the hip and buttock (Fig. 2). Another common myofascial pain condition is piriformis syndrome. The piriformis muscle attaches from the inner ileum and sacrum to the greater trochanter (Fig. 3) and rotates the hip externally, thereby contributing to the stability of the hip and back. Active piriformis trigger points also refer to the hip and buttock (Fig. 4). When hypertrophied, the piriformis may compress the sciatic nerve, which usually travels beneath it, resulting in additional leg pain or sciatica.

Table 1
Criteria for Distinguishing Between Myofascial Pain and Fibromyalgia

Criteria	Myofascial pain	Fibromyalgia
Pain location	Localized	Widespread
Physical examination		
Tenderness	Trigger point: discrete tenderness over painful muscle spasm; may or may not refer pain areas of pain complaints.	Tender points: tenderness to palpation over pre-specified points that may not be within areas of pain complaints.
Range of motion	Passive range of motion shows normal joint movement. Active range of motion is limited by pain.	Full passive and active range of motion.
Somatic complaints	Disturbances in sleep and mood are common. Irritable bowel syndrome, paresthesias, and other somatic complaints are infrequent.	Fatigue, mood disturbance, and somatic complaints are typical and are often as severe as pain.
Treatment		
Physical therapy	Focus on muscle stretching.	Focus on stretching plus aerobic exercise.
Injections	Trigger-point injections temporarily relieve pain and improve active range of motion.	Local injection of tender points is not beneficial.

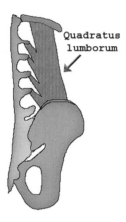

Fig. 1. Anatomy of the quadratus lumborum muscle.

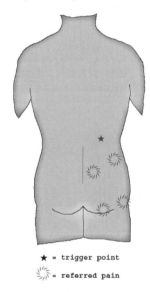

★ = trigger point

✷ = referred pain

Fig. 2. Referral pattern of active quadratus lumborum trigger points.

Several muscle groups in addition to the quadratus lumborum and piriformis are commonly affected in patients with myofascial pain. These include the upper trapezius, scalene, rhomboids, levator scapulae, and serratus anterior muscles. Areas of common trigger points and their referral patterns are shown in Figs. 5–9. Identifying typical pain referral patterns in myofascial pain helps the clinician recognize these common pain syndromes.

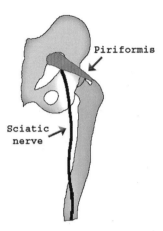

Fig. 3. Anatomy of the piriformis muscle.

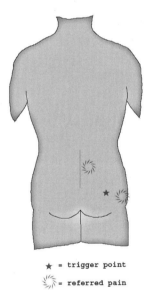

★ = trigger point

= referred pain

Fig. 4. Referral pattern from active piriformis trigger point.

3. EVALUATION

Localized chronic pain is generally caused by muscles and their surrounding tissue (myofascial pain), joints (mechanical pain), or nervous system structures (neuropathic pain). Patient evaluations should be designed to test each of these systems (Table 2).

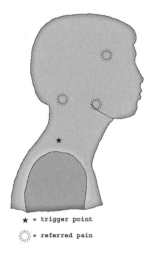

★ = trigger point

\~ = referred pain

Fig. 5. Referral pattern for upper trapezius trigger points.

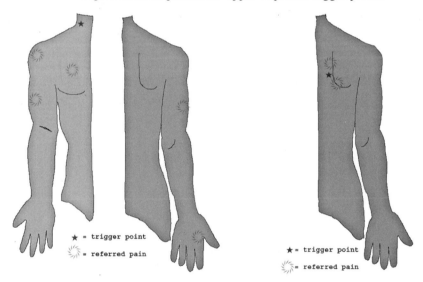

★ = trigger point

\~ = referred pain

★ = trigger point

\~ = referred pain

Fig. 6. Referral pattern for scalene muscle.

Fig. 7. Referral pattern for rhomboids.

Evaluation should include a detailed musculoskeletal examination to assess posture (which may be abnormal in all three types of pain), range of motion, muscle tone and tenderness, joint motion, and neurological function. Passive range of motion is evaluated by an examiner manipulating a joint through its full range in the relaxed patient. Active range of motion, on the other hand,

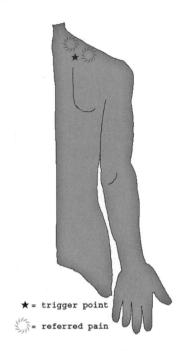

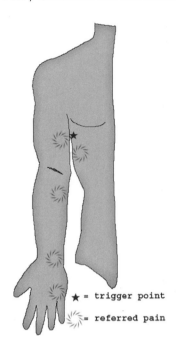

Fig. 8. Referral pattern for levator scapulae.

Fig. 9. Referral pattern for serratus anterior

requires the patient to voluntarily activate muscles to move each joint through its range of motion. An examiner can record the extent of active range of motion, as observed through patient performance. Greater restriction of active range of motion compared with passive range of motion suggests a myofascial restriction or reduced patient effort.

The presence of myofascial features can be identified by directly visualizing painful areas for increased muscle bulk, which suggests a spasm, and by palpating for taut bands and trigger points. Identification of taut bands is best performed by examining the stretched muscle with the fingertips. The taut band should feel like a tight cord or rope in the muscle. In addition, as seen in Mr. Duffy, palpation of taut bands demonstrates tenderness and may cause involuntary muscle contraction locally (a local twitch response), flinching and vocalizing pain, or both. This flinch response should occur exclusively when the trigger point is palpated and not as a response to palpation of other areas. Tenderness cannot be assessed in patients who do not permit even the gentlest touch of areas distant to the painful area.

Table 2
Evaluation of Patient With Localized Pain

System to test	Physical exam findings	Supplemental tests	Diagnostic label (if abnormal)
Muscles and soft tissues	Muscle spasm and tenderness. Taut bands and trigger points.	Physical therapy assessment.	Myofascial
	AROM restricted; PROM normal.		Mechanical
Joints	PROM restricted. Joint crepitus.	X-ray.	
	Joint inflammation. Joint instability.		
Nerves	Numbness, weakness, reflex changes in distributions consistent with spine, spinal root, or nerve abnormality.[a] Abnormal SLR.	EMG/NCV; MRI for suspected myelopathy or radiculopathy.	Neuropathic

[a]See Chapters 5 and 8. AROM, active range-of-motion; EMG/NCV, electromyography with nerve conduction velocity; MRI, magnetic resonance imaging; PROM, passive range-of-motion; SLR, straight-leg raise test.

Myofascial pain should not be diagnosed unless these abnormal clinical examination findings are identified. If patients cannot cooperate with testing because of extreme pain, the clinician should reschedule them for another visit when they may be more amenable to testing. Myofascial pain cannot be diagnosed unless a detailed assessment of range of motion, posture and gait, and strength and sensory testing has been completed. Myofascial pain should not be diagnosed in patients with no physical findings.

No laboratory or radiographic abnormalities are associated with myofascial pain. The diagnosis is generally based on a history of an inciting event or injury, physical examination findings of tight and tender muscles, and the absence of mechanical instability or neurological deficits. X-rays should be performed in patients with suspected joint abnormality, inflammation, or instability. Plain X-rays also provide a useful screening tool for patients with chronic pain over bony structures to rule out underlying bone disease. Magnetic resonance scans should be reserved for patients with evidence of myelopathy, radiculopathy, or another specific type of pathology that would be identified with this testing.

4. TREATMENT

Physical therapy is the cornerstone of myofascial pain therapy. A careful evaluation by a trained physical therapist is invaluable for correctly identifying trigger points and areas of muscle shortening. The exercise program needs to be tailor-made for each patient to specifically address postural abnormalities and myofascial changes contributing to the pain complaints. Therapy must focus on active stretching and range-of-motion exercises, although supplemental passive treatment modalities (administered by the therapist) may also be utilized. Patients should be instructed in a home-exercise routine to be performed at least twice daily, in addition to their physical therapy sessions. Temporarily isolated muscle stretching during a 1-hour therapy session, with no additional exercise to maintain stretches between appointments, will not be effective for most patients. The addition of targeted trigger-point injections, medications, or other physical therapy modalities are all designed in improve the ability to achieve an effective muscle stretch during active exercise (*see* Box 2).

4.1. Physical Therapy

Physical therapy treatment begins with a gentle stretching program and active range-of-motion exercises. Although passive stretching (stretching performed by a therapist on a relaxed patient) may be soothing, myofascial pain is most likely to improve in patients who perform active exercise (stretching performed by the patient). Patients should perform both whole-body stretches and stretches targeted to the painful area twice daily. Muscles should be

---

Box 2
Treatment of Myofascial Pain

- Primary treatment
  - Physical therapy
    - Posture correction
    - Stretching exercises
    - Active range of motion exercises
- Secondary treatment
  - Pharmacological therapy
    - Analgesics for pain flares
      - Acetaminophen
      - Nonsteroidal anti-inflammatory drugs
      - Tramadol
    - Tizanidine
      - Initially 1–2 mg at bedtime. May increase slowly to 24 mg/day in divided doses
    - Trigger point injections
  - Nonpharmacological therapy
    - Occupational therapy
      - Pacing skills
      - Work simplification/modification
    - Pain management psychology
      - Relaxation techniques
      - Stress management
      - Coping skills

---

stretched until a stretched sensation is first felt. Patients should not over-stretch their muscles or attempt to achieve maximal stretch. Stretching exercises help return shortened muscles to a more normal length, inactivating the taut band and trigger points. Several weeks after beginning a stretching program, patients should start using light weights to incorporate strengthening into the exercise routine. In one study, physical therapy that included active exercise (and incorporated a home-exercise program) and passive trigger point massage over 4 weeks significantly reduced both the number of trigger points and trigger point severity score (Fig. 10) *(4)*.

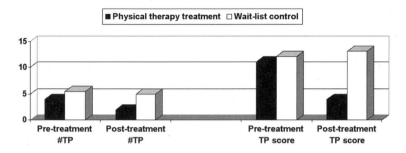

Fig. 10. Reduction in trigger point number and pain severity with physical therapy. Reduction in trigger point count (#TP) and trigger point severity score (TP score) were both significantly reduced in patients treated with physical therapy compared with controls ($p < 0.05$). (Based on ref. *4*.)

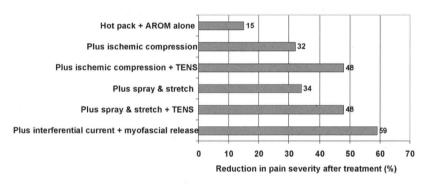

Fig. 11. Comparison among treatment modalities for myofascial pain. AROM, active range of motion; TENS, transcutaneous electrical nerve stimulation. All patients received hot packs plus AROM treatment. Pain reduction was significantly decreased after treatment for all treatment groups ($p < 0.05$) in these patients with myofascial trapezius pain. (Based on ref. *5*.)

A variety of treatment modalities may be added to myofascial stretching (Table 3). In a study comparing techniques used in patients with cervical myofascial pain, investigators observed significant pain reduction from all tested treatment modality combinations (Fig. 11) *(5)*. The addition of any therapy to hot packs plus active range-of-motion exercises resulted in significantly better pain reduction. The most effective forms of therapy were those that included transcutaneous electrical nerve stimulation or interferential current therapy. Notably, neither modality was administered in isolation in this study. Rather, both therapies were appropriately used as adjunctive therapy to improve the benefit that could be achieved from active range-of-motion exercises.

Table 3
Supplemental Treatment Modalities Used in Conjunction
With a Physical Therapy Stretching Exercise Program

Treatment	Description
Injections	
• Trigger-point injections	Local anesthetic (e.g., 0.5–1% lidocaine or 0.25–0.5% bupivacaine) injected into trigger point.
• Dry needling	Insertion of a solid, acupuncture-type needle into trigger point.
Physical therapy modalities	
• Ischemic compression	Application of pressure to trigger points for 90 seconds. Force is halfway between that which produces any pain and that which produces intolerable pain.
• Hot packs	Moist heating pads placed over the painful area for 20 minutes before exercise.
• Active range-of-motion	Five repetitions of actively moving painful area through full range-of-motion.
• Spray and stretch	Vasocoolant fluorimethane spray is applied to the entire painful area (not just the trigger point) prior to stretching.
• TENS	Electrodes placed around painful area and current applied for approximately 20 minutes.
• Interferential current therapy	Electrodes placed around painful area and current applied for approximately 20 minutes. Minimal skin resistance with interferential current therapy allows a maximum amount of energy to penetrate to deeper tissues. Used in patients who fail TENS.
• Myofascial release	Passive stretching and traction techniques, applied by a trained therapist.

TENS, transcutaneous electrical nerve stimulation.

4.2. Injections

Trigger-point injections require infiltration of a local anesthetic into myofascial trigger points. A 22- to 25-gauge needle is inserted into the skin approximately 1 cm away from the trigger point, then advanced to the trigger point. After verification of its placement outside the blood vessels, 0.1 to 0.2 mL of anesthetic is injected. The needle is then partially withdrawn, redirected, and advanced toward another area within the trigger point. This process is repeated until a local twitch response is no longer elicited, muscle tautness is reduced, or 0.5 to 1.0 mL of anesthetic has been injected around the trigger point. Pressure is maintained over the area after the injection to minimize hematoma development. Trigger-point injections are contraindicated in patients with a risk for coagulopathy or bleeding. It is not clear whether the addition of steroids to trigger-point injections lengthens the duration of pain relief.

Superficial dry needling involves the insertion of a solid thin needle (resembling an acupuncture needle) into trigger points. This method can also help deactivate myofascial trigger points when used in conjunction with stretching exercises *(6)*. Hong demonstrated significant reduction of myofascial shoulder girdle pain after either trigger point injections with local anesthetic or dry needling *(7)*. In both cases, benefit was derived only when a local twitch response was generated with the needle insertion. Soreness was less likely to occur after local anesthetic trigger point injections. The benefits of dry needling are supported by studies showing similar benefits after trigger point injections, regardless of the injected substance (including saline) *(8)*.

4.3. Pharmacological Therapy

Pharmacological therapy is designed to supplement physical therapy. Patients who fail to benefit from stretching programs alone may be treated with adjunctive tizanidine, a muscle relaxant with analgesic properties *(9)*. Unlike most muscle relaxants, which are ineffective in chronic pain, tizanidine effectively reduces chronic myofascial pain for many patients *(10)*. Tizanidine is also mildly sedating and can improve sleep disturbance in some patients when administered in low doses at bedtime. Analgesics may be used on an intermittent basis to treat pain flares. Daily analgesics are rarely helpful and chronic use may produce significant gastric and renal toxicity *(11,12)*.

4.4. Comprehensive Pain Management

Patients with prolonged myofascial pain complaints often report significant psychological distress, social restrictions, and work disability, in addition to myofascial pain. A survey of patients receiving trigger point injections identified prolonged duration of pain, change in social activities, and work disability as independent predictors of failure to respond to trigger point therapy *(13)*. In these patients, psychological pain management techniques and occupational therapy interventions are necessary in addition to physical therapy treatment.

5. SUMMARY

Myofascial pain is a unique pain syndrome, characterized by tight, tender muscles, with taut bands and tender trigger points. Myofascial pain syndrome is distinguished from mechanical pain by the absence of joint pathology, from neuropathic pain by the absence of neurological dysfunction, and from fibromyalgia by the absence of widespread body pain. Myofascial pain should be considered in patients with localized pain complaints. Knowledge of typical myofascial pain referral patterns (e.g., quadratus lumborum and piriformis syndromes) facilitates the identification of these common pain syndromes.

The focus of treatment for myofascial pain is active stretching and range-of-motion exercises. Passive physical therapy modalities, injections, and medications may be used adjunctively. Patients with long-standing myofascial pain may have additional psychological distress, disability, or both that will require additional, targeted therapy, including psychological interventions and occupational therapy.

REFERENCES

1. Simons DG, Travell JG, Simons LS. Myofascial Pain and Dysfunction: The Trigger Point Manual, vol 1., 2nd Ed. Baltimore, Md: Lippincott, Williams, & Wilkins; 1999.
2. Hubbard DR, Berkoff GM. Myofascial trigger points show spontaneous needle EMG activity. Spine 1993; 18:1803–1807.
3. Shootsky SA, Jaeger B, Oye RK. Prevalence of myofascial pain in general internal medicine practice. West J Med 1989; 151:157–160.
4. Gam AN, Warming S, Larsen LH, et al. Treatment of myofascial trigger-points with ultrasound combined with massage and exercise: a randomized controlled trial. Pain 1998; 77:73–79.
5. Hou CR, Tsai L, Cheng K, Chung K, Hong C. Immediate effects of various physical therapeutic modalities on cervical myofascial pain and trigger-point sensitivity. Arch Phys Med Rehabil 2002; 83:1406–1414.
6. Edwards J, Knowles N. Superficial dry needling and active stretching in the treatment of myofascial pain: a randomized controlled trial. Acupuncture Med 2003; 21:80–86.
7. Hong CZ. Lidocaine injection versus dry needling to myofascial trigger point: the importance of the local twitch response. Am J Phys Med Rehabil 1994; 73: 256–263.
8. Cummings TM, White AR. Needling therapies in the management of myofascial trigger point pain: a systematic review. Arch Phys Med Rehabil 2001; 82:986–992.
9. Hord AH, Chalfoun AG, Denson DD, Azevedo MI. Systemic tizanidine hydrochloride (Zanaflex) relieves thermal hyperalgesia in rats with an experimental mononeuropathy. Anesth Analg 2001; 93:1310–1315.
10. Malanga GA, Gwynn MW, Smith R, Miller D. Tizanidine is effective in the treatment of myofascial pain syndrome. Pain Physician 2002; 5:422–432.
11. Matzke GR. Nonrenal toxicities of acetaminophen, aspirin and nosteroidal anti-inflammatory agents. Am J Kidney Dis 1996; 28(Suppl 1):S63–S70.
12. Gambaro G, Perazella MA. Adverse renal effects of anti-inflammatory agents: evaluation of selective and nonselective cyclooxygenase inhibitors. J Intern Med 2003; 253:643–652.
13. Hopwood MB, Abram SE. Factors associated with failure of trigger point injections. Clin J Pain 1994; 10:227–234.

CME QUESTIONS—CHAPTER 9

1. What percentage of patients in a general medical practice may be diagnosed with myofascial pain?
   a. 3
   b. 10
   c. 30
   d. 90

2. Hallmarks of myofascial pain include:
   a. Tight muscle bands
   b. Muscular trigger points
   c. Restricted joint motion
   d. A and B
   e. All of the above

3. Choose the most accurate statement:
   a. The terms myofascial pain and fibromyalgia are both used to describe chronic pain experienced by patients with no real abnormalities.
   b. Myofascial pain and fibromyalgia may be considered synonymous.
   c. Myofascial pain is characterized by localized pain and trigger points; fibromyalgia is characterized by widespread pain with positive tender points.
   d. All of the above

4. Effective treatment for myofascial pain include:
   a. Stretching exercises
   b. Interferential current therapy
   c. Spray and stretch
   d. All of the above

CASE HISTORY

Ms. Colegrove is a 23-year-old elementary school teacher who reported persistent widespread body aching since falling while roller-blading 3 years earlier. She had not missed work because of the pain, but reported that she had curtailed her previously active evening sports, like roller-blading 5 miles or participating in an adult basketball league. She reported pain affecting different areas of her body on different days, with pain occurring at different times in all extremities, neck, and back. She also reported incapacitating migraine headaches two or times weekly. In addition to pain complaints, Ms. Colegrove reported difficulty with sleep and extreme fatigue, as well as intermittent numbness in nondermatomal areas. Examination showed a vivacious, attractive woman with a brisk gait and full active range of motion of her neck, back, and all extremities. Her strength and sensory examinations were completely normal, despite complaints of feeling weak and having numbness in her right leg. After completing the examination, she opened a spiral notebook, in which she recorded a daily log of all of her symptoms and another notebook containing materials from the Internet on fibromyalgia for her doctor to review. Her primary care physician (PCP) was struck with the stark contrast between Ms. Colegrove's severe complaints and reports of physical limitations and her perfect work attendance and her completely normal examination. The PCP suspected the absence of marriage and children had resulted in excessive focus on bodily sensations and recommended she increase her participation in social activities to provide additional distractions. No treatment was recommended in light of her lack of work disability and absence of physical dysfunctions on examination.

* * *

Ms. Colegrove embodies many of the features of the typical patient with fibromyalgia. She is young, intelligent, high-achieving, and highly motivated to improve. In addition, most patients with fibromyalgia will maintain required work activities, while curtailing additional enjoyable activities because of both pain and fatigue. Patients with fibromyalgia are highly cooperative with their

From: *Chronic Pain: A Primary Care Guide to Practical Management*
Edited by: D. A. Marcus © Humana Press, Totowa, NJ

examination and often cause the doctor to remark, "You did those tests better than I could do!" Instead of interpreting lack of physical limitations as a sign of a highly cooperative patient, health care providers often falsely assume patients' reports of disability must be exaggerated. As suspected by her PCP, most patients with fibromyalgia do tend to be very "tuned in" to bodily sensations and experience stress as somatic rather than emotional symptoms. This, along with a strong desire to improve, often results in patients with fibromyalgia recording copious, detailed information about their symptoms and scouring available literature for suggested treatments. PCPs must understand that patients with fibromyalgia are not seeking to maintain their disability by these actions, but are exceptionally eager to improve. This makes patients with fibromyalgia ideal candidates for self-management pain rehabilitation.

KEY CHAPTER POINTS

- Fibromyalgia describes a diverse symptom complex, including widespread body pain, tenderness to palpation, and somatic complaints.
- Fibromyalgia affects approximately 2% of adults, with women affected six times more frequently than men. Prevalence increases with age.
- Patients with fibromyalgia report significant disability, psychological distress, and reduced physical and mental health quality of life.
- Most patients with fibromyalgia report reduced pain and medication use over a 3-year period.

Fibromyalgia is best treated with multidisciplinary treatment, using therapies to specifically target individual patient symptoms

1. DEFINITION

The term *fibromyalgia* has been used to describe a wide variety of non-localized pain complaints, particularly pain syndromes in women with no identifiable pathology. In 1990, the American College of Rheumatology (ACR) established specific criteria to allow identification of fibromyalgia as a unique pain syndrome, rather than a wastebasket diagnosis for patients who failed to meet criteria for other pain syndromes *(1)*. The ACR requires both widespread pain and the presence of at least 11 of 18 painful tender points to meet diagnostic criteria for fibromyalgia *(see* Box 1 and Fig. 1).

Tender points are predetermined areas throughout the body that tend to be painful with pressure in patients with fibromyalgia (Fig. 2). Interestingly, firm palpation of these specific points tends to be perceived as painful in fibromyalgia patients, but not patients with other types of chronic pain. Positive tender points discriminate between fibromyalgia patients and other pain patients when using a cut-off score of at least 2 on a 0 to 10 severity scale (0 = *no pain or pressure*; 10 = *excruciating pain*) after application of 4 kg of pressure *(2)*. Digital palpation more effectively discriminates fibromyalgia patients than dolorimeter testing, making testing at the bedside easy *(1)*.

Box 1
Diagnosis of Fibromyalgia

- Widespread body pain
  - ○ Pain on both left and right sides of the body
  - ○ Pain above and below the waist
  - ○ Axial pain present
- Pain persisting at least 3 months
- At least 11 of 18 tender points painful to 4 kg pressure

Based on ref. *1.*

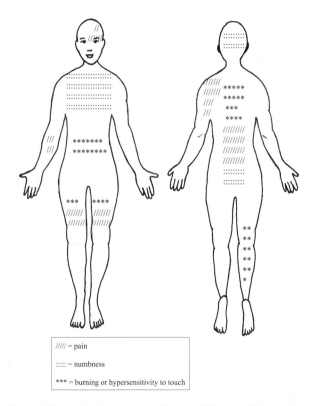

///// = pain

::::: = numbness

*** = burning or hypersensitivity to touch

Fig. 1. Typical pain drawing from a fibromyalgia patient.

Pressing with the thumb results in approximately 4 kg of pressure when the nail bed blanches. Higher scores reported for tender points correlate with greater levels of disability *(3).*

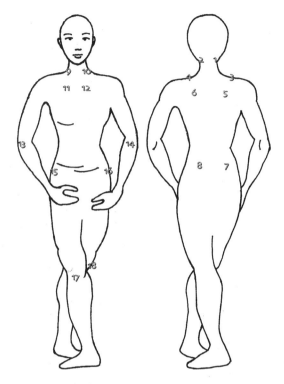

Fig. 2. Location of 18 possible fibromyalgia tender points. Location of tender points (right and left): 1 and 2: occiput; 3 and 4: trapezius; 5 and 6: supraspinatus; 7 and 8: gluteal; 9 and 10: lower lateral cervical; 11 and 12: 2nd costochondral junction; 13 and 14: lateral epicondyle; 15 and 16: greater trochanter; 17 and 18: medial knee fat pad.

Although the presence of these pain features defines fibromyalgia, fibromyalgia patients typically describe a variety of additional somatic and psychological complaints (*see* Box 2). Fatigue, sleep disturbance, morning stiffness, and headache are reported by the majority of fibromyalgia patients. Paresthesias, irritable bowel syndrome (IBS), depression, and anxiety are also common. Ms. Colegrove typifies fibromyalgia patients by reporting a variety of somatic complaints in addition to widespread pain.

IBS is a diagnosis of exclusion, with the diagnosis assigned in patients with no identifiable and correctable pathology. Patients with IBS report at least 12 weeks of abdominal pain during a year, with pain that is relieved with bowel movements and bowel movements that change in frequency and appearance (e.g., alternating diarrhea and constipation). It is important to ensure patients are not aggravating gastrointestinal complaints through excessive and/or alternating use of over-the-counter laxatives and diarrhea treatments.

Box 2
Common Associated Somatic and Psychological Symptoms
in Patients With Fibromyalgia

- Constitutional
  - Fatigue: 66–82%
  - Sleep disturbance: 66–75%
  - Sicca syndrome/dry eyes: 10–36%
  - Raynaud's syndrome: 17%
- Musculoskeletal
  - Morning stiffness: 76–77%
- Gastrointestinal
  - Irritable bowel syndrome: 30–48%

- Neurological
  - Headache: 53–82%
  - Paresthesias: 31–53%
- Genitourinary
  - Urinary urgency: 26–32%
  - Dysmenorrhea: 26%
- Psychiatric
  - Depression: 32–48%
  - Anxiety: 28–48%

Based on refs. *1,4,7.*

2. EPIDEMIOLOGY

Fibromyalgia affects approximately 2% of adults *(4–6)*. Fibromyalgia is more prevalent in women than men. A large community survey identified ACR-defined fibromyalgia in 3% of women versus 0.5% of men *(7)*. In addition, fibro-myalgia prevalence increases with age, reaching more than 7% of women aged 60 years or older. An evaluation for fibromyalgia symptoms in the general population revealed significantly higher reporting of fatigue, sleep disturbance, "pain all over," and IBS in women compared with men *(8)*. Similarly, a survey of fibromyalgia patients revealed that, although pain severity comparisons were similar between men and women, female patients more commonly endorsed fatigue, "pain all over," and IBS (Fig. 3) *(9)*.

2.1. Psychological Comorbidity

Depressive and anxious disorders occur comorbidly with fibromyalgia, although data of prevalence varies among different studies *(see* Box 3) *(10–13)*. Although chronic pain in general is associated with increased prevalence of depression and anxiety, these symptoms appear to be even more common in fibromyalgia patients (Fig. 4) *(10)*. Patients with fibromyalgia and comorbid anxiety or depression tend to have more physical symptoms and disability *(14)*.

Quality of life (QOL) is also reduced in patients with fibromyalgia. The Medical Outcomes Study Health Survey (SF-36) scores self-reported life quality for a variety of physical and emotional variables, with possible scores from 0 *(poorest QOL)* to 100 *(maximum QOL)*. Interestingly, fibromyalgia patients score significantly lower than rheumatoid arthritis patients for all measures, except for physical functioning (Fig. 5) *(10)*.

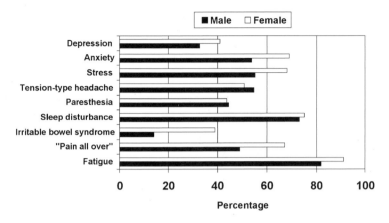

Fig. 3. Gender differences in fibromyalgia symptoms. (Based on ref. *9*.)

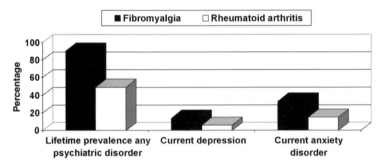

Fig. 4. Comparison of prevalence of psychiatric disorders in patients with fibromyalgia versus rheumatoid arthritis. (Based on ref. *10*.)

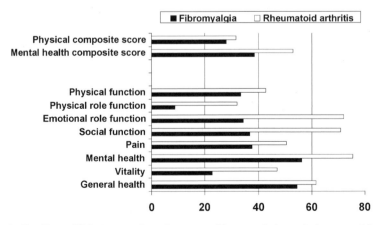

Fig. 5. Quality of life comparison between fibromyalgia and rheumatoid arthritis patients. (Based on ref. *10*.)

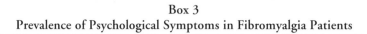

> **Box 3**
> **Prevalence of Psychological Symptoms in Fibromyalgia Patients**
>
> • Depression: 14–56% • Panic disorder: 7–25% • Generalized anxiety: 33%
>
> Based on refs. *10–13.*

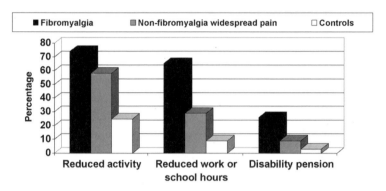

Fig. 6. Disability associated with fibromyalgia and other chronic pain. Reduced activity and reduced work or school hours were reported as occurring ≥1 day during a 2-week period. (Adapted from ref. *15.*)

2.2. Disability

Despite the presence of a generally unremarkable physical examination in fibromyalgia patients, fibromyalgia is associated with significant disability *(15)*. During a 2-week period, 74% of a community fibromyalgia sample endorsed reducing usual activities and 58% spent at least 1 day in bed because of health symptoms *(4)*. The mean number of days with reduced activities over a 2-week period was 4.7. Work activities were limited because of fibromyalgia for 65%, with 31% work disabled. A multicenter survey of fibromyalgia patients from diverse socioeconomic backgrounds similarly identified receipt of disability payments in 26% *(16)*.

Disability associated with fibromyalgia pain is greater than with other types of diffuse pain. A population survey of adults with fibromyalgia or widespread musculoskeletal (non-fibromyalgia) pain and no widespread pain controls identified significantly higher disability in the fibromyalgia group (Fig. 6) *(15)*. Widespread pain was differentiated as fibromyalgia or musculoskeletal based on the presence or absence, respectively, of tender points as performed by a rheumatologist. Disability was similar between genders and greater in patients with fibromyalgia compared with non-fibromyalgia pain or controls.

3. EVALUATION

Patients with widespread pain complaints should be assessed for somatic symptoms that occur comorbidly with fibromyalgia (Box 2). Although some symptoms, like paresthesias, cannot be individually treated beyond standard fibromyalgia therapy, others (e.g., migraine, sleep disturbance, and IBS) can be addressed directly. In addition, because fibromyalgia is comorbid with somatic complaints, patients seeking treatment for fatigue, sleep disturbance, or IBS should also be screened for pain complaints.

3.1. Assessment Measures

Patients reporting pain in several body regions should be screened for fibromyalgia with a tender point examination. Figure 7 provides a recording sheet for scoring tender points in the clinic. Scores should be recorded at baseline and again during and after treatment. The number of positive tender points (score ≥2) is the tender point count, with a possible range of 0 (*no tender points are positive*) to 18 (*all tender points are positive*). The total numeric score obtained from adding each individual tender point score is the total tender point score. Monitoring tender point count and total tender point score can serve as useful treatment efficacy markers.

In addition to pain assessments, patients identified with fibromyalgia should be screened for commonly associated somatic and psychological complaints (*see* Box 4). Treatment can be targeted to those symptoms that limit the patient's daily routine. Identifying those symptoms that occur, but are not disabling helps both patients and their doctors acknowledge the occurrence of somatic symptoms, but also prioritize those most in need of treatment.

All patients with fibromyalgia should be screened for depression and anxiety because of their high prevalence in fibromyalgia and the reluctance of many patients to discuss psychological symptoms with their treating clinicians, for fear of being labeled as a psychiatric patient, with all fibromyalgia symptoms attributed to emotional problems. Also, unless symptoms are severe, many patients do not recognize symptoms of anxiety or depression. Finally, patients often believe that their mood or anxiety symptoms are a consequence of suffering with chronic pain and that these symptoms will resolve once the pain severity has improved. Identifying severity of psychological distress can help motivate patients to address psychological symptoms separate from pain reduction. Screening tools for anxiety and depression are available online (Table 1).

The effect of fibromyalgia can be evaluated using the Fibromyalgia Impact Questionnaire (FIQ) (Box 5) *(17)*. This questionnaire may be used to determine severity of disability and follow patient progress through treatment. The FIQ correlates well with work disability *(4)* and is available at Website: www.myalgia.com/fig.pdf.

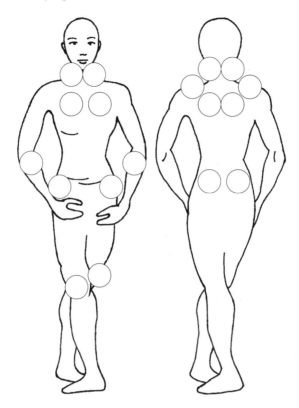

Fig. 7. Recording sheet for fibromyalgia examination. Record pain score from 0 to 10 (0 = *pressure or no pain*; 10 = *excruciating pain*) produced by exerting 4 kg pressure with the thumb (nail bed blanches).

Box 4 **Assessment of Fibromyalgia Patients**			
Which of the following problems limit your daily activities?			
Problem	Not a problem	Problem occurs but does NOT limit daily routine	Problem limits daily routine
Fatigue	☐	☐	☐
Sleep disturbance	☐	☐	☐
Frequent constipation	☐	☐	☐
Frequent diarrhea	☐	☐	☐
Depressed or blue mood	☐	☐	☐
Anxiety or nervousness	☐	☐	☐
Headache	☐	☐	☐

Box 5
Fibromyalgia Impact Questionnaire

Question 1. Rate how frequently you were able to perform each of the following
tasks *during the past week*. If you would not normally perform one of
these tasks, mark N/A for not applicable.

	Always 0	Mostly 1	Occasionally 2	Never 3	N/A
Do shopping	☐	☐	☐	☐	☐
Do laundry with washer and dryer	☐	☐	☐	☐	☐
Prepare meals	☐	☐	☐	☐	☐
Wash dishes/cooking utensils by hand	☐	☐	☐	☐	☐
Vacuum a rug	☐	☐	☐	☐	☐
Make beds	☐	☐	☐	☐	☐
Walk several blocks	☐	☐	☐	☐	☐
Visit friends or relatives	☐	☐	☐	☐	☐
Do yard work	☐	☐	☐	☐	☐
Drive a car	☐	☐	☐	☐	☐
Climb stairs	☐	☐	☐	☐	☐

Question 2. In the *past week*, how many days did you *feel good*?
(Circle a number from 0–7 days.)

0   1   2   3   4   5   6   7

Question 3. How many days in the *past week* did you *miss work* (including housework) because on your fibromyalgia?
(Circle a number from 0–7 days.)

0   1   2   3   4   5   6   7

Question 4. For each question below, circle the number on each scale that best
describes how you felt overall during the *past week*.

A. When working (including housework), how much did pain or other fibromyalgia symptoms interfere?

0   1   2   3   4   5   6   7   8   9   10
No problem with work   Great difficulty with work

B. How bad has your pain been?

0   1   2   3   4   5   6   7   8   9   10
No pain   Very severe pain

C. How tired have you been?

0   1   2   3   4   5   6   7   8   9   10
No tiredness   Very tired

Continued

Box 5
Fibromyalgia Impact Questionnaire *(Continued)*

D. How have you felt when you got up in the morning?

0	1	2	3	4	5	6	7	8	9	10

Awoke well rested   Awoke very tired

E. How bad has your stiffness been?

0	1	2	3	4	5	6	7	8	9	10

No stiffness   Very stiff

F. How nervous or anxious have you felt?

0	1	2	3	4	5	6	7	8	9	10

Not anxious   Very anxious

G. How depressed or blue have your felt?

0	1	2	3	4	5	6	7	8	9	10

Not depressed   Very depressed

Scoring the FIQ

Possible score ranges from 0 (no impact) to 100 (severe impact)

---

1. Add the numbers for each checked item in Question 1 and divide by the number of scored items. Number of scored items will be 11 unless some are not applicable. Multiply this average score by 0.33.
2. Score items in Question 2 in reverse order: 7 = 0, 6 = 1, 5 = 2, etc. Multiply the score for the selected item by 1.43.
3. Multiply selected number in Question 3 by 1.43.
4. Add all circled numbers together in Question 4.
5. Add numbers obtained for scoring questions 1–4 for the total FIQ score. Scores >70 represent severe impact.

Adapted from ref. *17.*

4. TREATMENT

The first step in treating fibromyalgia patients is to make the diagnosis. Once patients have received a diagnosis of fibromyalgia, they often become stereotyped by other health care providers, so the fibromyalgia label should never be used unless patients meet ACR criteria. Fibromyalgia patients need to be reassured that fibromyalgia is not a disease, but a symptom complex. Fibromyalgia symptoms are not progressive and will not lead to loss of muscle strength, paralysis, dementia, and so on.

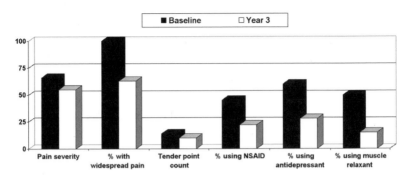

Fig. 8. Long-term outcome in fibromyalgia patients: comparison of pain and medication use at baseline and after 3 years. NSAID, nonsteroidal anti-inflammatory drug. (Based on ref. *18*.)

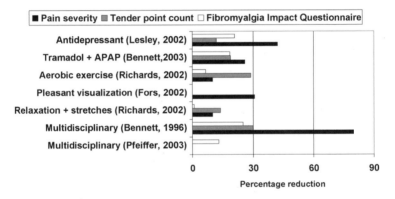

Fig. 9. Responses to fibromyalgia therapies. APAP, acetaminophen.

Most patients with fibromyalgia improve over time. Pöyhiä and colleagues *(18)* followed 59 patients with fibromyalgia who were treated in university and community practices for 3 years. During that time, patients experienced a significant ($p < 0.01$) decrease in pain scores (visual analog scale score: 66 at baseline vs 55 at 3 years) and tender-point count (14 vs 10). Most importantly, both pain and medication use decreased over 3 years (Fig. 8). This study offers encouragement that fibromyalgia patients and their healthcare providers can expect both symptomatic improvement and reduced reliance on medications over time.

Numerous studies have evaluated treatment efficacy in fibromyalgia, using a variety of endpoints. Studies most commonly measure FIQ scores, tender-point count, and pain severity. A comparison among different treatment types shows benefits from most types of therapy, including medications, education, aerobic exercise, and psychological pain management skills (Fig. 9) *(19–24)*.

4.1. Pharmacological Treatment

Most pharmacological trials in fibromyalgia patients have evaluated antidepressants. Studies show that antidepressants effectively reduce symptoms in fibromyalgia *(25)*. Most trials, however, show only modest superiority of antidepressants over placebo, with short-term efficacy exceeding long-term efficacy. A meta-analysis of 10 short-term studies with antidepressants (treatment duration: 3–24 weeks) showed an odds ratio for improvement of 4.2, with a number-needed-to-treat of four patients *(26)*. Although tricyclic antidepressants (TCAs) have been the most widely studied antidepressants for fibromyalgia, this latter meta-analysis included studies with TCAs, selective serotonin reuptake inhibitors (SSRIs), and *S*-adenosylmethionine. The authors concluded that both TCAs and SSRIs were effective for fibromyalgia.

Other medications used in chronic pain may also be beneficial for patients with fibromyalgia. Gabapentin is an antiepileptic drug with antinociceptive properties. Gabapentin has been most extensively studied in patients with neuropathic pain, although anecdotal reports suggest a benefit in some fibromyalgia patients. Gabapentin can reduce pain, sleep disturbance, and some anxiety symptoms. The antispasticity agent tizanidine has also shown promise for both myofascial pain and fibromyalgia *(27,28)*. Tizanidine can improve pain, muscle spasm, and sleep disturbance.

Analgesics have limited benefit for fibromyalgia patients. A review of four placebo-controlled trials testing nonsteroidal anti-inflammatory medications in patients with fibromyalgia failed to find superiority of analgesics over placebo *(25)*.

A recent, double-blind study comparing the combination of 37.5 mg tramadol with 325 mg acetaminophen (one to two tablets four times a day), however, did report significant improvements in pain, disability, and QOL *(24)*.

4.2. Individualized, Symptom-Focused, Multidisciplinary Treatment

Treatment outcome may be maximized in an individual patient by identifying specific symptom targets and prescribing a variety of treatments (Table 2). Some therapies, such as antidepressants, may be useful to treat a variety of possible symptoms, including fibromyalgia pain, migraine, sleep disturbance, and mood disturbance and anxiety.

Fibromyalgia patients benefit from education about their condition. Several valuable online references are available (*see* Box 6). These sites inform patients that they are not unique in their complaints and help legitimize fibromyalgia for patients and their families. Recording exercise and relaxation practices in a daily diary or calendar can also serve as an educational tool to assist with scheduling and compliance. (Exercise program logs are available in Chapter 16.)

Table 1
Online Psychiatric Screening Tools

Website address	Symptom tested
http://www.healthyplace.com/site/tests/psychological.asp	Separate tests screen for depression, anxiety, personality traits, and stress
http://www.psychcorp.com	Standard depression assessment tool: Beck Depression Inventory
http://www.mindgarden.com/Assessments/Info/staiinfo.htm	Standard anxiety assessment: State-Trait Anxiety Inventory

Table 2
Individualized, Symptom-Focused Fibromyalgia Treatment

Troublesome symptom	Therapist	Treatment
Body pain	Physician	Antidepressant; Gabapentin; Tizanidine
	Physical therapist	Aerobic exercise/reconditioning; Stretching exercises
	Occupational therapist	Work station modification; Body mechanics
	Psychologist	Stress management; Cognitive–behavioral therapy; Relaxation training
Fatigue	Physical therapist	Aerobic exercise
	Occupational therapist	Pacing skills
	Nursing	Nutritional counseling
Irritable bowel syndrome	Physician	Laxatives; Anti-diarrhea agents; Antidepressants
	Physical therapist	Aerobic exercise
	Psychologist	Stress management
	Nursing	Dietary counseling: high-fiber, good hydration, low-fat, frequent small meals
Sleep disturbance	Physician	Antidepressants
	Psychologist	Relaxation training
	Nursing	Sleep hygiene
Depression/anxiety	Physician	Antidepressants
	Psychologist	Counseling; Psychotherapy
Headache	Physician	Antidepressants or other standard headache therapy
	Psychologist	Stress management; Biofeedback

Note: Choose possible treatments based on the presence of troublesome symptoms.

Box 6
Online Fibromyalgia Resources

- National Fibromyalgia Association web page
  fmaware.org
- Arthritis Foundation
  arthritis.org/conditions/diseasecenter/fibromyalgia/fibromyalgia.asp
- National Fibromyalgia Partnership, Inc.
  fmpartnership.org
- John Hopkins Arthritis web page
  www.hopkins-arthritis.som.jhmi.edu/other/fibromyalgia.html

---

5. SUMMARY

Fibromyalgia is a common, chronic pain condition affecting approximately 3% of women and 0.5% of men. Patients with fibromyalgia report a wide variety of troublesome somatic complaints, including fatigue, sleep disturbance, pares-thesias, headache, and digestive complaints. Fibromyalgia is diagnosed by the presence of widespread body pain and at least 11 of 18 possible tender points that are painful to digital palpation. Recording and monitoring the tender point examination aids both in the establishment of a diagnosis and assessment of treatment efficacy.

Symptoms of fibromyalgia are not progressive and tend to improve over time. Symptom improvement can be maximized by identifying, targeting, and treating troublesome symptoms in each individual patient. Antidepressants are the most beneficial types of medication for individuals with fibromyalgia, as they help reduce pain, depression, and headache and help improve sleep. Aerobic exercise and learning proper activity pacing skills, body mechanics, and sleep hygiene techniques are also beneficial.

REFERENCES

1. Wolfe F, Smythe HA, Yunus MB, et al. The American College of Rheumatology 1990 criteria for the classification of fibromyalgia: report of the Multicenter Criteria Committee. Arthritis Rheum 1990; 33:160–172.
2. Okifuji A, Turk DC, Sinclair JD, Starz TW, Marcus DA. A standardized manual tender point survey. I. Development and determination of a threshold point for the identification of positive tender points in fibromyalgia syndrome. J Rheumatol 1997; 24:377–383.
3. Lundberg G, Gerdle B. Tender point scores and their relations to signs of mobility, symptoms, and disability in female home care personnel and the prevalence of fibromyalgia. J Rheumatol 2002; 29:603–613.

4. White KP, Harth M, Speechley M, Ostbye T. Testing an instrument to screen for fibromyalgia syndrome in general population studies: the London Fibromyalgia Epidemiology Study Screening Questionnaire. J Rheumatol 1999; 26: 880–884.

5. Carmona L, Ballina J, Gabriel R, Laffon A. The burden of musculoskeletal diseases in the general population of Spain: results from a national survey. Ann Rheum Dis 2001; 60:1040–1045.

6. Maquet D, Croisier JL, Crielaard JM. Fibromyalgia in the year 2000. Rev Med Liege 2000; 55:991–997.

7. Wolfe F, Ross K, Anderson J, Russell IJ, Hebert L. The prevalence and characteristics of fibromyalgia in the general population. Arthritis Rheum 1995; 8:19–28.

8. Wolfe F, Ross K, Anderson J, Russell IJ. Aspects of fibromyalgia in the general population: sex, pain threshold, and fibromyalgia symptoms. J Rheumatol 1995; 22:151–156.

9. Yunus MB, Inanici F, Aldag JC, Mangold RF. Fibromyalgia in men: comparison of clinical features with women. J Rheumatol 2000; 27:485–490.

10. Walker EA, Keegan D, Gardner G, et al. Psychological factors in fibromyalgia compared with rheumatoid arthritis: I. Psychiatric diagnoses and functional disability. Psychosomatic Med 1997; 59:565–571.

11. Offenbaecher M, Glatzeder K, Ackenheil M. Self-reported depression, familial history of depression and fibromyalgia (FM), and psychological distress in patients with FM. J Rheumatol 1998; 57(Suppl 2):94–96.

12. Epstein SA, Kay G, Clauw D, et al. Psychiatric disorders in patients with fibromyalgia: a multicenter investigation. Psychosomatics 1999; 40:57–63.

13. Okifuji A, Turk DC, Sherman JJ. Evaluation of the relationship between depression and fibromyalgia syndrome: why aren't all patients depressed? J Rheumatol 2000; 27:212–219.

14. White KP, Nielson WR, Harth M, Ostbye T, Speechley M. Chronic widespread musculoskeletal pain with or without fibromyalgia: psychological distress in a representative community adult sample. J Rheumatol 2002; 29:588–594.

15. White KP, Speechley M, Harth M, Ostbye T. Comparing self-reported function and work disability in 100 community cases of fibromyalgia syndrome versus controls in London, Ontario: the London Fibromyalgia Epidemiology Study. Arthritis Rheum 1999; 42:76–83.

16. Wolfe F, Anderson J, Harkness D, et al. Work and disability status of persons with fibromyalgia. J Rheumatol 1997; 24:1171–1178.

17. Burckhardt CS, Clark SR, Bennett RM. The Fibromyalgia Impact Questionnaire: development and validation. J Rheumatol 1991; 18:728–734.

18. Pöyhiä R, Da Costa D, Fitzcharles MA. Pain and pain relief in fibromyalgia patients followed for three years. Arthritis Rheum 2001; 45:355–361.

19. Bennett RM, Burckhardt CS, Clark SR. Group treatment of fibromyalgia: a 6 month outpatient program. J Rheumatol 1996; 23:521–528.

20. Arnold LM, Hess EV, Hudson JI, et al. A randomized, placebo-controlled, double-blind, flexible dose study of fluoxetine in the treatment of women with fibromyalgia. Am J Med 2002; 112:191–197.

21. Richards SM, Scott DL. Prescribed exercise in people with fibromyalgia: parallel group randomised controlled trial. BMJ 2002; 325:185–189.

22. Fors EA, Sexton H, Götestam KG. The effect of guided imagery and amitriptyline on daily fibromyalgia pain: a prospective, randomized, controlled trial. J Psychiatr Res 2002; 36:179–187.
23. Pfeiffer A, Thompson JM, Nelson A, et al. Effects of a 1.5-day multidisciplinary outpatient treatment program for fibromyalgia: a pilot study. Am J Phys Med Rehabil 2003; 82:186–191.
24. Bennett RM, Kamin M, Kamin R, Rosenthal N. Tramadol and acetaminophen combination tablets in the treatment of fibromyalgia pain: a double-blind, randomized, placebo-controlled study. Am J Med 2003; 114:537–545.
25. Lautenschläger J. Present state of medication therapy in fibromyalgia syndrome. Scand J Rheumatol 2000; 29(Suppl 113):32–36.
26. O'Malley PG, Balden E, Tomkins G, et al. Treatment of fibromyalgia with antidepressants: a meta-analysis. J Gen Intern Med 2000; 15:659–666.
27. Longmire DR. Bimodal dose-response to adjunctive use of tizanidine HCL in control of myofascial pain. Abstract 869. October 21–24, 1999; Fort Lauderdale, FA: Program Book of the 18th Annual Scientific Meeting of the American Pain Society.
28. Russell IJ, Michalek JE, Xiao Y, et al. Cerebrospinal fluid substance P in fibromyalgia syndrome is reduced by tizanidine therapy. Poster presentation. March 14–17, 2002; Baltimore, MD: 21st Annual Scientific Meeting of the American Pain Society.

CME QUESTIONS—CHAPTER 10

1. Fibromyalgia is diagnosed in patients with the following pain characteristics:
   a. Pain occurs on both sides of the body
   b. Pain is present above and below the waist
   c. 11 or more tender points are painful to firm pressure
   d. All of the above

2. Which of the following statements about fibromyalgia epidemiology is/are true?
   a. Fibromyalgia occurs six times more often in women than men.
   b. Fibromyalgia prevalence increases with advancing age.
   c. Fibromyalgia is associated with better quality of life and less disability than other types of widespread pain or rheumatologic disease.
   d. A and B
   e. All of the above

3. Typical associated symptoms with fibromyalgia include:
   a. Fatigue
   b. Irritable bowel syndrome
   c. Bleeding disorder
   d. A and B
   e. All of the above

4. The class of medications that is most effective for treating fibromyalgia symptoms consists of:
   a. Opioids
   b. Antidepressants
   c. Analgesics
   d. Muscle relaxants

IV
Special Groups

11
Pediatric Pain

CASE HISTORY

Sarah is a 12-year-old girl who comes to the pediatrician with her mother, who reports that Sarah has been missing school because of abdominal pain. The pain is located in the center of her abdomen around the belly button. She has had no change in weight or bowel habits, and eating does not affect her pain. The abdominal pain began approximately 2 weeks after Sarah started seventh grade. Sarah's mother is particularly concerned about school absences because Sarah is now attending junior high school, where the curriculum is more demanding than in elementary school. Sarah is a quiet girl who has always performed well academically, but does not participate in extracurricular activities and tends to have only one or two close friends. Significant stressors for Sarah are parental conflicts over an impending custody hearing and the recent loss of her best friend, whose family relocated to another state. Sarah's examination is unremarkable. She describes diffuse, periumbilical tenderness. There is no organomegaly. The remainder of her physical examination is normal. Sarah is questioned about sexual activity or abuse, both of which she denies. Sarah's doctor reassures her mother that she's probably just having "growing pains," which will resolve on their own.

* * *

Children, like adults, may also suffer from chronic pain syndromes, especially musculoskeletal pain, headaches, and, as in Sarah's case, abdominal pain. When these pain complaints occur in children with no identifiable pathology, they may be termed "growing pains," and expected to resolve spontaneously if disregarded. Treating pediatric pain complaints like a bad behavior that can be extinguished by ignoring it can result in persistent discomfort and school disability. In addition, psychosocial stressors are frequently associated with pediatric pain. Identification and management of those stressors can reduce the expression of stress as somatic symptoms in childhood and, hopefully, provide useful skills for managing stresses in later life.

From: *Chronic Pain: A Primary Care Guide to Practical Management*
Edited by: D. A. Marcus © Humana Press, Totowa, NJ

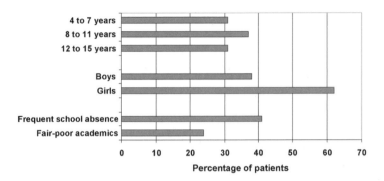

Fig. 1. Demographics of children reporting frequent aches and pains. Frequent pain was reported by 5% of pediatric patients. Girls and children 8–11 years old were more likely to report frequent pain. (Based on ref. *2*.)

KEY CHAPTER POINTS

- Most chronic pain syndromes in children are not associated with significant, identifiable pathology or serious illness.
- Common pain syndromes in children and adolescents include musculoskeletal pain, headache, stomach ache, and chest pain.
- Chronic pain complaints in childhood tend to persist for at least 1 year and, therefore, require treatment.
- Pain in children and adolescents results in significant disability, including school absence.
- Psychosocial factors, including changes in family and school stress, are significant aggravating factors for pediatric pain.

Sarah's complaints of troublesome, chronic pain are not unusual for adolescents, who often have associated with school disability. In a community survey, the majority of students in grades 4, 7, and 9 reported usually experiencing pain somewhere in the body, although more girls responded positively than boys (82 vs 64%; *p* < 0.001) *(1)*. A survey of more than 21,000 pediatric patients from 200 outpatient practices in the United States, Puerto Rico, and Canada identified "frequent aches and pain" in 5% of children, with girls affected more often than boys (Fig. 1) *(2)*. Frequent aches and pain were associated with frequent school absences and academic difficulty (*p* < 0.0001). Pain in childhood is also associated with emotional distress and sleep disturbance *(1)*.

Although there may be a tendency to expect children to "outgrow" their pain complaints, a survey of 1756 third and fifth grade students evaluated at study initiation and again 1 year later showed persistence of pain complaints (Fig. 2) *(3)*. After 1 year, nonspecific musculoskeletal pain was still reported occurring either weekly or monthly in 82% who had reported weekly pain at their initial assessment and 73% who had initially reported monthly pain. These data suggest

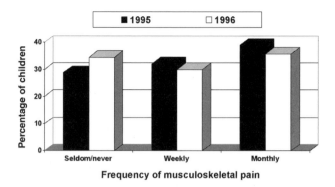

Fig. 2. Prevalence and persistence of nonspecific musculoskeletal pain in third and fifth graders. Students were evaluated for pain complaints initially in 1995 and again 1 year later in 1996. (Based on ref. *3*.)

that pain symptoms are likely to persist in children reporting recurring or chronic pain, suggesting a need for initial evaluation and intervention rather than observation. Sarah's consultation for chronic pain provides an important opportunity to develop strategies for minimizing both the discomfort and impact from her pain, as well as the important influence of psychosocial stressors, such as her feelings of isolation and abandonment with her parents' impending divorce and the loss of her closest friend. Because, in most circumstances, children don't readily "outgrow" pain complaints, failure to address these issues initially will likely result in prolonged dysfunction in school and social relationships, possibly setting the stage for chronic pain disability in adulthood.

1. COMMON CHRONIC PAIN SYNDROMES IN CHILDREN AND ADOLESCENTS

Common chronic pain syndromes in children include musculoskeletal pain, headache, abdominal pain, and chest pain. Musculoskeletal pain was reported in 71% of children in the third and fifth grade *(3)*. A survey of children aged 7 to 17 years identified recurrent headache in 15%, stomach pain in 8%, and back pain in 5% (Fig. 3) *(4)*. All pain complaints occurred more often in girls. Headache and back pain increased with age. Frequent episodes of pain in the head, stomach, and back occur in a significant minority of children (Fig. 4) *(5)*.

1.1. Musculoskeletal Pain

Only 6% of all office visits to a general pediatric clinic are for musculoskeletal pain complaints *(6)*. There is no gender preference for pediatric musculoskeletal pain (Fig. 5). The most commonly affected pain region is the knee.

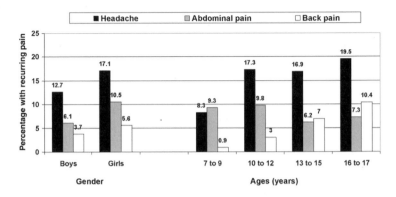

Fig. 3. Prevalence of recurring pain in children and adolescents. All pain complaints were more frequent in girls ($p < 0.001$) and were affected by age ($p < 0.01$). (Based on ref. *4*.)

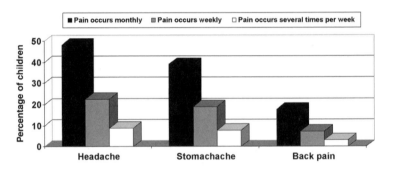

Fig. 4. Prevalence of frequent, recurring pain in young children (aged 6–13 years). (Based on ref. *5*.)

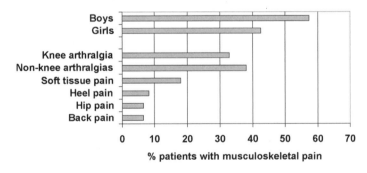

Fig. 5. Musculoskeletal pain complaints in children aged 3–14 years seen in a general pediatrics clinic. Musculoskeletal pain was reported by 6.1% of patients. Among children with musculoskeletal pain, the knee was most commonly affected and there was no gender preference. (Based on ref. *6*.)

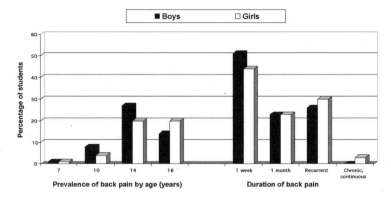

Fig. 6. Prevalence of low back pain in students. A total of 1171 students in grades 1, 4, 8, and 10 were asked about the occurrence of low back pain that interfered with school or leisure during the preceding 12 months. (Based on ref. *7*.)

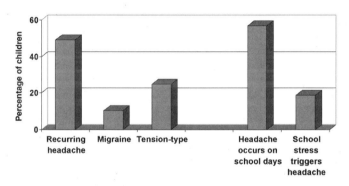

Fig. 7. Prevalence of recurring headache and relation to school in children aged 8–16 years old. (Based on ref. *8*.)

Back pain is one of the most common pain complaints in adulthood, and also affects a significant minority of children. A survey of students identified back pain that interfered with school or leisure activities during the preceding year in 10% of boys and 9% of girls (Fig. 6) *(7)*. Prevalence increased in adolescence. In almost half of cases, pain resolved within 1 week. Recurrent or chronic low back pain was reported by more often by girls than boys (33 vs 26%; $p < 0.01$).

1.2. Headache

Chronic headache often begins in childhood and adolescence and continues into adulthood. A survey of 5562 children aged 8 to 16 years identified recurring headache in almost half of respondents, with most headaches occurring during school hours (Fig. 7) *(8)*. Similar to adults, migraine was diagnosed in 10% of

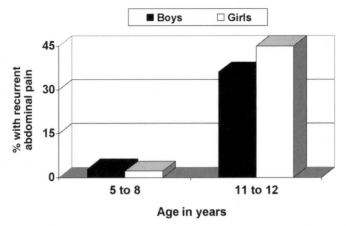

Fig. 8. Prevalence of recurrent abdominal pain There is no sex preference for recurrent abdominal pain in early childhood. A female predominance develops in adolescence. (Based on refs. *10* and *11*.)

children, with a female preponderance. Tension-type headache is much less common in children than adults.

Childhood headache is important because children with headache lose an average of 7.8 days per school year, compared to 3.7 days per year for children without headaches *(9)*. Frequent school absenteeism is a significant stressor, resulting in loss of academic performance, social interaction with peers, and self-esteem. These factors, themselves, often aggravate pain perception. Low self-esteem and depressive symptoms are premorbid predictors of adolescent headache in girls *(2)*.

1.3. Recurrent Abdominal Pain

Recurrent abdominal pain is defined as chronic pain (>3 months) with three or more episodes of abdominal pain that are severe enough to interfere with activities *(9a)*. Recurrent abdominal pain increases in prevalence during childhood, with a female predominance after adolescence (Fig. 8) *(10,11)*. As seen in Sarah, recurrent abdominal pain is typically experienced as episodic pain around the umbilicus that is unrelated to eating or activities. In addition, there should be no interference with nutrition or growth. Recurrent abdominal pain is often not associated with any identifiable pathology, although several treatable conditions may cause recurrent abdominal pain (*see* Box 1). In a recent evaluation of 107 children with recurrent abdominal pain, irritable bowel syndrome was identified in 45% of respondents, functional dyspepsia in 16%, and abdominal migraine in 5% *(12)*.

Recurrent abdominal pain and migraine are comorbid and may share common underlying pathological mechanisms. Compared with headache-free children, the risk of stomach ache in 5-year-olds with headache was almost nine

---

Box 1
Identifiable Causes of Some Cases of Recurrent Abdominal Pain

---

- Irritable bowel syndrome
- *Helicobacter pylori* gastritis
- Constipation
- Lactose intolerance
- Inflammatory bowel disease
  (especially during early stages
  of Crohn's disease)

- Gynecologic pathology
  - Endometriosis
  - Pelvic inflammatory disease
  - Ovarian cysts
- Abdominal migraine

---

times greater in children reporting infrequent headache and 14 times greater in children with frequent headache *(13)*. In addition, migraine is more likely to develop in adults who had childhood recurrent abdominal pain; 36% with recurrent abdominal pain develop migraine compared with 14% without a recurrent childhood abdominal pain *(14)*. Further support for a relationship between migraine and recurrent abdominal pain is the effectiveness of anti-migraine therapy for treating recurrent abdominal pain, including propranolol, cyproheptadine, and biofeedback *(15,16)*.

Approximately 25% of children with recurrent abdominal pain will continue to experience symptoms into adulthood, when they are often diagnosed with irritable bowel syndrome *(17)*. Therefore, as with other types of chronic abdominal pain, recurrent abdominal pain in childhood should be treated to prevent continuation of symptoms into adulthood.

1.4. Chest Pain

Chronic chest pain in pediatrics is typically caused by costochondritis or some other musculoskeletal condition (Table 1). An evaluation of 50 children referred to a cardiologist for chest pain revealed noncardiac conditions in every patient, mainly musculoskeletal pain or costochondritis (76%) *(18)*. In a similar survey of 161 pediatric patients seen in the emergency department with a chief complaint of chest pain, investigators found cardiac pathology (extrasystole) in only one patient *(19)*. In addition, the absence of associated symptoms (e.g., shortness of breath, palpitations, digestive complaints, and weight loss) correlated with musculoskeletal, idiopathic, or psychogenic causes of chest pain.

2. ASSESSMENT

Assessment of children and adolescents with pain focuses or ensuring absence of specific pathology (e.g., rheumatologic disease, fractures, or tumors) and identification of psychosocial contributors (e.g., school stress, bullying, depression, or major life changes). A thorough history and physical examination are necessary. Both patient and family should be included when obtaining a history. Historical reports of pain, risk behaviors, trauma, and possible abuse will also need to be asked of the child separately. Dissimilar reports of pain symptoms or severity between patient and parent should warrant further evaluation of family dynamics and psychosocial influences. Physical examination should include a screen for systemic illness (lymphadenopathy, organomegaly, livedo reticularis, or subcutaneous nodules), as well as a targeted evaluation of the painful area. Assessment of weight and height are also needed to ensure adequate nutritional status, especially in adolescent girls at risk for anorexia nervosa. As in adults, the presence of nonlocalized pain, superficial skin tenderness, sensory loss not affecting typical neurological patterns (e.g., dermatomes), and giveaway weakness suggest a nonspecific cause of pain complaints, with reduced need for extensive testing *(20)*.

2.1. Musculoskeletal Pain

Children with musculoskeletal pain should be evaluated for evidence of joint disease, such as arthritis or fracture, and neurological impairment. Musculoskeletal pain may be difficult to diagnose in children, who often misinterpret the origin of their pain. For example, children with hip pathology often describe thigh or knee pain. Therefore, the entire extremity needs to be thoroughly evaluated in children describing any joint area pain. Myofascial pain in children shares the same features seen in adult patients (*see* Chapter 9). Physical therapy evaluations may be helpful in patients with complex symptoms or reports of mechanical pain.

2.2. Headache

In children presenting with acute headache, infectious etiologies, like viral illness and sinusitis, are common and should be considered *(21)*. Imaging studies of the head are best reserved for children who have experienced traumatic or progressive headache, have a history of neurological illness (e.g., hydrocephalus), or have an abnormal neurological examination *(22)*. As in adult populations, children who experience a significant change in chronic headache pattern, chronic progressive headaches, or failure to respond to standard therapy may also need additional medical and neurological evaluations, including an imaging study.

The diagnosis of migraine in children differs from adults (Table 2). Children with migraine are less likely to endorse adult hallmark characteristics of migraine (Fig. 9) *(23)*. Although both children and adults report disabling headaches, migraine is more likely to be bilateral, shorter in duration, and lack reports of photophobia and phonophobia in children *(24)*. Children often fail to verbally express migrainous features, such as sensitivities to noises and lights.

Table 1
Causes of Pediatric Chest Pain (%) in Patients Referred to Cardiologist or Evaluated in an Emergency Department

Type of symptom	Referred to a cardiologist	Seen in emergency department		
	Total	Total	No associated symptoms	Associated symptoms
Musculoskeletal, idiopathic, or psychogenic	80	86	97	72
Infectious	0	9	1	8
Asthma	12	3	0.6	2
Gastrointestinal	8	0.6	0	0.6
Cardiac	0	0.6	0	0.6

Based on refs. 18,19.

Table 2
Diagnostic Distinctions Between Pediatric and Adult Migraine

Characteristic	Adult	Pediatric
Location	Unilateral	Usually bilateral; occipital migraine is rare and warrants additional evaluation.
Duration	4–72 hours	1–72 hours
Associated symptoms	Photophobia and phonophobia are usually present	Children rarely verbalize sensitivity to noise and lights; photo- and phonophobia may be inferred from behavior (e.g., retreating to dark, quiet room; turning off television or computer).

Based on ref. 24.

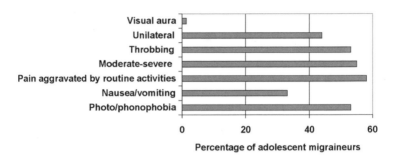

Fig. 9. Prevalence of migrainous features in adolescents with migraine. (Based on ref. *23*.)

A variety of migraine features that are not identified during clinical interview may first be recognized when headache diaries are reviewed. Migraine features that were initially unrecognized on interview but later identified after diary review in one study included aura (46%), vomiting (50%), nausea (31%), unilateral location (38%), throbbing quality (29%), photophobia (11%), and phonophobia (11%) *(25)*. Thus, the use of diaries that instruct children to focus on certain symptoms improves the description of those headaches as migraine.

Headache diaries are important not only to establish headache diagnosis, but also to identify headache frequency in children. A comparison of impressions identified at a medical interview vs review of a headache diary showed identification of frequent (weekly) headache in only 18% during interviews compared with 48% when diaries were reviewed *(26)*.

Asking children to draw a picture of their headaches is another useful diagnostic tool. In one study, diagnostic accuracy from children's headache drawings was compared to a standard clinical assessment *(27)*. Headache drawings were very effective in representing migraine features, with a diagnostic sensitivity of 93%, specificity of 83%, and positive predictive value of 87% (Fig. 10).

2.3. Recurrent Abdominal Pain

Surveys of children with recurrent abdominal pain reveal specific abdominal pathology in 38 to 45% (Fig. 11) *(28,29)*. History should try to identify features associated with specific pathologies *(see* Box 2). Patients with these symptoms will require additional laboratory, stool, or radiographic testing *(see* Box 3). In general, imaging studies and endoscopy are reserved for patients with symptoms and signs suggesting specific pathology, such as inflammatory bowel disease or peptic ulcer disease. History of sexual activity should also be sought, with pregnancy or pregnancy complications considered as a cause for abdominal pain in adolescent girls. Interestingly, pain

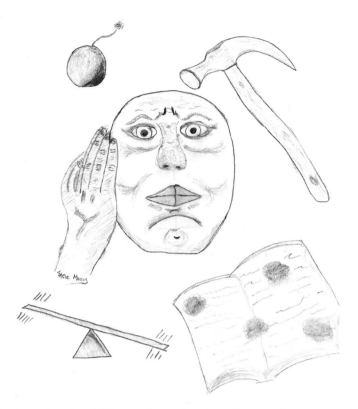

Fig. 10. Example of a child's headache drawing. This boy left class during an examination to go to the nurse, telling his teacher he couldn't take his test and felt like he was going to pass out. He vomited in the nurse's office and was tentatively diagnosed with a viral illness. His drawing of the episode tells a clear story of migraine. Severe pain on the side of his head felt like a hammer pounding and bomb exploding. His genuine inability to complete his test is shown by the drawing of visual scotomas, which obscured his view of the test paper. In addition, he noticed imbalance or vertigo with his episode, as shown by the teeter-totter, although he verbalized this as "feeling like I'm going to pass out."

located at or near the umbilicus, as seen in Sarah, is less likely to be caused by a specific condition compared with pain located distant from the umbilicus *(9a)*.

Abdominal migraine and, less commonly, abdominal epilepsy should also be considered in the differential diagnosis of recurrent abdominal pain in patients with additional features of migraine or epilepsy. Anti-migraine prophylaxis may be useful for abdominal migraine. An electroencephalogram may help confirm the diagnosis of abdominal epilepsy.

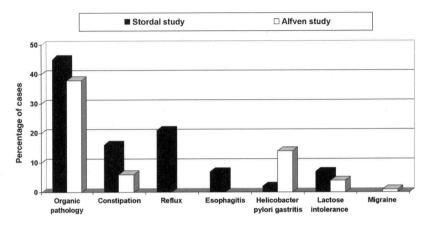

Fig. 11. Prevalence of organic pathology in children with recurrent abdominal pain. (Based on refs. *28* and *29*.)

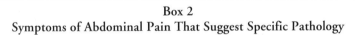

Box 2
Symptoms of Abdominal Pain That Suggest Specific Pathology

- Pain location distant from the umbilicus
- Association with diarrhea and/or constipation
- Weight loss

- Relationship to diet or eating
- Vomiting
- Fever

Box 3
Evaluation for Recurrent Abdominal Pain

- Physical examination
  ○ Weight and height
  ○ Organomegaly
  ○ Focal abdominal tenderness
  ○ Rectal examination
  ○ Joint screen for inflammation

- Laboratory testing
  ○ Complete blood count
  ○ Urinalysis
  ○ Stool guiac
  ○ Stool for ova and parasites
    if diarrhea is present

2.4. Chest Pain

In addition to history and physical examination, additional testing may be ordered in children with chest pain with associated symptoms *(19)*. Testing is most likely to identify nonmusculoskeletal pathology in children with associated symptoms (e.g., respiratory distress or palpitations) or signs (e.g., fever, respiratory distress, reduced breath sounds, wheezing, heart murmur, or abnormal rhythm) or the history of trauma. Chest X-rays and electrocardiograms, as indicated, are beneficial in these patients to clarify the diagnosis.

2.5. Psychosocial Factors

Although psychosocial factors alone are unlikely to entirely explain chronic pain complaints, they often are significant aggravating factors that can markedly enhance pain perception. For example, a review of 100 cases of recurrent abdominal pain identified a significant role for stress in aggravating nonspecific abdominal pain complaints in 48% of cases *(29)*. The most common stress-provoking events included those seen in Sarah, starting school and parents' divorce.

Significant personal stressors (e.g., family separation, moving, and death) also occur within 12 months of headache onset in 73% of adolescents *(30)*. Migraine occurs more often in children reporting unhappiness, fear of failure at school, or fear of a teacher *(31)*. Depressive symptoms are identified on clinical interview in 86% of teenagers with daily headache *(32)*. In addition, being the victim of bullying is associated with frequent headache episodes in children aged 7 to 10 years *(33)*.

Quality of life may be significantly affected by chronic pain in children, as it is in adults. Impairments in quality of life in pediatric patients can be assessed using the Pediatric Quality-of-Life Inventory (PedsQoL), which is available online at Website: www.pedsql.org. The PedsQoL has been used in pediatric patients with arthritis or migraine *(34–36)*.

3. TREATMENT

The same pharmacological and nonpharmacological treatments used for adult pain are generally effective in pediatric pain, although dosage adjustment is necessary. Chronic musculoskeletal, abdominal, and chest pain should be treated primarily with physical therapy exercises and psychological pain management skills, like stress management and relaxation therapies. For example, treatment of 57 adolescents with chronic pain (mean duration: 4 years) with combined physical therapy and cognitive therapy resulted in significantly improved physical function and reduced catastrophizing, anxiety, and disability *(37)*. In addition, prior to treatment, only 55% of the adolescents were attending school, with 25% attending full time. Three months after treatment, 84% were attending school, with 52% attending full time.

The primary goal for treating any chronic pain syndrome in children is to ensure school attendance. In most circumstances, attending school will not aggravate the pain complaints and will serve as distraction from pain and the sick role. Prolonged school absence results in isolation and fear of both academic and social deficiencies, additional stressors that may further aggravate pain complaints. The social and emotional development advantages of attending school cannot be duplicated with a homebound education environment. The longer school absence is maintained, the more difficult it is for children to

Table 3
Migraine Treatments With Proven Efficacy in Pediatric Migraine

	Pharmacological therapies	
Nonpharmacological therapies	Acute care	Prevention
Relaxation plus stress management	Ibuprofen	Antidepressants
		Amitriptyline
		Trazadone
Biofeedback	Triptans	Antiepileptics
	Sumatriptan	Valproate
	Zolmitriptan	Topiramate
	Rizatriptan	

Based on ref. *38.*

return to school because of failure to maintain academic work and fear of isolation from peers on return to school. Treatment begins with resuming a regular routine. Good school participation must be the top priority. School is important for social and emotional development, in addition to intellectual growth. Homebound education cannot equal the experience of the classroom environment. Family therapy will be necessary when parents are hesitant to insist on school attendance to help parents develop strategies for ensuring school participation, as well as identification of manipulative behaviors that erode parents' resolve to encourage activity normalization.

3.1. Headache Therapy

Both nonpharmacological and pharmacological therapies can effectively manage chronic headaches in children and adolescents (Table 3). Relaxation, stress management, and biofeedback are effective nonpharmacological headache therapies in pediatric patients *(39,40)*. Analgesics and triptans are also effective in pediatric patients, although dose adjustments are needed *(41–44)*. Generally, triptans are administered at approximately half of the starting adult dose in adolescents. Orally disintegrating triptans may be particularly useful in children. Preventive therapy with antidepressants and antiepileptics is also effective in children *(44–48)*. Controlled trials have not evaluated selective serotonin reuptake inhibitors (SSRIs) for migraine prevention in pediatric patients. Anecdotally, SSRIs may be effective and are generally better tolerated, with fewer cognitive effects, than other antidepressants.

4. SUMMARY

Common pain syndromes in children and adolescents include musculoskeletal pain, headache, stomach ache, and chest pain. In general, increased overall prevalence and a female predominance develop once children reach adolescence.

Fortunately, most chronic pain syndromes in children are not associated with significant, identifiable pathology or serious illness. Similar to adult patients with pain, lack of obvious pathology in pediatric patients does not suggest that the pain is imaginary. Untreated pain in children and adolescents can result in significant disability, including school absence and social isolation. Because chronic pain complaints in childhood tend to persist for at least 1 year and often into adulthood, treatment of pediatric pain is necessary to minimize impact on academic, social, physical, and emotional development. Disability in children with pain should be minimized by requiring school attendance, as well as participation in physical education programs, unless significant structural pathology precludes specific activities. Psychosocial factors, including changes in family and school stress, are significant aggravating factors for pediatric pain and need to be identified and openly addressed as part of the treatment plan.

REFERENCES

1. Bruusgaard D, Smedbråten BK, Natvig B. Bodily pain, sleep problems and mental distress in schoolchildren. Acta Paediatr 2000; 89:597–600.
2. Campo JV, Comer DM, Jansen-McWilliams L, Gardner W, Kelleher KJ. Recurrent pain, emotional distress, and health service use in childhood. J Ped 2002; 141:76–83.
3. Mikkelsson M, Salminen JJ, Kautiainen H. Non-specific musculoskeletal pain in preadolescents. Prevalance and 1-year persistence. Pain 1997; 73:29–35.
4. Grøholt E, Stigum H, Nordhagen R, Köhler L. Recurrent pain in children, socioeconomic factors and accumulation in families. Eur J Epidemiol 2003; 18:965–975.
5. Petersen S, Bergstrom E, Brulin C. High prevalence of tiredness and pain in young schoolchildren. Scand J Public Health 2003; 31:367–374.
6. De Inocencio J. Musculoskeletal pain in primary pediatric care: analysis of 1000 consecutive general pediatric clinic visits. Pediatrics 1998; 102:E63.
7. Taimela S, Kujala U, Salminen J, Viljanen T. The prevalence of low back pain among children and adolescents: a nationwide, cohort-based questionnaire survey in Finland. Spine 1997; 22:1132–1136.
8. Ozge A, Bugdayci R, Sasmaz T, et al. The sensitivity and specificity of the case definition criteria in diagnosis of headache: a school-based epidemiological study of 5562 children in Mersin. Cephalalgia 2003; 23:138–145.
9. Abu-Arafeh I, Russell G. Prevalence of headache and migraine in schoolchildren. BMJ 1994; 309:765–769.
9a. Apley J. The child with abdominal pains. 2nd Ed. Oxford, UK: Blackwell Scientific; 1975.
10. Bode G, Brenner H, Adler G, Rothenbacher D. Recurrent abdominal pain in children. Evidence from a population-based study that social and familial factors play a major role but not Helicobacter pylori infection. J Psychosom Res 2003; 54: 417–421.
11. Boey CM, Yao SB. An epidemiological survey of recurrent abdominal pain in a rural Malay school. J Paediatr Child Health 1999; 35:303–305.

12. Walker LS, Lipani TA, Greene JW, et al. Recurrent abdominal pain: symptom subtypes based on the Rome II criteria for pediatric functional gastrointestinal disorders. J Pediatr Gastroenter 2004; 38:187–191.
13. Sillanpaa M, Piekkala P, Kero P. Prevalence of headache at preschool age in an unselected child population. Cephalalgia 1991; 11:239–242.
14. Campo JV, Di Lorenzo C, Chiappetta L, et al. Adult outcomes of pediatric recurrent abdominal pain: do they just grow out of it? Pediatrics 2001; 108:e1.
15. Russell G, Abu-Arafeh I, Symon DN. Abdominal migraine: evidence for existence and treatment options. Paediatr Drugs 2002; 4:1–8.
16. Weydert JA, Ball TM, Davis MF. Systemic review of treatments for recurrent abdominal pain. Pediatrics 2003; 111:e1–e11.
17. Jarrett M, Heitkemper M, Czyzewski DI, Shulman R. Recurrent abdominal pain in children: forerunner to adult irritable bowel syndrome? J Spec Pediatr Nurs 2003; 8:81–89.
18. Evangelista JK, Parsons M, Rennenburg AK. Chest pain in children: diagnosis through history and physical examination. J Ped Health Care 2000; 14:3–8.
19. Gastesi-Larranaga M, Fernandez Landaluce A, Mintegi Raso S, Vazquez Ronco M, Benito Fernandez J. Dolor torácico en urgencies de pediatría: un proceso habitualmente benigno. An Pediatr (Barc) 2003; 59:234–238.
20. Song K, Morton AA, Koch KD, Herring JA, Browne RH, Hanway JP. Chronic musculoskeletal pain in childhood. J Ped Orthop 1998; 18:576–581.
21. Burton LJ, Quinn B, Pratt-Cheney JL, Pourani M. Headache etiology in a pediatric emergency department. Pediatr Emerg Care 1997; 13:1–4.
22. Kan L, Nagelberg J, Maytal J. Headaches in a pediatric emergency department: etiology, imaging, and treatment. Headache 2000; 40:25–29.
23. Shivpuri D, Rajesh MS, Jain D. Prevalence and characteristics of migraine among adolescents: a questionnaire survey. Indian Pediatr 2003; 40:665–669.
24. Headache Classification Committee of the International Headache Society. The International Classification of Headache Disorders, 2nd Ed. Cephalalgia 2004; 24(Suppl 1):24–25.
25. Metsähonkala L, Sillanpää M, Tuominen J. Headache diary in the diagnosis of childhood migraine. Headache 1997; 37:240–244.
26. Laurell K, Larsson B, Eeg-Olofsson O. Headache in schoolchildren: agreement between different sources of information. Cephalalgia 2003; 23:420–428.
27. Stafstrom CE, Rostasy K, Minster A. The usefulness of children's drawings in the diagnosis of headache. Pediatrics 2002; 109:460–472.
28. Stordal K, Nygaard EA, Bentsen B. Organic abnormalities in recurrent abdominal pain in children. Acta Paediatr 2001; 90:638–642.
29. Alfvén G. One hundred cases of recurrent abdominal pain in children: diagnostics procedures and criteria for a psychosomatic diagnosis. Acta Paediatr 2003; 92: 43–49.
30. Kaiser RS, Primavera JP. Failure to mourn as a possible contributory factor to headache onset in adolescence. Headache 1993; 33:69–72.
31. Anttila P, Metsähonkala L, Helenius H, Sillanpää M. Predisposing and provoking factors in childhood headache. Headache 2000; 40:351–356.
32. Kaiser R. Depression in adolescent headache patients. Headache 1992; 32:340–344.

33. Williams K, Chambers M, Logan S, Robinson D. Association of common health symptoms with bullying in primary school children. BMJ 1996; 313:17–19.
34. Varni JW, Seid M, Smith Knight T, Burwinkle T, Brown J, Szer IS. The PedsQL in pediatric rheumatology: reliability, validity, and responsiveness of the Pediatric Quality of Life Inventory Generic Core Scales and Rheumatology Module. Arthritis Rheum 2002; 46:714–725.
35. Sawyer MG, Whitman JN, Robertson DM, Taplin JE, Varni JW, Baghurst PA. The relationship between health-related quality of life, pain and coping strategies in juvenile idiopathic arthritis. Rheumatology (Oxford) 2004; 43:325–330.
36. Powers SW, Patton SR, Hommel KA, Hershey AD. Quality of life in paediatric migraine: characterization of age-related effects using PedsQL 4.0. Cephalalgia 2004; 24:120–127.
37. Eccleston C, Malleson PN, Clinch J, Connell H, Sourbut C. Chronic pain in adolescents: evaluation of a programme of interdisciplinary cognitive behaviour therapy. Arch Dis Child 2003; 88:881–885.
38. Marcus DA, Loder E. Migraine in female children and adolescents. In Migraine in Women. Loder E. Marcus DA (eds.) BC Decker, Ontario, 2004.
39. Sartory G, Muller B, Metsch J, Pothmann R. A comparison of psychological and pharmacological treatment of pediatric migraine. Behav Res Ther 1998; 36: 1155–1170.
40. Scharff L, Marcus D, Masek BJ. A controlled study of minimal-contact thermal biofeedback in children with migraine. J Pediatr Psychol 2002; 27:109–119.
41. Lewis DW, Kellstein D, Dahl G, et al. Children's ibuprofen suspension for the acute treatment of pediatric migraine. Headache 2002; 42:780–786.
42. Hershey AD, Powers SW, LeCates S, Bentti AL. Effectiveness of nasal sumatriptan in 5- to 12-year-old children. Headache 2001; 41:693–697.
43. Linder SL, Dowson AJ. Zolmitriptan provides effective migraine relief in adolescents. Int J Clin Pract 2000; 54:466–469.
44. Winner P, Lewis D, Visser WH, et al. Rizatriptan 5 mg for the acute treatment of migraine in adolescents: a randomized, double-blind, placebo-controlled study. Headache 2002; 42:49–55.
45. Battistella PA, Ruffilli R, Cernetti R, et al. A placebo-controlled crossover trial using trazadone in pediatric migraine. Headache 1993; 33:36–39.
46. Hershey AD, Powers SW, Bentti A, Degrauw T. Effectiveness of amitriptyline in the prophylactic management of childhood headache. Headache 2000; 40:539–549.
47. Serdaroglu G, Erhan E, Tekgul H, et al. Sodium valproate prophylaxis in childhood migraine. Headache 2002; 42:819–822.
48. Hershey AD, Powers SW, Vockell AB, et al. Effectiveness of topiramate in the prevention of childhood headaches. Headache 2002; 42:810–818.

CME QUESTIONS—CHAPTER 11

1. Common pain syndromes in pediatrics include:
   a. Musculoskeletal pain
   b. Headache
   c. Abdominal pain
   d. Chest pain
   e. All of the above

2. Which of the following statements is true?
   a. Most complaints of musculoskeletal pain should be considered growing pains.
   b. Musculoskeletal pain reports in elementary school children usually persist for at least 1 year.
   c. Musculoskeletal pain is usually endorsed to avoid unpleasant activities or homework.
   d. None of the above.

3. Which statistic is/are true?
   a. About 6% of all visits to a pediatric clinic are for complaints of musculoskeletal pain.
   b. About 10% of children have migraine headaches.
   c. About 25% of children with recurrent abdominal pain will report chronic abdominal pain as an adult.
   d. All of the above
   e. None of the above

4. Effective therapies for pediatric migraine include:
   a. Relaxation therapy
   b. Acupuncture
   c. Ibuprofen
   d. A and C
   e. All of the above

12

Pregnancy and Pain

CASE HISTORY

Ms. Rogers is a healthy 29-year-old primigravida in her seventh month of pregnancy. Her pregnancy has been uncomplicated, except for a weight gain of 40 lb. Over the last 4 weeks, she reports a pain in her left thigh. Initially, this would only occur with prolonged sitting or riding in the car, or when waiting in exceptionally long lines in the store. Now she finds that she has nearly constant pain in her upper, outer thigh. Additionally, this painful area feels prickly when she touches it. This week, she has also noticed pain and tingling in her right thumb when she wakes up in the morning or scrubs the counters at her home. Her mother told her that these are the symptoms of multiple sclerosis, just like in a character on the mother's soap opera television show. A distraught and tearful Ms. Rogers shares her concerns with her primary care physician, who reassures her that pain, including compressive neuropathy, occurs in a significant number of women during pregnancy and that these symptoms usually go away after delivery.

* * *

New pain, neurological complaints, or both during pregnancy are accompanied by special concerns for patient and doctor, both of whom worry about the risks of testing and treatment to the fetus, as well as the effects of any new health problem on the ability of the new mother to care for her baby. Alterations in hormones, water distribution, and weight are all important factors in changing risk for pain from new and preexisting pain syndromes during pregnancy. Understanding typical changes in common problems during pregnancy—such as headache, back pain, and compressive neuropathy—can allay fears and minimize the use of unnecessary testing.

KEY CHAPTER POINTS

- Pain complaints occur in the majority of pregnant women.
- The lower back is the most common pain location during pregnancy.

From: *Chronic Pain: A Primary Care Guide to Practical Management*
Edited by: D. A. Marcus © Humana Press, Totowa, NJ

- Compressive neuropathies occur more commonly during pregnancy because of changes in water retention, weight, and posture; they include Bell's palsy, carpal tunnel syndrome, and meralgia paresthetica.
- Premorbid headache, especially migraine, improves in the majority of women in early pregnancy. Headache does persist, however, throughout pregnancy for a significant minority of women.
- Persistent pain during pregnancy may require treatment with safe nonpharmacologic and pharmacological therapies to minimize disability and the need to self-medicate.

Pregnancy is associated with increased risk for a variety of musculoskeletal and neuropathic pain complaints. In a prospective study of 200 pregnant women, investigators identified pain occurring during pregnancy in 166 (85%), with new pain beginning during pregnancy in 137 (70%) *(1)*. The most common body area affected by pain was the back, especially in the lumbar and sacral areas (Fig. 1). In addition to the development of new pain during pregnancy, preexisting pain conditions—such as low back pain and headache—are also often modified during pregnancy.

In this chapter, several commonly occurring painful conditions that occur in pregnancy are reviewed. Evaluating and treating pain during pregnancy offers unique challenges because of concerns for the effects of testing and treatment interventions on the developing baby. Increased ability of the patient to identify common, self-limited, pregnancy-related pain complaints reduces the need to perform unnecessary testing during pregnancy and helps distinguish atypical conditions that may warrant additional evaluations.

1. COMMON PAIN SYNDROMES IN PREGNANCY

Important pain syndromes during pregnancy include conditions that occur commonly in women of childbearing age (e.g., migraine) and pain complaints that occur more frequently during pregnancy (e.g., low back pain and compressive neuropathy). Pregnancy can change the severity of premorbid pain and the risk for developing new pain complaints. Understanding expected changes during pregnancy allows women with pre-existing chronic pain conditions to prepare for expected changes and develop safe and effective treatment strategies. Ready identification of common pain syndromes in pregnant women, as seen in Ms. Rogers, results in the alleviation of concern for both patient and healthcare provider.

1.1. Headache

In addition to providing reproductive functions, sex hormones, including estrogen, act as important pain modulators *(2,3)*. The dramatic rise in estrogen during the early stages of pregnancy offers a protective effect against common headaches (e.g., migraine and tension-type headache). Therefore,

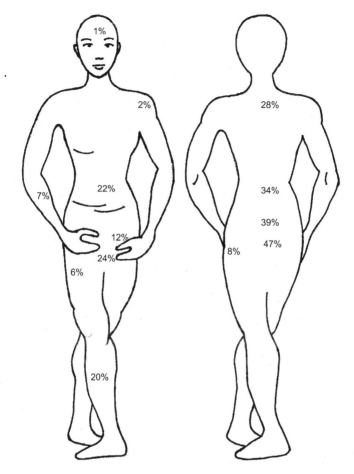

Fig. 1. Pain during pregnancy. Proportion of women reporting pain in different body regions of the body during pregnancy. (Based on ref. *1*.)

many women experience relief from preexisting chronic headache during pregnancy. Headache is most likely to improve during the first trimester, when the rise in estrogen is greatest. As estrogen levels plummet after delivery, protection against headaches is lost and headaches tends to increase in frequency. A prospective study of 47 pregnant migraineurs (average week of gestation at study initiation: 11) showed that headache frequency decreased by at least 50% in more than half of the women during their first trimester and almost 90% by their third trimester (Fig. 2) *(4)*. After delivery, migraine returned within 2 days for 4% of the study participants, within 1 week for 34%, and within 1 month for 55%. Bottle-feeding increased the risk for headache.

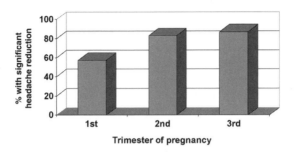

Fig. 2. Percentage of migraineurs with a significant (≥50%) reduction in headache activity during pregnancy. (Based on ref. *4*.)

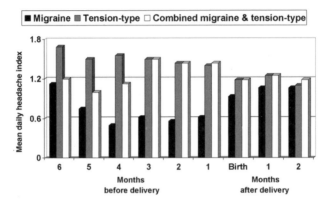

Fig. 3. Headache activity in women who report headaches at the end of the first trimester. The headache index is calculated as an average daily headache severity score and recorded four times daily. *No headache* has a score of 0; *incapacitating headache* has a score of 10. Headache activity decreased in migraineurs during pregnancy, returning to higher levels postpartum. Headache activity for tension-type and combined headaches was fairly stable throughout pregnancy. (Based on ref. *5*.)

Headache, however, does continue during pregnancy for a minority of women. This was demonstrated in another prospective study of women who were still reporting headache at the end of their first trimester (*5*). Between the second and third trimesters, headache frequency was reduced by only 30%. Migraineurs were more likely to experience headache improvement than women with tension-type headache (Fig. 3). These data suggest that headaches will probably continue without significant improvement in women who report ongoing headache activity at the end of the first trimester (typically around the time of the first visit to the obstetrician). In addition, improvement in headache symptoms during one pregnancy does not predict headache relief in subse-

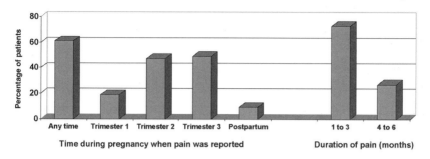

Fig. 4. New-onset back pain reported during pregnancy. (Based on ref. *1*.)

quent pregnancies. Differences in age, sleep deprivation when caring for other young children, and stress may all contribute to these differences.

Breastfeeding is unlikely to influence headache. In a large series of 2500 migraineurs followed for 6 years, investigators noted only five pregnancies in which nursing resulted in changes in headache frequency *(6)*. These data strongly suggest that women should not be discouraged from breastfeeding because of concerns about aggravating headache.

In addition to changes in benign headache, pregnancy also increases the risk for headache related to intracranial pathology. Acute strokes, cerebral venous thrombosis, symptomatic brain tumor, and benign intracranial hypertension (pseudotumor cerebri) occur with increased frequency during pregnancy *(7)*. Pituitary adenomas and meningiomas also develop with increased frequency during pregnancy *(8,9)*. Some autoimmune disorders, such as systemic lupus erythematosus, are aggravated by pregnancy and may result in headache. Eclampsia is another cause of pregnancy-related headache. A thorough history with detailed medical and neurological examinations, including a bedside fundoscopic examination, will usually help the clinician identify women who need additional testing to rule out pathological causes of headache.

1.2. Back Pain

Changes in posture of the spine and pelvis, along with increased joint laxity, result in increased risk for mechanical back pain during pregnancy. A community survey of more than 1500 women identified back pain that was at least moderately severe in 35.5% during pregnancy *(10)*. A prospective study of 200 obstetrical patients identified back pain as a complaint during pregnancy in 149 (76%), with pain beginning during pregnancy in 119 (61%) *(1)*. The prevalence of back pain was highest during the second and third trimesters and generally self-limited (Fig. 4).

In general, similar to the evaluation of back pain in the nonpregnant patient, imaging should be reserved during pregnancy for women with neurological loss or symptoms suggesting radiculopathy, myelopathy, or other nonmusculoskeletal types of pain. Electromyographic and nerve conduction velocity testing can be safely performed during pregnancy and can help localize pathology.

1.3. Neuropathy

Neuropathy may occur or be aggravated during pregnancy by changes in weight, posture, and fluid balance. Common types of compressive neuropathy that can arise during pregnancy include facial neuropathy (Bell's palsy), median neuropathy (carpal tunnel syndrome) and lateral femoral cutaneous neuropathy (meralgia paresthetica). Ms. Rogers describes symptoms typical for two types of compressive neuropathy—meralgia paresthetica causing thigh pain and carpal tunnel syndrome causing thumb pain.

Bell's palsy occurs from compression of the facial nerve, typically near the stylomastoid foramen or within the bony facial canal. Patients describe facial pain, followed by weakness. Bell's palsy is characterized by a wide-open eye on the affected side at rest, and weakness of facial muscles during attempted movement. Facial weakness is evident by lack of wrinkling of the forehead, inability to close the eye, and poor movement of the mouth. Bell's palsy is typically treated with eye protection (e.g., drops and patching) and prednisone. The incidence of Bell's palsy during pregnancy and the puerperium is about 0.04%, which is more than three times the incidence in nonpregnant women of comparable age *(11)*. Nearly 80% of cases occur during the third trimester, and most cases occur unilaterally. Fortunately, 72% of women experience complete resolution of symptoms within 10 weeks of symptom onset. A retrospective chart review compared Bell's palsy outcome in pregnant vs nonpregnant women of comparable age. Most patients recovered from facial weakness, although the recovery was inferior in patients who had developed complete facial weakness and in pregnant women (Fig. 5) *(12)*. Treatment with prednisone did not affect the likelihood for recovery significantly. Expectation for good recovery from Bell's palsy suggests that treatment should be primarily supportive.

The median nerve supplies sensation to the lateral aspect of the hand, over the thumb and first two fingers. This nerve also supplies motor function to the thenar eminence, allowing opposition of the thumb (Fig. 6). Median nerve compression at the wrist under the carpal tunnel may occur during pregnancy. Pain and dysesthesia are typically aggravated by stretching the wrist, such as during hyperextension when scrubbing counters or floors. Reported prevalence of carpal tunnel syndrome during pregnancy varies widely in the literature from 2 to 62% *(13,14)*. A survey of obstetrical patients in the eighth and ninth months of pregnancy identified preexisting carpal tunnel syndrome symptoms in 12% and pregnancy-related carpal tunnel syndrome in 50% *(13)*.

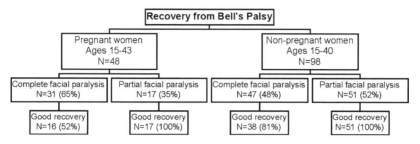

Recovery from Bell's Palsy			
Pregnant women Ages 15-43 N=48		Non-pregnant women Ages 15-40 N=98	
Complete facial paralysis N=31 (65%)	Partial facial paralysis N=17 (35%)	Complete facial paralysis N=47 (48%)	Partial facial paralysis N=51 (52%)
Good recovery N=16 (52%)	Good recovery N=17 (100%)	Good recovery N=38 (81%)	Good recovery N=51 (100%)

Fig. 5. Outcome of Bell's palsy in pregnant vs nonpregnant women of childbearing age initially evaluated within 6 weeks of symptom onset. (Based on ref. *12*.)

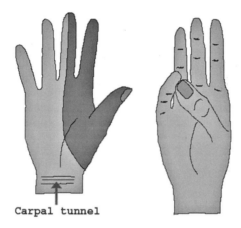

Carpal tunnel

Fig. 6. Carpal tunnel syndrome. Area of sensation (dark gray in the left picture) and motor function (opposition of the thumb in the right picture) supplied by the median nerve.

Carpal tunnel syndrome symptoms during pregnancy usually include bilateral sensory and motor symptoms, with the most common time of onset during the third trimester (Fig. 7) *(14)*.

In addition, carpal tunnel syndrome symptoms usually resolve after delivery (Fig. 8). Postural correction and nighttime splints typically improve symptoms. Local steroid injections may also be considered, especially when motor loss is present.

The lateral femoral cutaneous nerve arises from the second and third lumbar roots. After passing under the inguinal ligament, the lateral femoral cutaneous nerve supplies sensation to the upper, outer thigh. Compression of this nerve may occur in the inguinal canal, often due to obesity or shifts in pelvic

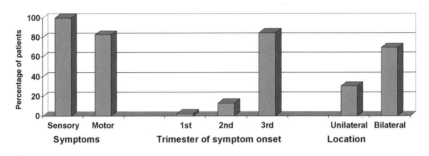

Fig. 7. Carpal tunnel symptoms during pregnancy. (Based on ref. *14*.)

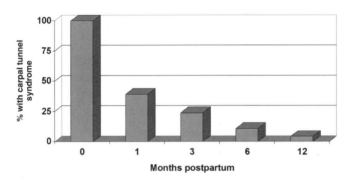

Fig. 8. Resolution of pregnancy-related carpal tunnel syndrome. Of 46 women who developed carpal tunnel syndrome during pregnancy, only 18 (39%) still had symptoms 1 month after delivery and 2 (4%) had them 1 year after delivery. Two women required decompressive surgery; the rest were treated conservatively. (Based on ref. *14*.)

posture, with increased lumbar lordosis during pregnancy. Symptoms are typically unilateral and usually begin in gestational week 31 *(15,16)*, although meralgia paresthetica has been reported during the first trimester *(17)*. Compression results in pain (meralgia) and numbness (paresthetica) in the upper, outer thigh (Fig. 9). During pregnancy, meralgia paresthetica is treated with postural exercises, anti-inflammatory analgesics (between gestational weeks 4 and 32), and, if necessary, local steroid injections.

2. TESTING DURING PREGNANCY

A thorough medical history and complete physical examination, including bedside neurological testing, are the best examination tools for distinguishing among the causes of pain complaints during pregnancy and in nonpregnant women. Women with a suspicious history or examination may need to be evalu-

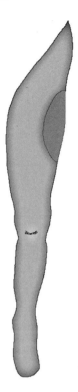

Fig. 9. Meralgia paresthetica: pain and numbness in the distribution of the lateral femoral cutaneous nerve. Area of sensory supply by the lateral femoral nerve is shaded in darker gray.

ated with laboratory or radiographic studies, as warranted by their signs and symptoms. In general, screening should be performed for medical conditions that would be treated during pregnancy. Laboratory testing and electromyography or nerve conduction tests (to identify neuropathy or radiculopathy) can be safely performed throughout pregnancy.

It is safe to obtain cerebral spinal fluid (CSF) for examination during pregnancy and reliable results can be expected. Davis compared the CSF in asymptomatic women undergoing spinal anesthesia for delivery ($n = 44$) and tubal ligation ($n = 22$) *(18)* and found no differences in opening pressure, cell count, or protein levels between the two groups. In addition, active labor, length of gestation, and type of delivery (vaginal vs Cesarean section) did not influence CSF evaluation results. Abnormal CSF test results obtained during pregnancy, therefore, should not be attributed to the pregnancy itself, but must be further evaluated as they are in the nonpregnant patient.

Radiological studies are limited during pregnancy because of concerns for the developing baby. Ultrasonography is considered safe throughout pregnancy and is preferred to radiographic testing. Magnetic resonance imaging (MRI) is also considered relatively safe during pregnancy. Studies have failed to identify any specific sequelae of exposure to MRI during pregnancy *(19)*, including evaluations of the offspring of female MRI technicians and 3-year-olds who had been exposed to MRI *in utero (20,21)*. Based on these data, the American College of Radiology recommends MRI as a preferred imaging study during pregnancy to avoid exposure to ionizing radiation when imaging studies are need and the results of testing may change patient care *(22)*. Gadolinium crosses the placenta and is generally to be avoided during pregnancy. Traditional radiographic studies should be considered when diagnostic information is necessary and cannot be obtained through ultrasonography or other safe testing, and may produce information that will change patient care. The maximum tolerated cumulative fetal dose exposure during pregnancy is 5 rad *(23)*. Most common radiographic studies, including plain X-rays and computed tomography, provide radiation doses well below this level.

3. TREATMENT

Although most women assert a desire to avoid medications during pregnancy, up to one-third self-medicate health symptoms, especially with analgesics *(24–26)*. The therapeutic benefit can be maximized by and the risk to the infant minimized by providing the safest treatments (Table 1). Nonpharmacological treatments—such as relaxation, biofeedback, and exercises—are safe during pregnancy. Under some circumstances, women will need additional medical therapy, particularly for chronic pain owing to a problem that predates the pregnancy. Risks from medications must be balanced against the risks of nontreatment, which may result in pain, distress, deconditioning, and disability.

3.1. Nonpharmacological Therapy

Pain management skills—such as relaxation, biofeedback, and stress management—effectively reduce pain during pregnancy *(27,28)*. Exercise should be low impact and focus on stretching. Transcutaneous electrical nerve stimulation and acupuncture are often restricted during pregnancy because of theoretical concerns about excessive nerve stimulation.

Women with pre-existing problems causing chronic pain who intend to attempt conception should maximize nonpharmacological therapy. The development of effective pain management skills (e.g., relaxation, stress management, and therapeutic exercises) before conception may minimize the need for medication. Pregnancy planning is also an excellent time to adopt healthy

Table 1
Safe Pain Treatments During Conception and Pregnancy

Nonmedical therapy	Medications for pain flares	Daily medications

Psychological skills
• Relaxation
• Biofeedback
• Stress management
• Cognitive restructuring
	Nonopioid analgesics
	• Acetaminophen
	• NSAIDs
	  (between 4 and 32 weeks)
		Antidepressants
		• Selective serotonin
		  reuptake inhibitors
		• Bupropion

Physical therapy • Postural correction • Modalities • Stretching exercises	Opioid analgesics • Limit to intermittent use	Antiepileptics • Gabapentin[a]
Occupational therapy • Body mechanics • Work station simplification	Antiemetics • For migraine with nausea	β-Blockers for migraine prevention
Other • Nicotine cessation		

[a] Gabapentin should be discontinued in third trimester because of negative effects on fetal bony growth. NSAID, nonsteroidal anti-inflammatory drug.

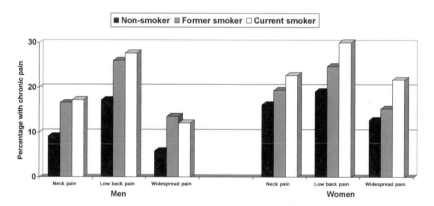

Fig. 10. Relationship between smoking and chronic pain. Differences in prevalence were significant for neck, back, and widespread pain (pain in more than three body areas) for both men and women ($p < 0.05$). (Based on ref. *33*.)

lifestyle habits that reduce chronic pain, such as weight reduction for obese patients (*see* Chapter 16) and regular exercise, activity-pacing skills, body mechanics, and work simplification. Because nicotine affects the activity of a variety of pain modulators (including endorphins) and thus alters pain transmission *(29–31)*—thereby contributing to musculoskeletal pain, fibromyalgia, headache, and other chronic pain conditions *(32–36)* (Fig. 10)—smoking cessation should also be strongly recommended.

3.2. Medications During Pregnancy

Severe pain flares may be treated with acetaminophen and opioids. Medications that inhibit prostaglandin synthesis (e.g., nonsteroidal anti-inflammatory drugs [NSAIDs]) hamper implantation and should be avoided while conception is being attempted *(37,38)*. NSAID use during later stages of pregnancy is associated with premature closure of the fetal ductus arteriosus, and thus should be avoided after gestational week 32 *(39–41)*. Codeine has been linked with the risk for cleft palate and inguinal hernia *(42–44)*, although this association has not been confirmed in recent studies. Codeine is rarely useful during pregnancy because of its constipating effects; hydrocodone is usually better tolerated. Opioids are best limited to infrequent, intermittent use. Patients who have been using opioids daily during mid to late pregnancy must continue to use them because of the risks of fetal mortality and premature labor associated with intrauterine fetal opioid withdrawal *(45)*.

Acute migraine may also be treated safely with antiemetics. Triptan was not associated with a risk for malformations in a recent review of available literature or in data from voluntary registries collected by pharmaceutical companies *(46)*. In two European studies, investigators reported trends toward early delivery and lower birth weight in the offspring of women who use triptan *(47,48)*. Therefore, although significant concern is not warranted when triptans are inadvertently used during pregnancy, additional data are needed before the regular use of triptans during pregnancy can be recommended for most women. Injectable sumatriptan can be used during breastfeeding if the woman pumps and discards milk obtained during the first 4 hours after a sumatriptan injection and supplements feedings with stored or bottled milk.

Some antidepressants and antiepileptic medications may be used during pregnancy for long-standing neuropathic pain and chronic headache. β-Blockers may be used daily to prevent headache. Pregnancy-related compressive neuropathy is usually self-limited and should initially be treated with postural correction. Neuropathic medications are generally not needed.

4. SUMMARY

Pain complaints are reported by the majority of women during pregnancy. The most common area of the body affected is the low back. Various types of compressive neuropathy—e.g., Bell's palsy, carpal tunnel syndrome, and meralgia paresthetica—also occur more frequently during pregnancy. By identifying common complaints, the health care provider can alleviate fears of serious illness, provide advice about the expected course of pain, and recommend effective and safe types of treatment. Pain complaints occurring during pregnancy should be evaluated with testing that minimizes risks to the baby while information necessary to direct patient care during pregnancy is obtained.

Patients with premorbid chronic pain that continues or worsens during pregnancy will often need to use nonpharmacological and pharmacological therapies. Pain complaints that develop during pregnancy are generally self-limited and resolve postpartum.

REFERENCES

1. Kristiansson P, Svärdsudd K, von Schoultz B. Back pain during pregnancy: a prospective study. 1996; 21:702–708.
2. Marcus DA. Interrelationships of neurochemicals, estrogen, and recurring headache. Pain 1995; 62:129–139.
3. Marcus DA. Sex hormones and chronic headache. Exp Opin Pharmacother 2001; 2:1839–1848.
4. Sances G, Granella F, Nappi RE, et al. Course of migraine during pregnancy and postpartum: a prospective study. Cephalalgia 2003; 23:197–205.
5. Marcus DA, Scharff L, Turk D. Longitudinal prospective study of headache during pregnancy and postpartum. Headache 1999; 39:625–632.
6. Wall VR. Breastfeeding and migraine headaches. J Hum Lact 1992; 8:209–212.
7. Marcus DA. Headache in pregnancy. Curr Pain Headache Rep 2003; 7:288–296.
8. Azpilcueta A, Peral C, Giraldo I, Chen FJ, Contreras G. Meningioma in pregnancy. Report of a case and review of the literature. Ginecol Obstet Mex 1995; 63:349–351.
9. Saitoh Y, Oku Y, Izumoto S, Go J. Rapid growth of a meningioma during pregnancy: relationship with estrogen and progesterone receptors –case report. Neurol Med Cir (Tokyo) 1989; 29:440–443.
10. Stapleton DB, MacLennan AH, Kristiansson P. The prevalence of recalled low back pain during and after pregnancy: a South Australian population survey. Aust NZ J Obstet Gynaecol 2002; 42:482–485.
11. Cohen Y, Lavie O, Granovsky-Grisaru S, Aboulafia Y, Diamant Y. Bell palsy complicating pregnancy: a review. Obstet Gynecol Surv 2000; 55:184–188.
12. Gillman GS, Schaitkin BM, May M, Klein SR. Bell's palsy in pregnancy: a study of recovery outcomes. Otolaryngol Head Neck Surg 2002; 126:26–30.
13. Padua L, Aprile I, Caliandro P, et al. Symptoms and neurophysiological picture of carpal tunnel syndrome in pregnancy. Clin Neurophysiol 2001; 112:1946–1951.
14. Turgut F, Çetinsahinahin M, Turgut M, Bölükbasi O. The management of carpal tunnel syndrome in pregnancy. J Clin Neurosci 2001; 8:332–334.
15. Peterson PH. Meralgia paresthetica related to pregnancy. Am J Obstet Gynecol 1952; 64:690–691.
16. Rhodes P. Meralgia paresthetica in pregnancy. Lancet 1957; 273:831.
17. Ferra Verdera M, Ribera Leclerc H, Garrido Pastor JP. Two cases of paresthetic meralgia of the femoral cutaneous nerve. Rev Esp Anestesiol Reanim 2003; 50:154–156.
18. Davis LE. Normal laboratory values of CSF during pregnancy. Arch Neurol 1979; 36:443.
19. Levine D, Barnes PD, Edleman RR. Obstetric MR imaging. Radiology 1999; 211:609–617.

20. Kanal E, Gillen J, Evans J, Savitz D, Shellock F. Survey of reproductive health among female MR workers. Radiology 1993; 187:395–399.

21. Baker P, Johnson I, Harvey P, Mansfield P: A three-year follow-up of children imaged in utero using echo-planar magnetic resonance. Am J Obstet Gynecol 1994; 170:32–33.

22. ACR standards: MRI safety and sedation. (Available at Website: www.acr.org, accessed 02/24/04.)

23. Toppenberg KS, Hill A, Miller DP. Safety of radiographic imaging during pregnancy. Am Fam Physician 1999; 59:1813–1818, 1820.

24. Gomes KR, Moron AF, Silva R, Siqueira AA. Prevalence of use of medicines during pregnancy and its relationship to maternal factors. Rev Saude Publica 1999; 33:246–254.

25. Fonseca MR, Fonseca E, Bergsten-Mendes G. Prevalence of drug use during pregnancy: a pharmacoepidemiological approach. Rev Saude Publica 2002; 36: 205–212.

26. Damase-Michel C, Lapeyre-Mestre M, Moly C, Fournie A, Montastruc JL. Drug use during pregnancy: survey in 250 women consulting at a university hospital center. J Gynecol Obstet Biol Repro (Paris) 2000; 29:77–85.

27. Marcus DA, Scharff L, Turk DC. Nonpharmacologic management of headaches during pregnancy. Psychosomatic Medicine, 1995; 57:527–533.

28. Scharff L, Marcus DA, Turk DC. Maintenance of effects in the nonmedical treatment of headaches during pregnancy. Headache 1996; 36:285–290.

29. Pomerleau OF. Endogenous opioids and smoking –a review of progress and problems. Psychoneuroendocrinolgy 1998; 23:115–130.

30. Mansbach RS, Rovetti CC, Freeland CS. The role of monoamine neurotransmitters system in the nicotine discriminative stimulus. Drug Alcohol Depend 1998; 23:115–130.

31. Wewers ME, Dhatt RK, Snively TA, Tejwani GA. The effect of chronic administration of nicotine on antinociception, opioid receptor binding and met-enkephalin levels in rats. Brain Res 1999; 822:107–113.

32. Payne TJ, Stetson B, Stevens VM, Johnson CA, Penzien DB, Van Dorsten B. Impact of cigarette smoking on headache activity in headache patients. Headache 1991; 31:329–332.

33. Andersson H, Ejlertsson G, Leden I. Widespread musculoskeletal chronic pain associated with smoking. An epidemiological study in a general rural population. Scan J Rehabil Med 1998; 30:185–191.

34. Yunus MB, Arslan S, Aldag JC. Relationship between fibromyalgia features and smoking. Scand J Rheumatol 2002; 31:301–305.

35. Luo X, Edwards CL, Richardson W, Hey L. Relationships of clinical, psychological, and individual factors with the functional status of neck pain patients. Value Health 2004; 7:61–69.

36. Omokhodion FO, Sanya AO. Risk factors for low back pain among office workers in Ibadan, Southwest Nigeria. Occup Med (Lond) 2003; 53:287–289.

37. Carp HJ, Fein A, Nebel L. Effect of diclofenac on implantation and embryonic development in the rat. Eur J Obstet Gynecol Reprod Biol 1988; 28:273–277.

38. Kanayama K, Osada H, Nariai K, Endo T. Inhibitory effects of indomethacin on implantation and its related phenomena. J Int Med Res 1996; 24:258–262.

39. Momma K, Hagiwara H, Konishi T. Constriction of fetal ductus arteriosus by non-steroidal anti-inflammatory drugs: study of additional 34 drugs. Prostaglandins 1984; 28:527–536.

40. Rein AJ, Nadjari M, Elchalal U, Nir A. Contraction of the fetal ductus arteriosus induced by diclofenac. Case report. Fetal Diagn Ther 1999; 14:24–25.

41. Zenker M, Klinge J, Kruger C, Singer H, Scharf J. Severe pulmonary hypertension in a neonate caused by premature closure of the ductus arteriosus following maternal treatment with diclofenac: a case report. J Perinat Med 1998; 26:231–234.

42. Bracken MB, Holford TR. Exposure to prescribed drugs in pregnancy and association with congenital malformations. Obstet Gynecol 1981; 58:336–344.

43. Saxen I. Association between oral cleft and drugs taken during pregnancy. Int J Epidemiol 1975; 4:37–44.

44. Saxen I. Epidemiology of cleft lip and palate: an attempt to rule out chance correlations. Br J Prev Soc Med 1975; 29:103–110.

45. Drug use and dependence. The Merck Manual of Diagnostics and Therapeutics, 17th Ed., Section 15, chapter 195. (Available at Website: www.merck.com/pubs; accessed 02/24/04.)

46. Loder E. Safety of sumatriptan in pregnancy: a review of the data so far. CNS Drugs 2003; 17:1–7.

47. Olesen L, Steffensen FH, Sorensen HT, et al. Pregnancy outcome following prescription for sumatriptan. Headache 2000; 40:20–24.

48. Kallen B, Lygner PE. Delivery outcome in women who used drugs for migraine during pregnancy with special reference to sumatriptan. Headache 2001; 41: 351–356.

CME QUESTIONS—CHAPTER 12

1. What percentage of women will typically report pain during pregnancy?
    a. 70–80%
    b. 30–40%
    c. 15–25%
    d. 2–5%

2. Which chronic pain syndrome typically improves during pregnancy?
    a. Migraine
    b. Low back pain
    c. Carpal tunnel syndrome
    d. All of the above

3. Safe testing during pregnancy includes:
    a. Physical examination
    b. Blood tests
    c. Ultrasound
    d. Electromyography/nerve conduction studies
    e. A–C
    f. A–D

4. Safe treatments during pregnancy include:
    a. Bupropion
    b. Valproate for migraine prevention
    c. Relaxation and biofeedback
    d. A and C
    e. All of the above

13

Geriatrics and Chronic Pain

CASE HISTORY

Mr. Williams is a healthy, active 72-year-old who plays par golf 3 days a week. He is also a regular volunteer in his church and at a local nursing home. He comes to the doctor complaining of pain in his low back, buttock, and leg when he walks approximately two blocks. Often, the leg goes numb as well. Once he gets the pain, it only goes away after he sits down. Because of the pain, he has had to discontinue golfing and most of his volunteer activities. He recently started riding a bicycle to keep up his activity level, and reports he can ride for several miles without any pain. The only time he can walk without developing severe buttock and leg pain is when he helps his wife by pushing the shopping cart in the grocery store. Mr. Williams also notes that the residents at the nursing home where he helps serve meals have begun to tease him, saying, "You're getting old, Bob. You're looking more and more like an old man everyday. Look how you stoop when you walk!" Mr. Williams' physical examination shows excellent forward flexion of his back, although he reports discomfort with back extension. His neurological examination is normal and he briskly walks up and down the hallway in the office without complaint. Mr. Williams is reminded that he's "not a kid anymore," and his doctor suggests developing an interest in more sedentary activities.

* * *

Mr. Williams presents a common history of the healthy, active senior patient who develops a pain complaint. Often, reports of pain in elderly patients are misinterpreted as expressions of depression or are considered to represent the normal aging process. Mr. Williams' story is typical of spinal stenosis, a treatable and usually reversible cause of pain. Failure to address pain complaints in the elderly can result in unnecessary restrictions in activity that may result in increased disability and reduced independence long-term. Although many of the same pain complaints that affect younger patients may also occur in older individuals, prevalence of pain conditions changes with aging. Understanding common pain syndromes in the elderly, such as spinal stenosis, can improve diagnosis and reduce unnecessary restrictions in activities.

From: *Chronic Pain: A Primary Care Guide to Practical Management*
Edited by: D. A. Marcus © Humana Press, Totowa, NJ

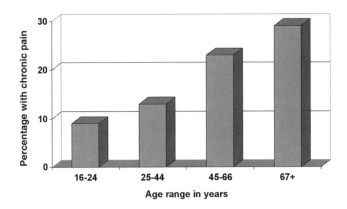

Fig. 1. Prevalence of chronic pain in a population-based survey. (Based on ref. *1*.)

KEY CHAPTER POINTS

• Chronic pain affects almost one-third of the elderly.
• Risk of musculoskeletal pain syndromes increases with aging, and include arthritis, osteoporosis with fractures, and lumbar stenosis.
• Migraine becomes less prevalent with aging.
• Headache beginning after age 50 should be fully evaluated to rule out important causes of secondary headache, including temporal arteritis, intracranial tumor, subdural hematoma, and cervical spine disease.
• Pharmacological and nonpharmacological therapies used in younger patients are effective in older patients, although drug selection and dosage must be adjusted to minimize adverse events and drug interactions.

The prevalence of chronic pain increases with age, affecting nearly 30% of the elderly (Fig. 1) *(1)*. Chronic pain in elderly patients should not be considered "a normal part of the aging process." As seen with Mr. Williams, untreated chronic pain can result in decreased functional ability, loss of independence, reduced quality of life, and depression. Therefore, pain complaints in elderly patients should be accorded the same importance as similar complaints in younger patients.

Over the next several decades, pain management practices will need to shift to increase emphasis on addressing pain in the elderly. A United Nations' survey has identified a worldwide aging trend in both developed and less developed regions (Fig. 2) *(2)*. The percentage of the world population aged 60 or older was 8% in 1950 and 10% in 2000, and is projected to reach 21% by 2050. In addition, individuals aged 80 or older represent the fastest growing age group worldwide. As the population continues to age, health care providers will be increasingly confronted with chronic pain complaints and will need to be knowledgeable about pain syndromes that commonly occur in elderly patients (*see* Box 1).

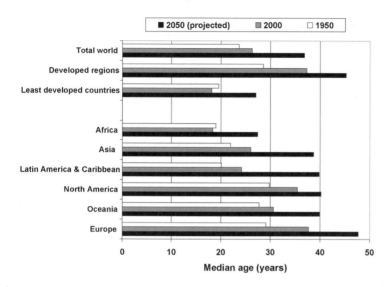

Fig. 2. Aging trends in world populations. (Based on ref. 2.).

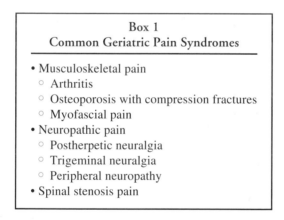

1. COMMON CHRONIC PAIN COMPLAINTS

Patients may continue to describe long-standing chronic pain complaints that persist into their elder years or, like Mr. Williams, develop new pain complaints with aging. Although many elderly individuals will not have work disability related to pain, losing the ability to maintain a healthy, active lifestyle and participate in social activities significantly impairs the quality of life for seniors. Recognition of common pain syndromes in elderly patients improves the chance for an accurate diagnosis and reduces the risk for disability. Two of the most important types of pain that are significantly modified in elderly patients are musculoskeletal pain and headache.

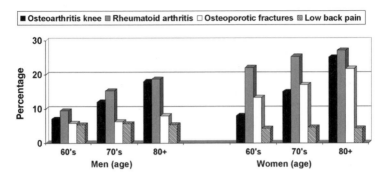

Fig. 3. Prevalence of musculoskeletal abnormalities in the elderly in developed countries. (Based on ref. *3.*)

1.1. Musculoskeletal Pain

Musculoskeletal abnormalities become more prevalent with advancing age, representing a significant risk for pain, disability, and loss of independence *(3)*. As seen with Mr. Williams, musculoskeletal pain can significantly restrict household, employment, or volunteer activities, as well as leisure and social activities. Common painful musculoskeletal conditions include arthritis and osteoporosis with resultant fractures (Fig. 3). These conditions occur more commonly in women than men. Interestingly, the prevalence of chronic low back pain does not increase with aging.

1.1.1. Osteoporosis and Fractures

The prevalence of osteoporosis increases with advancing age in both men and women (Fig. 4) *(4)*. The relative risk of a hip fracture is nearly five times greater in both older men and women with osteoporosis compared with individuals without osteoporosis (Fig. 4). Osteoporosis also increases the risk for vertebral compression fractures, which occur in 23% of ambulatory women age 75 years or older *(5)*.

1.1.2. Lumbar Stenosis

Lumbar spinal stenosis is characterized by pain in the back, buttocks, and leg that occurs with standing or walking. Because the diameter of the lumbar canal compresses with back extension and opens with flexion, patients like Mr. Williams tend to stoop while walking to minimize pain, and report pain relief after sitting (which is also associated with lumbar flexion). Vascular claudication also occurs with walking, but is related more to activity rather than posture. Although the pain of vascular claudication typically resolves while standing after discontinuing walking, patients with lumbar stenosis usually need to sit to achieve relief. Reports of longer walking tolerance when shopping in the gro-

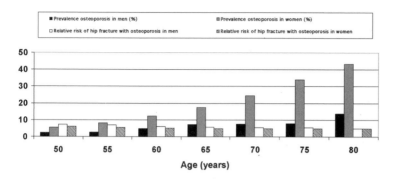

Fig. 4. Risk of osteoporosis and hip fracture with increasing age. Risk for osteoporosis is greater in women than men. The occurrence of osteoporosis in both men and women results in an approximately five times increased risk of hip fracture after age 50. (Based on ref. *4*.)

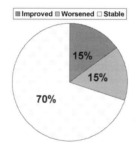

Fig. 5. Natural history of lumbar stenosis. Thirty-two untreated patients (mean age = 60 years) were followed long-term (mean = 4 years). (Based on ref. *6*.)

cery store (where stooping is assisted by using a shopping cart) suggest lumbar stenosis. Family members may also comment, "The longer Dad walks, the more he stoops forward." Neurological deficits in the extremities may occur in severe cases, although patients are typically normal when examined at rest. Lumbar stenosis symptoms tend to persist over time without treatment, although they infrequently worsen (Fig. 5) *(5)*.

1.2. Headache

The prevalence of headache continues to be higher in elderly women than men, although the prevalence of migraine decreases with advancing age. A survey of more than 1000 community-living adults 65 years or older revealed three or more headache episodes during the preceding year in 22% *(7)*. The overall prevalence of headache was higher in women. Migraine was particularly sensitive to reduction with advancing age, with a lower prevalence when compared to a similar survey of young adults (Fig. 6) *(8)*.

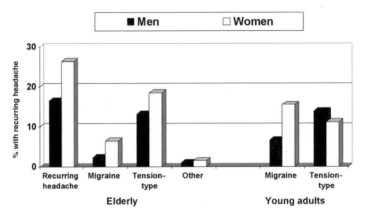

Fig. 6. Prevalence of recurring headache in elderly (mean age = 75 years) and young adults (mean age = 22 years). (Based on refs. 7 and 8.)

Table 1
Prevalence of Symptoms of Temporal Arteritis and Polymyalgia Rheumatica

Temporal arteritis	Polymyalgia rheumatica
Head pain/scalp tenderness: 66%	Proximal limb pain and stiffness
Fatigue with chewing (jaw claudication): 50%	70–95% shoulders
Polymyalgia rheumatica: 40%	50–70% hip and neck
Visual loss/disturbance: 20%	Systemic symptoms: 30%
Low grade fever: 15%	Fever
Cough: 10%	Fatigue
	Anorexia
	Weight loss

Based on ref. 9.

New-onset headache or head pain should always be fully investigated in older adults. It is unusual for common benign headaches seen in young adults, like migraine, to begin after age 50. The presence of intracranial pathology (e.g., tumors or subdural hematomas) and cervical disease (e.g., arthritis) should be considered in elderly patients with new-onset headache. Two other important head pains that typically affect elderly patients are temporal arteritis and trigeminal neuralgia.

1.2.1. Temporal or Giant-Cell Arteritis

Temporal arteritis or giant-cell arteritis may occur as an isolated head pain syndrome or as part of a more systemic picture of polymyalgia rheumatica (Table 1) *(9)*. Temporal arteritis is a medical emergency that should be considered in the differential diagnosis of new headache in elderly patients because of the significant risk for vision loss and stroke. Visual ischemic complications occur in 26% and irreversible blindness in 15% of patients with biopsy-proven temporal arteritis *(10)*. Stroke, usually in the vertebrobasilar distribution, occurs in approximately 3% of patients with temporal arteritis *(11)*.

Evaluation begins with a hematocrit and erythrocyte sedimentation rate (ESR). Patients with strong presumptive diagnoses of temporal arteritis or anterior ischemic neuropathy should be treated with steroids presumptively, immediately after blood work is obtained. Treatment should not be delayed until blood test results or a temporal artery biopsy has been obtained. Biopsy should, however, be performed within 2 to 3 days of initiating steroid therapy.

1.2.2. Trigeminal Neuralgia

Trigeminal neuralgia is an excruciating, lancinating facial pain, typically triggered by stimulating the skin over the affected area, such as by touching, talking, or chewing. Patients sometimes also report a dull facial pain between severe paroxysms. Pain most commonly affects the second or third divisions of the trigeminal nerve, causing pain over the cheek or jaw. Interestingly, the right trigeminal nerve is more likely to be involved than the left. The overall incidence of trigeminal neuralgia in the general population is 0.004% *(12)*. The risk increases with age, and women are twice as likely to be affected as men.

2. ASSESSMENT TOOLS

Although the same general pain assessments used in younger patients may be applied to elderly patients, additional tools have been developed to allow the convenient and appropriate assessment of pain severity and its impact in elderly populations. Tools that focus on disability for activities appropriate to the lifestyles of seniors are most appropriate. Two geriatric assessment tools that incorporate both pain severity and associated disability are the Geriatric Pain Measure questionnaire and the 6-minute walk test.

The Geriatric Pain Measure is a validated assessment tool of pain severity and impact that can be easily administered in the office (Table 2) *(13)*. After completion, this form may be placed in the patient's chart to serve as documentation of pain severity. Patients can complete additional questionnaires at follow-up appointments to document treatment response.

The 6-minute walk test is a standardized, easy-to-employ measure of functional ability in elderly patients *(14)*. After marking 100-foot distances in a hallway, patients are asked to walk back and forth in the hallway at a comfortable pace, with rest breaks permitted, while an examiner records the number of laps (i.e., total distance) completed in 6 minutes (mean: 362 meters [1188 feet] for men; 332 meters [1089 feet] for women). This test can help document functional impairment at baseline (based on walking less than the expected distance) and provide a follow-up efficacy response measure after treatment.

Table 2
Geriatric Pain Measure

I. Please put a "Yes" or "No" check for each item. Answer each question considering the impact that PAIN has on your ability to do or enjoy activities.

Question	Yes	No
Do or would you have pain with any of the following activities:		
Running, lifting heavy objects, or strenuous sports	☐	☐
Moving a heavy table, vacuuming, bowling, or golfing	☐	☐
Lifting or carrying groceries	☐	☐
Climbing more than one flight of stairs	☐	☐
Climbing only a few steps	☐	☐
Walking more than one block	☐	☐
Walking one block or less	☐	☐
Bathing or dressing	☐	☐
Does or would pain cause you to:		
Reduce work or other activities	☐	☐
Accomplish less than you expect	☐	☐
Limit the type of work or activities you do	☐	☐
Use extra effort for work or other actitivites	☐	☐
Have trouble sleeping	☐	☐
Miss attending religious functions	☐	☐
Lack enjoyment in nonreligious social or recreational activities	☐	☐
Be unable to travel or use standard transportation	☐	☐
Feel fatigued or tired	☐	☐
Do you have pain:		
That never goes away completely	☐	☐
Every day	☐	☐
At least several times a week	☐	☐
In the last week, has your pain caused you to feel sad or depressed?	☐	☐
Total	___	___

II. Rate your pain severity on a scale from zero (no pain) to 10 (the worst pain imaginable):

   a. How severe is your pain TODAY?

   0   1   2   3   4   5   6   7   8   9   10

   b. What was your average pain severity over the last week?

   0   1   2   3   4   5   6   7   8   9   10

Scoring:

Add total number of "Yes" checks and two numbers from Section II. Multiply sum by 2.38 to produce a score ranging from 0 to 100.

Interpretation: <30 is mild pain; 30–69 is moderate pain; >70 is severe pain.

Based on ref. *13*.

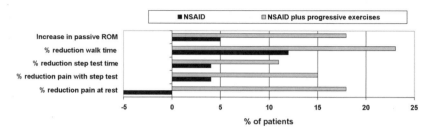

Fig. 7. Treatment of knee osteoarthritis with medication vs medication plus progressive exercise. Patients older than 65 years with painful knee osteoarthritis were randomized to 8 weeks of 1200 mg oxaprozin/day plus stretches without resistance or progression (NSAID) or oxaprozin plus progressive home range-of-motion and resistance exercises (NSAID plus progressive exercise). Pain and functional measures were all superior in patients treated with supplemental progressive exercise ($p < 0.05$). NSAID, nonsteroidal anti-inflammatory drug; ROM, range of motion. (Based on ref. *16*.)

3. TREATMENT

The same nonpharmacological and pharmacological therapies used in younger adults are also used for elderly patients with chronic pain. Medication selection and dosing are more complicated in older patients because of the increased prevalence of comorbid medical illness and increased sensitivity to medication side effects.

3.1. Nonpharmacological Therapy

Nonpharmacological therapy retains good efficacy in elderly patients. Effective pain control in elderly patients has been demonstrated with biofeedback, cognitive–behavioral therapy, progressive exercise, and Tai Chi *(15–18)*. Similar to findings in younger patients with chronic pain, the addition of nonpharmacological therapy to pharmacotherapy enhances both pain relief and functional improvement (Fig. 7) *(16)*.

Exercise recommendations for musculoskeletal pain in elderly patients are modified for comorbid illness and baseline physical capabilities. Exercises for chronic pain should include stretching exercises and reconditioning exercises. For example, stationary bicycling three times a week for 25 minutes each session resulted in reduced pain and improved functional ability in elderly patients with knee osteoarthritis, as indicated by the 6-minute walk test *(19)*.

A longitudinal study evaluated the effect of regular exercise at least 4 days/week in patients aged 70 years, specifically their ability to perform activities of daily living (ADLs) independently at age 77 *(20)*. Individuals who participated in regular exercise at age 70 years were significantly more likely to be able to perform ADLs with ease at age 77 years than those who did not do regular exercise.

This difference was still seen after adjusting for diabetes, hypertension, chronic back pain, loneliness, ease of performing ADLs at age 70 years, and health deterioration from age 70 to 77 years. Exercise is, therefore, an important recommendation for elderly patients to reduce pain and maximize long-term independence.

3.2. Medications

The same medications used in younger adults are used for pain syndromes in elderly individuals. Drug selection and dosage must be adjusted in elderly patients to minimize adverse events and drug interactions. A review of outpatient visits from two large national, ambulatory care surveys in the United States revealed the use of at least one inappropriate drug in elderly patients at 3.8% of visits *(21)*. The major categories of drug offenders were pain relievers and central nervous system drugs, which are routinely used for pain management in younger patients.

Focal pain complaints in the elderly may be treated with local treatments, which minimize systemic effects. These may include topical capsaicin or 5% lidocaine, trigger-point injections for myofascial pain, and epidural steroid injections for lumbar stenosis.

Diffuse pain complaints may require systemic medications. Analgesics are less tolerated in the elderly than in younger patients. Risk for gastric toxicity related to nonsteroidal anti-inflammatory agents (NSAIDs) increases in elderly patients, especially when long-acting NSAIDs are used *(22,23)*. Gastric toxicity may be reduced by limiting NSAID use to short-acting NSAIDs or selective cyclooxygenase-2 (COX-2) inhibitors *(24)*. Renal effects are also more problematic in older patients, including concerns about the interference of NSAIDs with the efficacy of diuretics. Opioids require careful monitoring to minimize sedating and cognitive effects, as well as constipation. High-fiber diets, regular exercise, and the use of lactulose and senna are appropriate for minimizing medication-induced constipation. Acetaminophen is well tolerated and is particularly useful in patients with comorbid medical illnesses. The combination of tramadol 37.5 mg and acetaminophen 325 mg is an effective and generally well-tolerated alternative for elderly patients to manage flare analgesia *(25)*.

Neuropathic medications should also be used in low doses. Use of tricyclic antidepressants (TCAs) should be limited in elderly patients. Trazodone has fewer cardiovascular effects than TCAs, as well as good efficacy for deafferentation pain *(26)*. Selective serotonin reuptake inhibitors (SSRIs) are less effective than TCAs, but provide superior tolerability *(27)*. Antiepileptic drugs (AED) are also effective therapy for neuropathic pain. Gabapentin is the most effective AED agent for neuropathic pain *(28,29)*, having fewer cognitive effects than other AEDs *(30,31)*.

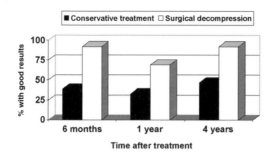

Fig. 8. Outcome for patients with lumbar stenosis randomized to conservative vs surgical treatment. (Based on ref. *35*.)

The drug dosage should be lower in older patients to minimize the risk for adverse events. For example, the muscle relaxant tizanidine is tolerated in an elderly population, but its sedating side effects limit the dosing level *(32)*. Low doses of tizanidine (1 mg) should be initiated at bedtime and increased slowly to a maximum of 2 to 4 mg twice daily, as tolerated.

3.3. Osteoporosis and Fractures

The results of large-scale controlled clinical trials indicate that the treatment of osteoporosis with bisphosphonates risedronate or alendronate consistently reduces the 3-year risk of developing vertebral and nonvertebral fractures by approximately 40% *(33)*. Muscle-strengthening exercises also reduce the risk for fractures in the elderly. Sinaki and colleagues randomized 65 healthy, post-menopausal women to an exercise program designed to promote progressive strengthening of the back extensor muscles or a control group *(34)*. After 2 years, exercise was discontinued. Participants were then reassessed 8 years later with radiographs. The incidence of vertebral compression fracture was significantly lower in women who performed the back exercises (1.6%) com-pared with controls (4.3%; $p = 0.03$).

3.4. Lumbar Stenosis

Lumbar stenosis is typically treated with extension exercises, epidural steroid injections, and, for more severe symptoms, surgical decompression. Recondi-tioning exercises should be performed in the flexed position (e.g., stationary bicycling, or as aqua therapy). In a prospective study, investigators followed 100 patients treated long-term for lumbar stenosis with sciatica (median age: 59 years). Patients with severe pain were treated surgically and those with mild symptoms were treated conservatively *(35)*. Thirty-one patients had moderately severe symptoms and were randomized to surgery or conservative therapy. Both short- and long-term outcomes were superior with surgery (Fig. 8). Patients initially

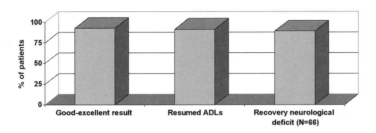

Fig. 9. Long-term outcome for 118 patients with lumbar stenosis aged 70 or older treated with surgery. Mean follow-up time: 7 years. Neurological deficits were present before surgery in 66 patients (56% of the total sample). ADL, activities of daily living. (Based on ref. *36*.)

assigned to conservative treatment later achieved relief with surgery similar to that of patients treated initially with decompression. Thus, initial treatment of mild to moderate symptoms with conservative measures is not harmful because a delay in surgery does not significantly hinder outcome. Surgical results are similarly good in elderly patients with lumbar stenosis (Fig. 9) *(36)*. In addition, surgical complications are not increased in elderly patients *(36)*. Conservative therapy should be used as first-line therapy in elderly patients with comorbid medical illnesses, because the surgical outcome is negatively influenced by comorbid disease, such as diabetes *(37)*.

3.5. Temporal or Giant-Cell Arteritis

Patients presenting with visual complaints are initially treated with intravenous steroids (e.g., 1000 mg methylprenisolone daily pulsed in two to four divided doses for several days). Otherwise, the initial treatment is typically prednisone 60 to 100 mg daily. Headache should resolve within several days after initiating steroids. The prednisone dosage should be gradually tapered during the first month of treatment; thus, most patients will be taking approximately 40 mg daily after 4 weeks. Prednisone should be continued for approximately 6 to 18 months, with the dosage decreased by 10% per week or 2.5 to 5.0 mg every 1 to 2 weeks until a maintenance dosage of 10 to 20 mg/day is reached. The tapering schedule is dependent on continuation of symptomatic control and reduction in ESR. Small increases in ESR often occur during steroid tapering and do not require an increase in steroids if the patient remains asymptomatic. Because treatment is started before a diagnosis is verified, the treating physician must not feel obligated to maintain a full 6- to 18-month course of treatment when the diagnosis has been ruled out (e.g., negative ESR and negative biopsy). This is particularly true because of the serious adverse events associated with chronic steroid use (including cataracts, glucose intolerance, osteoporosis, aseptic necrosis of the femoral head, myopathy, and infection risk).

Table 3
First-Line Pharmacological Therapy for Trigeminal Neuralgia

Drug	Initiation dosage	Dosage after titration
Carbamazepine	100 mg/day	200 mg four times a day
Phenytoin	200 mg/day	300–500 mg/day
Baclofen	5–10 mg three times a day	20 mg four times a day

3.6. Trigeminal Neuralgia

Trigeminal neuralgia may be treated with AEDs (e.g., phenytoin or carbamazepine), baclofen, peripheral glyercol injections, or microvascular decompression (Table 3). Gabapentin may also be used in patients who are unable to
tolerate other AEDs, although its efficacy is inferior. A review of 92 patients
with trigeminal neuralgia being treated with gabapentin showed complete or
nearly complete pain relief in 27% and partial pain relief in 20%; pain relief
was sustained in 63% *(38)*. A retrospective study of 157 patients treated with
glycerol injections and followed for 4 years revealed a good initial success rate
of 98% *(39)*. Pain recurred in 60 patients (39%), usually between 2 to 3 years
after the initial injection. Impaired sensation occurred after injection in 14 patients. A similar long-term follow-up of patients treated with microvascular
decompression showed that 71% of patients were pain-free long term and pain
recurred in 29% *(40)*. Recurrence typically occurred within 2 years of initial
surgery. γ-Knife radiosurgery offers an additional treatment option for
patients with trigeminal neuralgia. A study of refractory trigeminal neuralgia
in patients who had failed medical or surgical treatment showed that pain relief
was achieved following γ-Knife radiosurgery in 77% *(41)*. Long-term follow-
up showed a good or excellent response in 70% after 1 year, 60% after 2 years,
and 48% after 3 years.

4. SUMMARY

Chronic pain continues to be a significant problem in elderly patients, with
chronic pain affecting almost one third of seniors. Chronic pain is not an
expected symptom of aging and should be evaluated and treated in elderly
patients. Although chronic pain may not interfere with work performance in
an elderly population, important consequences of untreated chronic pain
may ensue, including discomfort, disability, depression, and possible loss of
independence. Most common pain problems can be effectively treated in this
age group. Exercise, cognitive restructuring, and biofeedback continue to be
effective pain management tools for older adults. Medications may also
enhance pain control, although drug selection and dosages need to be adjusted
to minimize the risk for adverse events and drug–drug interactions.

REFERENCES

1. Eriksen J, Jensen MK, Sjøgren P, Ekholm O, Rasmussen NK. Epidemiology of chronic non-malignant pain in Denmark. Pain 2003; 106:221–228.
2. United Nations Population Information Network. World population prospects: the 2002 revision. (Available at Website: http://www.un.org/popin, accessed February 11, 2004).
3. Woolf AD, Pfleger B. Burden of major musculoskeletal conditions. Bull World Health Organ 2003; 81:646–656.
4. Kanis JA, Johnell O, Oden A, Jonsson B, De Laet C, Dawson A. Risk of hip fracture according to the World Health Organization criteria for osteopenia and osteoporosis. Bone 2000; 27:585–590.
5. Grados F, Marcelli C, Dargent-Molina P, et al. Prevalence of vertebral fractures in French women older than 75 years from the EPIDOS study. Bone 2004; 34: 362–367.
6. Johnsson KE. The natural course of lumbar spinal stenosis. Clin Orthop 1992; 279:82–86.
7. Camarda R, Monastero R. Prevalence of primary headaches in Italian elderly: preliminary data from the Zabút Aging Project. Neurol Sci 2003; 24:S122–S124.
8. Deleu D, Khan MA, Humaidan H, Al Mantheri Z, Al Hashami S. Prevalence and clinical characteristics of headache in medical students in Oman. Headache 2001; 41:798–804.
9. Salvarani C, Cantini F, Boiardi L, Hunder GG. Medical progress: polymyalgia rheumatica and temporal arteritis. N Eng J Med 2002; 347:261–271.
10. Gonzalez-Gay MA, Garcia-Porrua C, Llorca J, et al. Visual manifestations of giant cell arteritis: trends and clinical spectrum in 161 patients. Medicine (Baltimore) 2000; 79:283–292.
11. Gonzalez-Gay MA, Blanco R, Rodriguez-Valverde V, et al. Permanent visual loss and cerebrovascular accidents in giant cell arteritis. Arthritis Rheum 1998; 41: 1497–1504.
12. Katusic S, Beard CM, Bergstralh E, Kurland LT. Incidence and clinical features of trigeminal neuralgia, Rochester, Minnesota, 1945–1984. Ann Neurol 1990; 27: 89–95.
13. Ferrell BA, Stein WM, Beck JC. The Geriatric Pain Measure: validity, reliability and factor analysis. J Am Geriatr Soc 2000; 48:1669–1673.
14. Enright PL, McBurnie MA, Bittner V, et al. The 6-min walk test: a quick measure of functional status in elderly adults. Chest 2003; 123:387–398.
15. Arena JG, Hannah SL, Bruno GM, Meador KJ. Electromyographic biofeedback training for tension headache in the elderly: a prospective study. Biofeedback Self Regul 1991; 16:379–390.
16. Petrella RJ, Bartha C. Home based exercise therapy for older patients with knee osteoarthritis: a randomized clinical trial. J Rheumatol 2000; 27:2215–2221.
17. Reid MC, Otis J, Barry LC, Kerns RD. Cognitive-behavioral therapy for chronic low back pain in older persons: a preliminary study. Pain Med 2003; 4:223–230.
18. Song R, Lee EO, Lam P, Bae SC. Effects of tai chi exercise on pain, balance, muscle strength, and perceived difficulties in physical functioning in older women with osteoarthritis: a randomized clinical trial. J Rheumatol 2003; 30:2039–2044.

19. Mangione KK, McCully K, Gloviak A, Lefebvre I, Hofmann M, Craik R. The effects of high-intensity and low-intensity cycle ergometry in older adults with knee osteoarthritis. J Gerontol A Biol Sci Med Sci 1999; 54:M184–M190.

20. Stessman J, Hammerman-Rozenberg R, Maaravi Y, Cohen A. Effect of exercise on ease in performing activities of daily living and instrumental activities of daily living from age 70 to 77: the Jerusalem Longitudinal Study. J Am Geriatr Soc 2002; 50:1934–1938.

21. Goulding MR. Inappropriate medication prescribing for elderly ambulatory care patients. Arch Intern Med 2004; 164:305–312.

22. Johnson AG, Day RO. The problems and pitfalls of NSAID therapy in the elderly: Part I. Drugs Aging 1991; 1:130–143.

23. Scharf S, Kwiatek R, Ugoni A, Christophidis N. NSAIDs and faecal blood loss in elderly patients with osteoarthritis: is plasma half-life relevant? Aust NZ J Med 1998; 28:436–439.

24. Bell GM, Schnitzer TJ. COX-2 inhibitors and other nonsteroidal anti-inflammatory drugs in the treatment of pain in the elderly. Clin Geriatr Med 2001; 17:489–502.

25. Rosenthal NR, Silverfield JC, Wu SC, Jordan D, Kamin M. Tramadol/acetaminophen combination tablets for the treatment of pain associated with osteoarthritis flare in an elderly patient population. J Am Geriatr Soc 2004; 52:374–380.

26. Ventafridda V, Caraceni A, Saita L, et al. Trazodone for deafferentation pain: comparison with amitriptyline. Psychopharmacology (Berlin) 1988; 95(Suppl): S44–S49.

27. Ansari A. The efficacy of newer antidepressants in the treatment of chronic pain: a review of current literature. Harv Rev Psychiatry 2000; 7:257–277.

28. Harden RN. Gabapentin: a new tool in the treatment of neuropathic pain. Acta Neurol Scand Suppl 1999; 173:43–47.

29. Carter GT, Galer BS. Advances in the management of neuropathic pain. Phys Med Rehabil Clin N Am 2001; 12:447–459.

30. Martin R, Meador K, Turrentine L, et al. Comparative cognitive effects of carbamazepine and gabapentin in healthy senior adults. Epilepsia 2001; 42:764–771.

31. Martin R, Kuzniecky R, Ho S, et al. Cognitive effects of topiramate, gabapentin, and lamotrigine in healthy young adults. Neurology 1999; 52:321–327.

32. Vilming ST, Lyberg T, Lataste X. Tizanidine in the management of trigeminal neuralgia. Cephalalgia 1986; 6:181–182.

33. Ettinger MP. Aging bone and osteoporosis: strategies for preventing fractures in the elderly. Arch Intern Med 2003; 163:2237–2246.

34. Sinaki M, Itoi E, Wahner HW, et al. Stronger back muscles reduce the incidence of vertebral fractures: a prospective 10 year follow-up of postmenopausal women. Bone 2002; 30:836–841.

35. Amundsen T, Weber H, Nordal HJ Magnes B, Abdelnoor M, Lilleås F. Lumbar spinal stenosis: conservative or surgical management? A prospective 10-year study. Spine 2000; 25:1424–1436.

36. Ragab AA, Fye MA, Bohlman HH. Surgery of the lumbar spine for spinal stenosis in 118 patients 70 years of age or older. Spine 2003; 28:348–353.

37. Arinzon Z, Adunsky A, Fidelman Z, Gepstein R. Outcomes of decompression surgery for lumbar spinal stenosis in elderly diabetic patients. Eur Spine J 2004; 13:32–37.

38. Cheshire WP. Defining the role for gabapentin in the treatment of trigeminal neuralgia: a retrospective report. J Pain 2002; 3:137–142.
39. Erdem E, Alkan A. Peripheral glycerol injections in the treatment of idiopathic trigeminal neuralgia: retrospective analysis of 157 cases. J Oral Maxillofac Surg 2001; 59:1176–1180.
40. Mendoza N, Illingworth RD. Trigeminal neuralgia treated by microvascular decompression: a long-term follow-up study. Br J Neurosurg 1995; 9:13–19.
41. Petit JH, Herman JM, Nagda S, DiBiase SJ, Chin LS. Radiosurgical treatment of trigeminal neuralgia: evaluating quality of life and treatment outcomes. Int J Radiation Oncology Biol Phys 2003; 56:1147–1153.

CME QUESTIONS—CHAPTER 13

1. Common pain syndromes in elderly patients include:

   a. Arthritis
   b. Migraine
   c. Osteoporosis with fracture
   d. A and C
   e. All of the above

2. Which statement(s) about musculoskeletal pain in the elderly is/are true?

   a. Prevalence of low back pain increases with aging.
   b. Osteoporosis increases risk of hip fracture five times in elderly patients.
   c. Lumbar stenosis pain is relieved by back extension.
   d. All of the above

3. Which statement about headaches in elderly patients is true?

   a. Migraine becomes more frequent with aging.
   b. New-onset headache may be observed for 6 months before a work-up.
   c. Symptoms of temporal arteritis often include head pain, scalp tenderness, and jaw claudication.
   d. Gabapentin is the most effective treatment for trigeminal neuralgia.

4. Effective and tolerated pain management therapies in the elderly include:

   a. Stationary bicycling
   b. Tai Chi
   c. Biofeedback
   d. Tramadol
   e. All of the above

14

Gender and Ethnic Issues in Chronic Pain

CASE HISTORY

Mrs. Thomas is a 65-year-old Mexican-American woman who has lived in the United States with her family for the past 30 years. She is troubled with disabling arthritis in her lower extremities, which interferes with her ability to perform household chores and care for her three active grandchildren. She comes to the doctor in tears, asking if there is some additional therapy she can use besides ibuprofen. Mrs. Thomas' daughter and two of the grandchildren accompany her to the appointment and also describe Mrs. Thomas' severe pain, explaining that she is often heard praying for relief and moaning with pain. Her daughter also notes that Mrs. Thomas has talked about seeing a *curandero*, a traditional healer in their community, if the doctor can't offer any additional therapy. Mrs. Thomas' doctor feels annoyed at what he perceives to be a threat of seeking care with an additional practitioner, hearing the message, "Even someone with no real medical training would be better than you!" He is concerned that Mrs. Thomas is exaggerating the severity of her pain complaints in order to obtain opioid prescriptions, and recommends that she continue using ibuprofen.

* * *

Caring for patients with chronic pain requires knowledge of patient gender and cultural experiences, which may color the pain experience, presentation, and response to therapy. Physician biases can interfere with understanding the impact of pain complaints and the need for therapy. Research studies are available that explore differences in pain perception based on gender and ethnicity, with fewer studies exploring differences in physician responses and treatment practices. In addition, studies have shown important differences in medication response between genders, which should be considered when selecting treatment.

KEY CHAPTER POINTS

- Women are more sensitive to pain, with a lower pain threshold and tolerance than men.

From: *Chronic Pain: A Primary Care Guide to Practical Management*
Edited by: D. A. Marcus © Humana Press, Totowa, NJ

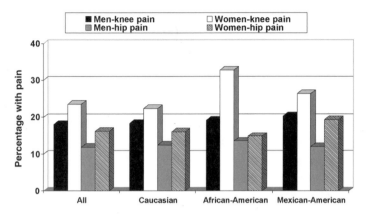

Fig. 1. Prevalence of severe knee or hip pain occurring on most days in adults ≥60 years old. Both gender and ethnicity influence likelihood of experiencing severe knee or hip pain. (Based on refs. *1,2*.)

- Women are less responsive than men to analgesic therapy, including therapy with ibuprofen and morphine.
- Pain perception is similar among ethnic groups; however, pain tolerance is reduced in Asians and African-Americans. Pain-related psychological distress and disability is also higher in African-Americans.
- Physicians are more likely to prescribe nonspecific analgesics and lower dosages of opioid analgesics to non-Caucasians.
- Patient selection of alternative or complementary therapy varies by ethnicity.

Large-scale samples of chronic pain sufferers show differences in pain based on gender and ethnicity. For example, review of severe knee and hip pain in older adults participating in the third National Health and Nutrition Examination Survey showed increased prevalence of severe pain in women overall, as well as non-Caucasian women (Fig. 1) *(1,2)*. Like Mrs. Thomas, older Mexican-American women have a higher prevalence of severe knee and hip pain compared with men and Caucasian women.

Understanding gender and ethnic differences in pain perception and treatment response helps doctors successfully tailor treatment programs to maximize treatment acceptability and efficacy. Invalid cultural stereotypes may color clinicians' views when selecting treatment, resulting in inadequate care. For example, doctors may misinterpret pain severity if they assume Asian patients are stoic, with a high pain tolerance, whereas Hispanics are dramatic, with a low pain tolerance. Although further studies are needed to fully understand pain perception and response differences between genders and among ethnic groups, current studies do provide a framework for beginning to understand that important gender and ethnic differences do exist.

1. GENDER DIFFERENCES IN PAIN EXPERIENCE

Epidemiological studies of community samples demonstrate important gender differences in chronic pain perception, with increased pain prevalence and severity in women. A statewide Australian health survey of more than 17,500 adults identified chronic pain in 20% of women and 17% of men *(3)*. Of the 13% of the sample reporting interference in activities of daily living (ADLs) from pain, 60% were female. In addition, females with chronic pain (with or without interference) reported increased psychological distress, compared to females without chronic pain. Men only reported increased psychological distress if they experienced both chronic pain and interference with ADLs. Similar findings were obtained in a cross-sectional survey of 1051 adults in Hong Kong *(4)*. Chronic pain was identified in 10.8%, with a female preponderance (56%). Female gender was identified as an independent risk factor for chronic pain (odds ratio [OR] = 1.5). In this sample, women did not report more pain interference than men; however, women were more likely to seek medical advice than men (81 vs 63%).

1.1. Pain Perception Differs Between Genders

Pain perception and response differ between men and women. Women have a lower pain threshold, pain tolerance, and analgesic response after exposure to experimental pain compared with men *(5,6)*. Women with acute pain report greater pain and analgesic use than males *(7)*, whereas women with chronic pain report greater pain severity, frequency, duration, and interference with ADLs and responsibilities *(8,9)*.

Gender differences in pain experience can be at least partially attributed to neural influences of sex hormones. In addition to providing reproductive functions, sex hormones, like estrogen, also act as important pain modulators. Chronic exposure to estrogen increases the risk for developing chronically painful conditions and results in increased pain sensitivity *(10)*. In addition to an overall pattern of increased pain susceptibility in women based on chronic hormonal exposure, cycling estrogen levels cause regular and predictable variations in pain perception.

As estrogen cycles, important pain-modulating neurotransmitters, including serotonin, γ-aminobutyric acid, endorphins, norepinephrine, and dopamine, change in response *(11)*. High estrogen results in an increase in pain-blocking neurochemicals, whereas pain-activating neurochemicals increase when estrogen falls to low levels (Fig. 2). This direct link between pain modulation and changing estrogen levels results in increases in pain threshold with rising estradiol in both rodents *(12)* and humans *(13)*. For example, pain threshold increases as estradiol levels rise during the normal menstrual cycle *(5)*. When estradiol levels drop with menstruation, 60% of women with chronic headache and 40% with irritable bowel syndrome will notice predictable aggravation of pain symp-

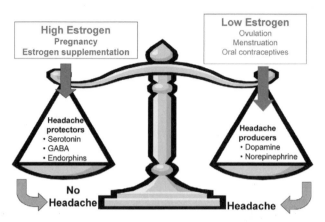

Fig. 2. Changing levels of pain-modulating neurochemicals in response to estradiol cycling. These neurochemicals change in response to cycling estradiol. Elevations in estradiol, such as during pregnancy or with estrogen supplementation (such as low-dose hormonal therapy of menstrual migraine [*see* Chapter 4]), results in increases in pain-blocking neurotransmitters. When estradiol drops from a high to a low level, such as with ovulation, menses, or during the placebo week of oral contraceptives, pain-activating neurotransmitter activity increases. GABA, γ-aminobutyric acid.

toms *(14)*. Rheumatoid arthritis (RA) symptoms also cycle with menstruation, with cyclical changes in joint swelling, morning stiffness, pain, and grip strength *(15,16)*.

Pregnancy is associated with consistently reduced chronic pain complaints when estrogen levels are high, and increased complaints following estrogen withdrawal postpartum (Fig. 3) *(12)*. Headache improvement occurs during pregnancy for 50 to 80% of migraineurs *(17–19)* and worsens in the early postpartum period for 50% *(20,21)*. Similarly, the incidence of RA decreases during pregnancy (OR = 0.64), and increases during the first 3 months postpartum (OR = 3.4) *(22)*. Joint improvement occurs during the third trimester with reduced pain in 66% and reduced swelling in 64% *(23)*. Joint pain worsens during the first 6 months postpartum for about 77%.

1.2. Psychological Differences in Pain Perception

Thoughts about the pain experience significantly influence pain perception and chronicity. Catastrophizing describes a tendency to exaggerate the impact of pain and the inability of the patient to cope with the pain. This would include feelings like, "My pain is never going to improve," "I am helpless to reduce my pain," and "Pain makes life so it's not worth living."

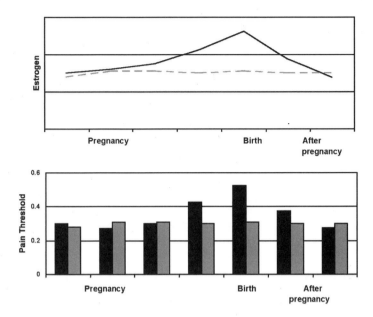

Fig. 3. Response of pain threshold to estradiol changes with pregnancy. In this novel experiment, rodents were treated with placebo (dotted line and gray bars) or changing doses of estradiol that simulated normally occurring levels during pregnancy (solid line and black bars). Pain threshold experiments were completed over the month of the normal rodent pregnancy. Pain threshold was constant in the placebo-treated rodents, but changed in conjunction with changing estradiol levels in the estradiol-treated rodents. Pain threshold reached its peak at maximum estradiol dosage, occurring at the time of birth, and decreased once estradiol levels dropped postpartum. (Based on ref. *12.*)

Unrealistic, negative thoughts about pain, like catastrophizing, increase pain severity and persistence *(24,25)*. Additionally, functional magnetic resonance imaging testing shows increased activation of sensory, attention, and emotional areas of the brain during exposure to pressure sensations in patients with higher catastrophic thinking, resulting in increased pain perception *(26)*. Scores on scales that measure catastrophic thinking in pain patients are one and one-half to more than twice as high in women compared with men *(27,28)*. These psychological differences in the cognitive response to the pain experience may also worsen pain perception in women.

1.3. Gender and Chronic Pain Treatment

Gender differences in chronic pain can perhaps be most easily noticed when spouses are interviewed together. Husbands and wives often report different pain reactions and severity after exposure to similar pain-provoking situations.

Additionally, they often report differing responses to common pain management strategies, like distracting themselves from pain or even common analgesic medications. These anecdotal reports reflect important physiological differences in pain processing between genders.

1.3.1. Gender Differences in Seeking Treatment

Women are overrepresented in chronic pain patient samples, with the female predominance in patient samples in excess of what would be predicted from community samples of gender differences in pain prevalence. Women are more likely than men to seek medical care for all medical problems, including chronic pain. Men are less likely to seek medical treatment overall *(29,30)* and they delay evaluation until symptoms become severe *(31,32)* Therefore, men seen in the clinic for pain complaints have greater pain severity, interference, and disability than men with the same condition evaluated in community samples *(33,34)*.

Psychological comorbidity also increases treatment-seeking behavior. For example, comorbid psychological distress associated with fibromyalgia is significantly greater in treatment-seeking compared with community samples *(35)*. Higher prevalence of psychological distress in women in general population samples may also increase likelihood of seeking treatment *(36)*.

1.3.2. Gender-Specific Response to Pain Therapy

Response to pain therapy is also modulated by gender. In an experimental pain model, ibuprofen effectively reduced pain threshold in men, while performing no better than placebo in women (Fig. 4) *(37)*. Additionally, response to opioids is also gender-specific. μ-opioids (e.g., morphine) provide a greater analgesic response in men, whereas κ-opioids (e.g., butorphanol) provide greater analgesic response in women *(38,39)*. A study comparing postoperative pain and analgesic response prospectively in 423 women and 277 men showed the requirement for 30% higher dosing with morphine in women to achieve an analgesic response comparable to men *(40)*. These studies are supported by positron emission tomography testing, which shows objective gender differences in activation of μ-opioid receptors in the brain after exposure to experimental pain *(41)*.

Response to nonpharmacological therapies also shows gender preferences *(42)*. For example, attentional focusing on experimental pain resulted in a 39% reduction in sensory pain score in men, with no reduction of pain in women *(43)*. Personality differences also dictate different responses to nonpharmacological therapy. For example, women often respond well to visualization and imagery techniques in relaxation training, whereas men typically prefer the use of an external monitoring device (e.g., biofeedback) to assess the relaxation response.

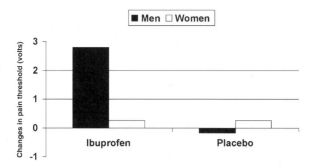

Fig. 4. Change in pain threshold after treatment with ibuprofen or placebo. Pain threshold was significantly reduced with ibuprofen in men ($p < 0.05$) and not different between ibuprofen and placebo in women. (Based on ref. *37.*)

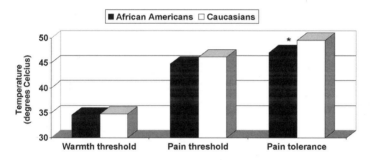

Fig. 5. Differences in pain tolerance by race. Experimental pain testing was completed in healthy college students. Warmth and pain thresholds were similar between races. Pain tolerance was significantly lower in African-Americans ($p < 0.05$). (Based on ref. *44.*)

2. ETHNIC/CULTURAL DIFFERENCES IN PAIN EXPERIENCE

Studies are beginning to identify important ethnic and cultural differences in pain tolerance, pain impact, and treatment response. Most studies have compared Caucasians and African-Americans, with fewer studies evaluating other ethnic groups. Recent studies are beginning to evaluate important differences in Hispanic and Asian populations, providing a broader context for understanding ethnic influences on the pain experience.

2.1. Pain Perception and Ethnicity

Although pain threshold is similar between ethnic groups, studies consistently show a lower pain tolerance and greater perception of pain stimuli as unpleasant in African-Americans compared with Caucasians (Fig. 5) *(44–46).*

Reduced pain tolerance in African-Americans to experimental pain supports findings in a population of patients with chronic pain that showed similar pain intensity but increased perception of pain unpleasantness in African–Americans *(47)*.

A similar study testing pain threshold in three Asian ethnic groups (Chinese, Malay, and Indian) likewise showed comparable pain thresholds among the ethnic groups *(48)*. Pain tolerance was not measured in this study. An older study did compare pain tolerance in Oriental and Occidental subjects to cold pressor pain *(49)*. Pain tolerance was reduced in Oriental subjects. In addition, analgesic response to acupuncture was not superior in Oriental subjects.

Studies comparing pain and associated symptoms in African-Americans and Caucasians show increased symptoms of depression and posttraumatic stress disorder in African-Americans *(50)*. Large samples of patients with chronic pain show increased pain-related depression, anxiety, anger, fear, and disability in African-Americans compared with Caucasians ($p < 0.05$) *(51,52)*. Fewer studies have evaluated other ethnic groups. A large study of 4700 participants in a health survey identified significantly higher scores on screening for depression in Hispanics, African-Americans, and American Indians in comparisons to Caucasians *(53)*. Further studies are needed to determine if this same trend would be seen in patients with chronic pain.

2.2. Treatment Selection and Ethnicity

Treatments may vary by ethnicity because of differences in physician prescribing practices, as well as variations in acceptability of treatments among different ethnic groups. For example, Mrs. Thomas described using prayer when pain was severe. Although the doctor interpreted prayer as a sign of hopelessness or catastrophizing, religion is an important coping tool for Hispanic patients *(54)*. Hispanics view prayer as an effective, active coping strategy that results in enhanced psychological well-being. Rather than negating the value of religion as a coping tool for Mrs. Thomas, her physician should reinforce this practice as a way to help minimize pain impact.

2.2.1. Medications

A study asking doctors to determine therapy for patients with different ethnic backgrounds based on clinical vignettes showed no difference based on patient ethnicity *(55)*. Similarly, a comparison of pain management for acute fracture in the emergency room showed similar use of analgesics in Caucasians, Hispanics, African-Americans, and Asians *(56)*. This study, however, only looked at whether analgesic therapy was prescribed and did not compare analgesic type or dosage.

Physician prescribing practices do show important ethnic differences (Fig. 6) *(57)*. A study assessing analgesic dosing in patients after surgery for fracture

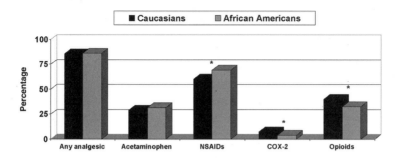

Fig. 6. Racial differences in treatment of osteoarthritis. Use of nonspecific nonsteroidal anti-inflammatory drugs (NSAIDs) was higher in African-Americans, whereas Caucasians were more likely to be prescribed selective cyclooxygenase inhibitors (COX-2) or opioids ($*p < 0.001$). (Based on ref. *57.*)

showed higher morphine-equivalent analgesic daily dosages in Caucasians (22 mg) compared with African-Americans (16 mg) and Hispanics (13 mg; $p < 0.01$) *(58)*. An earlier study of postoperative pain similarly showed that, although opioid self-administered through patient-controlled analgesia immediately after surgery was similar among ethnic groups, physician-prescribed dosing was lower after conversion to oral dosing in Hispanics and Asians compared to Caucasians and African-Americans *(59)*.

The role of ethnicity in selecting nonanalgesic therapy in patients with pain has been less well studied. One study evaluating the use of antidepressants for depression and chronic pain in Hispanic and non-Hispanic patients showed no significant ethnic differences *(60)*.

Ethnicity may also influence use of prescribed therapy. In one study, although Caucasian and African-American patients with osteoarthritis were prescribed the same number of medications, the number of prescriptions that were actually filled were significantly lower for African-Americans ($p < 0.001$) *(57)*. In another study, prescribed medications were not purchased by 11% of Caucasians, 16% of Hispanics, and 20% African-Americans *(61)*. Reasons for failure to obtain prescribed medications may include cost constraints, misunderstanding or fear about prescribed therapy, or failure of the prescribed therapy to correspond to treatment expectations.

2.2.2 Complementary and Alternative and Medicine

In a population-based survey of adults with chronic pain, 18% reported using an alternative therapist during the preceding year and 16% used alternative medications *(62)*. The use of complementary and alternative medicine (CAM) is highest in Caucasians, although selection of individual therapies varies by ethnic group (Figs. 7 and 8) *(63,64)*. For example, Hispanics, like Mrs. Thomas,

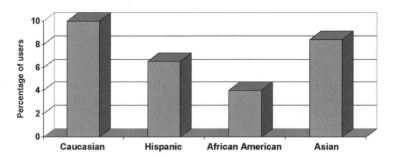

Fig. 7. Use of complementary and alternative medicine. Complementary and alternative medicine was used by 9% of the US adult population during 1996. Odds ratio for using these therapies was related to ethnic group: Caucasian = 1.0; Hispanic = 0.58; African-American = 0.46; and Asian = 0.66. (Based on ref. *63*.)

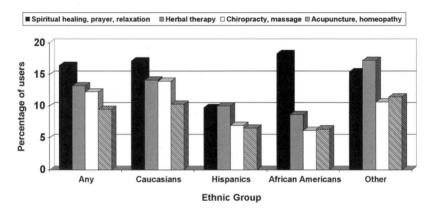

Fig. 8. Use of types of complementary and alternative medicine. (Based on ref. *64*.)

in comparison with non-Hispanics, are 10 times more likely to use traditional folk medicine *(65)*. A survey of Hispanic pediatric patients identified use of traditional healers by 20% of the children *(66)*.

Elderly have increased use of CAM. One survey identified use of CAM in 48% of the elderly, most frequently dietary supplements (47%), chiropracty (16%), home remedies (16%), acupuncture (15%), and Oriental medicine (13%) *(67)*. Choice of individual therapy was predicted by ethnic group, with Caucasians more likely to use chiropracty, massage, vitamins, diet, and psychospiritual therapy; Hispanics more likely to use dietary supplements, home remedies, and folk healers; and Asians more likely to use acupuncture and Oriental medicine.

3. SUMMARY

Gender and ethnicity significantly influence pain tolerance and therapeutic response. False gender and ethnic stereotypes can color health care providers' assessment and treatment practices, resulting, as in the case of Mrs. Thomas, in miscommunication, frustration, and poor pain control. Consistent, scientifically studied variations in the pain experience between men and women and among ethnic groups should be noted when making clinical practice decisions, so that pain evaluation and treatment is maximized for all patients.

Studies have shown that women are more sensitive to pain, with a lower pain threshold and tolerance. In addition, women are less responsive than men to analgesic therapy, including therapy with ibuprofen and morphine. These differences are mediated in part by estradiol, as demonstrated by similar pain differences in humans and rodent pain models in response to changing estradiol levels. Pain perception is similar among ethnic groups; however, pain tolerance is reduced in Asians and African-Americans. Pain-related psychological distress and disability is also higher in African-Americans.

Although physicians report using similar treatment strategies with case vignettes regardless of ethnicity, actual prescribing patterns identify important differences, with non-Caucasians more likely to receive prescriptions for nonspecific analgesics and lower dosages of opioids. The resultant possible undertreatment of chronic pain is further compounded by the fact that non-Caucasians are also less likely to fill prescriptions. This tendency to undertreat non-Caucasians who have greater pain distress and disability must be corrected in clinical practice.

REFERENCES

1. Christmas C, Crespo CJ, Franckowiak SC, Bathon JM, Bartlett SJ, Andersen RE. How common is hip pain among older adults? Results from the Third National Health and Nutrition Examination Survey. J Fam Pract. 2002; 51:345–348.
2. Andersen RE, Crespo CJ, Ling SM, Bathon JM, Bartlett SJ. Prevalence of significant knee pain among older Americans: results from the Third National Health and Nutrition Examination Survey. J Am Geriatr Soc. 1999; 47:1435–1438.
3. Blyth FM, March LM, Brnabic AM, et al. Chronic pain in Australia: a prevalence study. Pain 2001; 89:127–134.
4. Ng KJ, Tsui SL, Chan WS. Prevalence of common chronic pain in Hong Kong adults. Clin J Pain 2002; 18:275–281.
5. Hellstrom B, Lundberg U. Pain perception to the cold pressor test during the menstrual cycle in relation to estrogen levels and a comparison with men. Integr Physiol Behav Sci 2000; 35:1377–1379.
6. Keogh E, Herdenfeldt M. Gender, coping and the perception of pain. Pain 2002; 97:195–201.
7. Zeichner A, Loftin M, Panopoulos G, et al. Sex differences in pain indices, exercise, and use of analgesics. Psychol Rep 2000; 86:129–133.
8. Unruh AM. Gender variations in clinical pain experience. Pain 1996; 65:123–167.

9. Unruh AM, Ritchie J, Merskey H. Does gender affect appraisal of pain and pain coping strategies? Clin J Pain 1999; 15:31–40.

10. Coyle DE, Sehlhorst CS, Behbehani MM. Intact female rats are more susceptible to the development of tactile allodynia than ovariectomized female rats following partial sciatic nerve ligation (PSNL). Neurosci Lett 1996; 203:37–40.

11. Marcus DA. Interrelationships of neurochemicals, estrogen, and recurring headache. Pain 1995; 62:129–139.

12. Dawson-Basoa MB, Gintzler AR. 17-Beta-estradiol and progesterone modulate an intrinsic opioid analgesic system. Brain Res 1993; 601:241–245.

13. Cogan R, Spinnato JA. Pain and discomfort thresholds in late pregnancy. Pain 1986; 27:63–68.

14. Lee OY, Mayer EA, Schmulson M, Chang L, Naliboff B. Gender-related differences in IBS symptoms. Am J Gastroenterology 2001; 96:2184–2193.

15. Latman NS. Relation of menstrual cycle phase to symptoms of rheumatoid arthritis. Am J Med 1983; 74:957–960.

16. Rudge SR, Kowanko IC, Drury PL. Menstrual cyclicity of finger joint size and grip strength in patients with rheumatoid arthritis. Ann Rheum Dis 1983; 42:425–430.

17. Callaghan N. The migraine syndrome in pregnancy. Neurology 1968; 18:197–199.

18. Granella F, Sances G, Zanferrari C, et al. Migraine without aura and reproductive life events: a clinical epidemiological study in 1300 women. Headache 1993; 33:385–389.

19. Maggioni F, Alessi C, Maggino T, et al. Primary headaches and pregnancy. Cephalalgia 1995; 15:54.

20. Stein GS. Headaches in the first post partum week and their relationship to migraine. Headache 1981; 21:201–205.

21. Stein GS, Morton J, Marsh A, et al. Headaches after childbirth. Acta Neurol Scand 1984; 69:74–79.

22. Lansink M, de Boer A, Dijkmans BA, et al. The onset of rheumatoid arthritis in relation to pregnancy and childbirth. Clin Exp Rheumatol 1993; 1:171–174.

23. Barrett JH, Brennan P, Fiddler M, Silman AJ. Does rheumatoid arthritis remit during pregnancy and relapse postpartum? Results from a nationwide study in the United Kingdom performed prospectively from late pregnancy. Arthritis Rheum 1999; 42:1219–1227.

24. Jensen MP, Ehde DM, Hoffman AJ, Patterson DR, Czerniecki JM, Robinson LR. Cognitions, coping and social environment predict adjustment to phantom limb pain. Pain 2002; 95:133–142.

25. Haythornthwaite JA, Clark MR, Pappagallo M, Raja SN. Pain coping strategies play a role in the persistence of pain in post-herpetic neuralgia. Pain 2003; 106:453–460.

26. Gracely RH, Geisser ME, Giesecke T, et al. Pain catastrophizing and neural responses to pain among persons with fibromyalgia. Brain 2004; 127(Pt 4):835–843.

27. Keefe FJ, Lefebvre JC, Egert JR, Affleck G, Sullivan MJ, Caldwell DS. The relationship of gender to pain, pain behavior, and disability in osteoarthritis patients: the role of catastrophizing. Pain 2000; 87:325–334.

28. Sullivan ML, Tripp DA, Santor D. Gender differences in pain and pain behavior: the role of catastrophizing. Cognitive Ther Res 2000; 24:121–134.

29. Linet MS, Celentano DD, Stewart WF. Headache characteristics associated with physician consultation: a population-based survey. Am J Prev Med 1991; 7: 40–46.

30. Davies J, McCrae BP, Frank J, et al. Identifying male college students' health needs, barriers to seeking help, and recommendations to help men adopt healthier lifestyles. J Am Coll Health 2000; 48:259–267.

31. Ottesen MM, Kober L, Jorgensen S, Torp-Pedersen C. Determinants of delay between symptoms and hospital admission in 5978 patients with acute myocardial infarction. Eur Heart J 1996; 17:429–37.

32. Johansson E, Long NH, Diwan VK, Winkvist A. Gender and tuberculosis control. Perspectives on health seeking behaviour among men and women in Vietnam. Health Policy 2000; 52:33–51.

33. Marcus DA. Gender differences in treatment-seeking chronic headache sufferers, Headache 2001; 41:698–703.

34. Marcus DA. Gender differences in chronic pain in a treatment-seeking population. J Gend Specif Med 2003; 6:19–24.

35. Aaron LA, Bradley LA, Alarcon GS, et al. Psychiatric diagnoses in patients with fibromyalgia are related to health care-seeking behavior rather than to illness. Arthritis Rheum 1996; 39:436–445.

36. Carroll LJ, Cassidy JD, Cote P. The Saskatchewan Health and Back Pain Survey: the prevalence and factors associated with depressive symptomatology in Saskatchewan adults. Can J Public Health 2000; 91:459–464.

37. Walker JS, Carmody JJ. Experimental pain in healthy human subjects: gender differences in nociception and in response to ibuprofen. Anesth Analg 1998; 86: 1257–1262.

38. Gear RW, Miaskowski C, Gordon NC, et al. Kappa-opioid produce significantly greater analgesia in women than in men. Nat Med 1996; 2:1248–1250.

39. Miller PL, Ernst AA. Sex differences in analgesia: a randomized trial of mu versus kappa opioid agonists. South Med J 2004; 97:35–41.

40. Cepeda MS, Carr DB. Women experience more pain and require more morphine than men to achieve a similar degree of analgesia. Anesth Analg 2003; 97:1464–1468.

41. Zubieta JK, Dannals RF, Frost JJ. Gender and age influences on human brain mu-opioid receptor binding measured by PET. Am J Psychiatry 1999; 156:842–848.

42. Jensen IB, Bergstrom G, Ljungquist T, Bodin L, Nygren AL. A randomized controlled component analysis of a behavioral medicine rehabilitation program for chronic spinal pain: are the effects dependent on gender? Pain 2001; 91:65–78.

43. Keogh E, Hatton K, Ellery D. Avoidance versus focused attention and the perception of pain: differential effects for men and women. Pain 2000; 85:225–230.

44. Edwards RR, Fillingim RB. Ethnic differences in thermal pain responses. Psychosomatic Med 1999; 61:346–354.

45. Sheffield D, Biles PL, Orom H, Maixner W, Sheps DS. Race and sex differences in cutaneous pain perception. Psychosom Med 2000; 62:517–523.

46. Edwards RR, Doleys DM, Fillingim RB, Lowery D. Ethnic differences in pain tolerance: clinical implications in a chronic pain population. Psychosom Med 2001; 63:316–323.
47. Riley JL, Wade JB, Myers CD, Sheffield D, Papas RK, Price DD. Racial/ethnic differences in the experience of chronic pain. Pain 2002; 100:291–298.
48. Yosipovitch G, Meredith G, Chan YH, Goh CL. Do ethnicity and gender have an impact on pain thresholds in minor dermatologic procedures? A study on thermal pain perception thresholds in Asian ethnic groups. Skin Res Technol 2004; 10:38–42.
49. Knox VJ, Shum K, McLaughlin DM. Response to cold pressor pain and to acupuncture analgesia in Oriental and Occidental subjects. Pain 1977; 4:49–57.
50. Green CR, Baker TA, Smith EM, Sato Y. The effect of race in older adults presenting for chronic pain management: a comparative study of black and white Americans. J Pain 2003; 4:82–90.
51. McCracken LM, Matthews AK, Tang TS, Cuba SL. A comparison of blacks and whites seeking treatment for chronic pain. Clin J Pain 2001; 17:249–255.
52. Riley JL, Wade JB, Myers CD, Sheffield D, Papas RK, Price DD. Racial/ethnic differences in the experience of chronic pain. Pain 2002; 100:291–298.
53. Plant EA, Sachs-Ericsson N. Racial and ethnic differences in depression: the roles of social support and meeting basic needs. J Consult Clin Psychol 2004; 72:41–52.
54. Abraído-Lanza AF, Vásquez E, Echeverría SE. En las manos de Dios [in God's hands]: religious and other forms of coping among Latinos with arthritis. J Consult Clin Psychol 2004; 72:91–102.
55. Tamayo-Sarver JH, Dawson NV, Hinze SW, et al. The effect of race/ethnicity and desirable social characteristics on physicians' decisions to prescribe opioid analgesics. Acad Emerg Med 2003; 10:1239–1248.
56. Fuentes EF, Kohn MA, Neighbor ML. Lack of association between patient ethnicity or race and fracture analgesia. Acad Emerg Med 2002; 9:910–915.
57. Dominick KL, Dudley TK, Grambow SC, Oddone EZ, Bosworth HB. Racial differences in health care utilization among patients with osteoarthritis. J Rheumatol 2003; 30:2201–2206.
58. Ng B, Dimsdale JE, Shragg GP, Deutsch R. Ethnic differences in analgesic consumption for postoperative pain. Psychosom Med 1996; 58:125–129.
59. Ng B, Dimsdale JE, Rollnick JD, Shapiro H. The effect of ethnicity on prescriptions for patient-controlled analgesia for post-operative pain. Pain 1996; 66:9–12.
60. Sleath BL, Rubin RH, Huston SA. Antidepressant prescribing to Hispanic and non-Hispanic white patients in primary care. Ann Pharmacother 2001; 35:419–423.
61. Reed M, Hargraves JL. Prescription drug access disparities among working-age Americans. Issue Brief Cent Study Health Syst Change 2003; 73:1–4.
62. Haetzman M, Elliott AM, Smith BH, Hannaford P, Chambers WA. Chronic pain and the use of conventional and alternative therapy. Fam Pract 2003; 20:147–154.
63. Bausell RB, Lee W, Berman BM. Demographic and health-related correlates of visits to complementary and alternative medical providers. Med Care 2001; 39:190–196.
64. Ni H, Simile C, Hardy AM. Utilization of complementary and alternative medicine by United States adults. Results from the 1999 National Health Interview Survey. Med Care 2002; 40:353–358.

65. Palinkas LA, Kabongo ML. The use of complementary and alternative medicine by primary care patients: a SURF*NET study. J Fam Pract 2000; 49:1121–1130.
66. Risser AL, Mazur LJ. Use of folk remedies in a Hispanic population. Arch Pediatr Adolesc Med 1995; 149:978–981.
67. Najm W, Reinsch S, Hoehler F, Tobis J. Use of complementary and alternative medicine among the ethnic elderly. Altern Ther Health Med 2003; 9:50–57.

CME QUESTIONS—CHAPTER 14

1. In comparison to men tested with experimental pain, women have:
    a. A higher pain threshold
    b. A greater pain tolerance
    c. A lower response to analgesic medication
    d. A and B
    e. All of the above

2. Osteoarthritis of the knee and hip occur more commonly in elderly:
    a. Men
    b. Women
    c. Caucasians
    d. Hispanics
    e. A and C
    f. B and D

3. Which of the following statements is true?
    a. Physicians believe they prescribe similarly to different ethnic groups.
    b. Physicians are less likely to prescribe COX-2 specific anti-inflammatory medications to non-Caucasians.
    c. Physicians are more likely to prescribe lower doses of opioids to non-Caucasians.
    d. None of the above
    e. All of the above

4. Which statement is true:
    a. Non-Caucasians have a higher pain threshold.
    b. Because the pain threshold is higher in non-Caucasians, they require lower doses of analgesics.
    c. Acceptability of complementary and alternative medicine is similar among ethnic groups.
    d. None of the above
    e. All of the above

V
Comorbid Conditions

15

Psychological Comorbidity

CASE HISTORY

Ms. Malone is a 43-year-old nurse who works in a prenatal intensive care unit. She developed low back pain while lifting equipment at work 2 years earlier. She was initially work disabled for 6 months, but successfully returned to modified nursing duties after completing physical therapy and work hardening. She has continued to experience low back pain and comes to her primary care physician (PCP) to see if any additional therapy may help reduce the severity of her pain flares, which often interfere with her sleep. The PCP notices that Ms. Malone is fidgeting in the chair and becomes teary-eyed when describing her inability to perform all of the household chores because of limits resulting from pain. When asked if she is depressed, Ms. Malone begins to sob, "I knew you'd think it was all just in my head! I'm not depressed—I'm in pain! Why doesn't anyone understand that?!" Further gentle probing reveals frequent episodes of crying at work, difficulty with sleep, and a 25-lb unintentional weight loss. When not working, Ms. Malone tends to retreat to her bed at home and resents her family's efforts to get her involved in activities she used to enjoy. She also describes resentment that her teenage children now effectively perform many of the household and meal-preparation chores, leaving her to feel she has lost her position as household manager. Ms. Malone has also recently "lost interest" in her exercise program, which was previously very beneficial in managing her pain and pain flares.

* * *

Psychological distress occurs commonly in patients with chronic pain. Pain and psychological distress can produce a vicious cycle: pain results in increased depression and anxiety, and depression and anxiety increase pain complaints. Although Ms. Malone's pain started after a work injury, she describes current symptoms of significant depression that are aggravating her pain and interfering with her previously effective pain management program by affecting her sleep, activity level, and compliance with exercise therapy. In her case, effective treatment must include primary management of depression rather than simply the addition of pain medications or pain-relieving therapy.

From: *Chronic Pain: A Primary Care Guide to Practical Management*
Edited by: D. A. Marcus © Humana Press, Totowa, NJ

KEY CHAPTER POINTS

- Psychological distress occurs in about half of all chronic pain patients.
- Premorbid depression, anxiety, and history of childhood abuse increase risk for chronic pain in adults.
- Current depression and anxiety increase risk for developing persistent pain.
- Identifying and treating psychological distress is an important aspect of pain management.
- Psychological pain management skills, such as cognitive–behavioral therapy, relaxation, and stress management, are effective tools for reducing pain severity and impact.

Psychological symptoms commonly accompany chronic pain. Nearly half of all patients with a pain disorder have associated psychological or psychiatric comorbidity *(1)*. The National Comorbidity Survey identified mood and anxiety disorders in a community sample of 5877 individuals, aged 15 to 54 years old *(2)*. Chronic pain was endorsed by 6.5%. Both mood and anxiety disorders occurred more commonly in those with chronic pain ($p < 0.05$) (Fig. 1).

Patients like Ms. Malone often argue that their depression is not causing the pain, but the pain led to depression. There is a strong relationship between pain and psychological distress. Although pain is not usually a direct symptom of depression or anxiety, psychological symptoms do influence the pain experience. Data from the World Health Organization were analyzed to determine relationships between psychological symptoms and chronic pain *(3)*. The presence of psychological distress at baseline predicted the development and chronicity of pain complaints (Fig. 2). In addition, the persistence of pain complaints also predicted the onset of new symptoms of depression and anxiety.

1. PREMORBID PSYCHOLOGICAL FACTORS

Early life events and premorbid psychological factors can increase the risk for developing chronic pain after exposure to pain-producing situations, such as a work injury or automobile accident. Childhood exposure to traumatic or stressful events increases the risk for chronic pain in adulthood *(4)*. In addition, premorbid adult depression and anxiety also predict increased likelihood of pain chronicity *(5)*. Stress is another important factor for pain persistence. A longitudinal study of adults in the Canadian National Population Health Survey identified stress as an important predictor for the development of back pain in both men and women (odds ratio [OR]: 1.2) *(6)*. Similarly, a prospective study of newly employed workers linked several workplace psychological factors with increased risk for developing chronic pain *(7)*. Odds ratios for developing pain were 1.7 for exposure to stressful work, 1.6 for hectic work, and 1.7 for dissatisfaction with support from colleagues. Identifying premorbid psychological factors may help predict those patients at higher risk for developing more recalcitrant pain complaints, and suggest the need for more aggressive initial intervention.

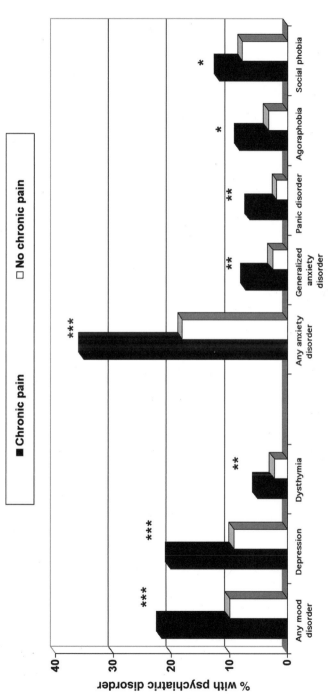

Fig. 1. Prevalence of mood and anxiety disorders in a community sample with and without chronic pain. All mood and anxiety disorders occurred more commonly in individuals with chronic pain: *$p < 0.05$; **$p < 0.01$; ***$p < 0.0001$. (Based on ref. 2.)

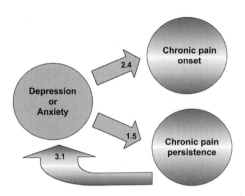

Fig. 2. Relationship between psychological distress and chronic pain, with odds ratios in directional arrows. Baseline depression or anxiety predicts both the development and persistence of pain. Persistent pain predicts the development of new-onset depression and anxiety. (Based on ref. *3*.)

1.1. Childhood Stressors and Adult Pain

Stressful, traumatic, and abusive experiences in childhood predispose patients to develop chronic pain as adults. A survey of 91 consecutive patients with chronic pain identified childhood abuse in 55%, with physical abuse in 37% and sexual abuse in 27% *(4)*. Stressful and traumatic childhood events also occurred frequently in these adults with chronic pain (Fig. 3).

1.1.1. Abuse and Chronic Pain

A comparison of studies seeking relationships between childhood abuse and chronic pain complaints showed stronger relationships when treatment-seeking patients rather than community surveys were evaluated *(8)*. This supports the hypothesis that abuse may be more closely linked to the development of treatment-seeking behavior than chronic pain. Because physicians treat patients and not community members, however, the reason for increased abuse in patients with chronic pain is probably less important than recognizing an increased risk. Abuse victims may be more likely to be seen for chronic pain complaints because abuse increases the prevalence of the pain complaint, abuse increases the likelihood that the victim will seek medical attention for a pain complaint, or a combination of both factors. In every possible scenario, patients with chronic pain are more likely to have histories of abuse, which are often unrecognized and untreated. For example, in one series, none of the men and only 4% of women who had been previously sexually abused had ever sought counseling for the abuse *(9)*. Evaluation for abuse must be part of the routine assessment of all patients with chronic pain.

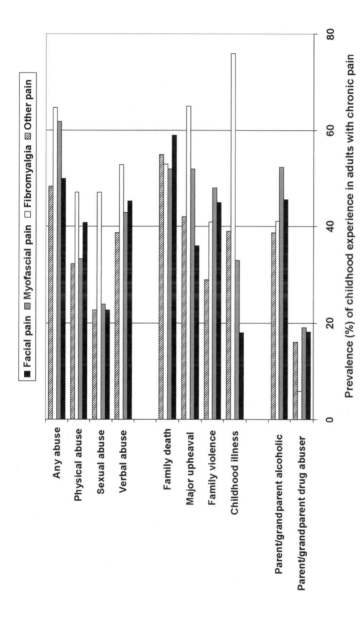

Fig. 3. Prevalence of childhood abuse, trauma, and stressors in adult chronic pain patients. (Based on ref. 4.)

A community survey of older adults identified a history of sexual assault in 5% of men and 13% of women, with repeated assaults in 10% of the sexually assaulted men and 22% of the assaulted women *(9)*. A history of sexual abuse increased risk for arthritis in women (OR = 1.8). A similar analysis of five community surveys identified increased risk for headache in victims of childhood abuse *(10)*. The odds ratio for adult headache was 1.89 in victims of childhood sexual abuse vs 1.03 for victims of sexual abuse in adulthood.

Reports of abuse are greater in treatment-seeking populations. A survey of 90 female patients with chronic pain identified abuse in nearly half, with sexual abuse alone in 18%, physical abuse alone in 11%, and both sexual and physical abuse in 19% *(11)*. Women who had been victims of abuse were more likely to report physical, pain, and anxiety somatic complaints in comparison to non-abused patients with pain ($p < 0.05$). Although visits to mental health professionals were higher for abused women, utilization of non-mental health medical services was not higher in abused women. Abuse has also been linked to increased reporting of chronic pelvic pain *(12)* and abdominal pain (*see* Chapter 6).

1.2. Depression and Anxiety

Premorbid depression and anxiety increase the risk for developing new chronic pain complaints. Workers in occupations that pose a high risk for back pain were followed after an acute back injury for the development of persistent complaints after 3 months *(5)*. Factors associated with an increased risk for chronic pain were evaluated. Both anxiety and depression predicted an increased risk for back pain chronicity (OR: 2.08 for anxiety/insomnia; 2.47 for severe depression).

2. CURRENT PSYCHOLOGICAL FACTORS

Current psychological factors are important variables in patients with chronic pain. Identification of psychological distress and primary and secondary gains are important to fully understand the patient with chronic pain. When psychological distress, such as depression in the case of Ms. Malone, or gain is very prominent, initial therapy may have to focus on these issues before pain management will be effective. For most medical patients, including patients with chronic pain, exposure to psychological symptoms or stress will aggravate the primary medical symptoms. Identifying and treating those factors that typically aggravate chronic pain—such as depressed mood, anxiety, and stress—are important aspects of patient care.

2.1. Stress

Mental stress is one of the most common triggers of chronic medical symptoms. Exposure to stress increases cardiac symptoms in patients with heart

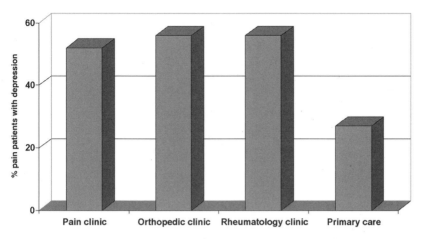

Fig. 4. Prevalence of depression in chronic pain patients. (Based on ref. *16.*)

disease, bowel symptoms in patients with gastrointestinal disorders, seizures in patients with epilepsy, and pain in chronic pain sufferers. Stress is identified as a usual trigger for pain flares by 31% of patients with chronic pain *(13)*. Pain flares triggered by stress exposure are no less "real" than the heart attack occurring during a stressful situation.

Stress aggravates chronic pain through a variety of physiological changes in the nervous system, specifically through changes in a variety of neurotransmitters important for pain transmission. For example, stress leads to hyperalgesia and changes in the activity of a variety of catecholamines that are important for pain transmission, including dopamine and norepinephrine *(14,15)*. These changes themselves will serve to aggravate pain perception.

2.2. Depression and Anxiety

A survey of 716 patients with chronic pain attending a specialty clinic identified depression in 59%, with anxiety in 56% *(13)*. Prevalence of depression is about twice as high in patients with pain who attend specialty clinics compared with primary care patients (Fig. 4) *(16)*. Depression prevalence is also higher in patients with greater pain severity (Fig. 5) *(17)*. As expected, the presence of psychological distress aggravates pain severity and impedes response to pain treatment (*see* Box 1).

Pain prevalence is also high in patients with the primary complaint of depression. A literature review identified pain in an average of 65% of individuals with depression *(16)*. Interestingly, more than 50% of depressed individuals described only somatic symptoms, with no emotional complaints.

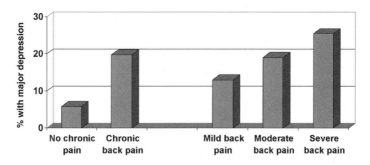

Fig. 5. Prevalence of major depression in individuals with chronic back pain. Data from the Canadian Community Health Survey–Cycle 1 (n = 118,533). Prevalence of chronic back pain was 9%. Prevalence of major depression increased with the presence of chronic back pain, as well as pain severity. (Based on ref. *17*.)

Box 1
Depression Predictions

Depression predicts:
• Onset of new pain
• Persistent pain after acute injury
• Poor response to pain treatment
• Long-term, pain-related disability

Based on ref. *16*.

Nearly 66% of these complaints were pain-related. These data further support the need to screen for depression in patients reporting chronic pain.

2.3. Primary and Secondary Gain

Primary gain is a sense of internal control or relief from anxiety that is associated with the occurrence of physical symptoms. Secondary gains are external rewards, such as financial compensation, release from unpleasant responsibilities, or increased personal attention. Patients with chronic pain rarely experience primary gain from their symptoms, usually experiencing increased conflict and anxiety from their pain complaints. In Ms. Malone's case, she feels anxious and out of control from her chronic pain, losing her work role as an intensive care nurse and home role as homemaker in charge of most household tasks. She did initially receive secondary gain after her back injury, with workers' compensation benefits.

Secondary gain issues should be evaluated in every patient with chronic pain. The presence of secondary gain does not, by itself, suggest pain symp-

---

Box 2
Internet Resources for Identification of Psychological Distress

Internet screening tools	Symptom assessed
http://mcrcr4.med.nyu.edu/Psych/screens/index.html	Depression
http://www.med.nyu.edu/Psych/screens/depres.html	Depression
http://www.freedomfromfear.org/screenrm.asp	Depression
http://www.stanford.edu/group/bipolar.clinic/what_is/primemd.htm	Depression
http://www.med.nyu.edu/Psych/screens/anx.html	Anxiety
http://www.freedomfromfear.org/screenrm.asp	Anxiety
http://www.anxietyhelp.org/information/sas_zung.html	Anxiety
http://www.anxietyhelp.org/information/hama.html	Anxiety
https://www.amihealthy.com/static/AboutSurveys.asp#SF36-v2	Quality-of-life

---

tom magnification. It is important to acknowledge, however, that patients with active litigation typically report greater pain severity and disability than similar patients without litigation *(18,19)*. Failure to identify possible conflicts with secondary gain results in a reduced understanding of the patient's needs. Open discussions about secondary gain—such as preinjury work conflicts or concerns about returning to work—facilitate the development of treatment designed to effectively address patient concerns and maximize successful reduction in pain and disability.

3. ASSESSMENT

General screening tools for depression and anxiety that are used in general medical populations are also useful in patients with chronic pain. For example, the Beck Depression Inventory and Center for Epidemiological Studies–Depression Scale effectively identify depression in patients with chronic pain *(20)*. A variety of easy-to-use screening tools are also available on the Internet (*see* Box 2). Quality-of-life (QOL) screening helps identify impact from pain on physical, social, and emotional functioning. Repeated QOL assessments can serve as monitors of treatment efficacy.

A variety of brief assessment tools are available to screen primary care patients for psychological distress. The PRIME-MD, for example is a short, 10-item questionnaire that screens for depression and is available on the Internet Website: (http://www.stanford.edu/group/bipolar.clinic/what_is/primemd.htm; accessed 3-16-04). The General Health Questionnaire-12 and Symptom Checklist-10 are also effective screening tools for mood and anxiety disorders in primary care *(21)*.

```
┌─────────────────────────────────────────────────────────┐
│                         Box 3                           │
│       Effective Psychological Pain Management Treatments │
├─────────────────────────────────────────────────────────┤
│    • Cognitive–behavioral therapy                       │
│    • Relaxation (may include biofeedback)               │
│    • Development of coping skills                        │
│    • Stress management                                  │
│    • Pain education                                     │
└─────────────────────────────────────────────────────────┘
```

4. TREATMENT

Management of patients with chronic pain needs to include reduction in psychological distress as an important treatment goal. Even in patients without significant psychological distress, a reduction in pain severity and disability are typically achieved using psychological pain management skills. Psychological forms of pain therapy are best utilized with other types of pain therapy, such as medications, physical therapy, and occupational therapy. Studies show a superior response when treatment includes both medication and psychological therapy *(22,23)*.

4.1. Treating Comorbid Psychological Symptoms

Patients with comorbid psychological disorders and chronic pain often insist that the psychological symptoms will resolve spontaneously once pain symptoms are controlled. Because psychological symptoms increase the risk for developing new and persistent pain while functioning as triggers for pain aggravation, specific treatment of psychological symptoms cannot be ignored. Patients with comorbid depression, anxiety, and so on, will need to have those symptoms addressed before or in conjunction with pain therapy. Patients with severe psychological symptoms are not able to effectively participate in rehabilitative therapy to reduce pain and will need to begin psychological therapy for the emotional disorder first. Patients who are severely depressed will have difficulty motivating themselves to comply with exercise therapy (as seen with Ms. Malone), whereas very anxious patients often tend to overuse pain medications in an effort to reduce feelings of inner agitation and distress.

4.2. Psychological Treatment of Chronic Pain

Psychological treatments of chronic pain—including education, relaxation with biofeedback, cognitive–behavioral therapy (CBT), and stress management—are uniformly effective for a wide variety of chronically painful conditions *(see* Box 3) *(24,25)*. CBT helps patients recognize distorted thinking about pain complaints and behavioral responses to pain. Strategies are then developed to replace counterproductive thoughts and behaviors with more adaptive views and responses to pain (Table 1). This type of problem-solving

Table 1
Replacing Cognitive and Behavioral Distortions With More Appropriate Thoughts and Responses

Maladaptive thoughts and responses	Adaptive thoughts and responses
Oh no. I have another migraine. Now I will never get my work done!	My migraines usually last about 6 hours. I know I can reduce the severity by taking my medicine and doing relaxation techniques. I will need to take a break to treat my migraine for about 30 minutes, but then I will be able to complete my work.
My low back pain flared when I was driving to my mother's house. I guess I'll never be able to visit her again.	I see that I can't just jump in the car and drive for 3 hours. Next time, I'd better do some stretching exercises before I start driving and schedule brief rest stops along the way.
My pain became intolerable when I returned to work after my injury. After one 8-hour day, I had to spend 2 weeks in bed. I don't plan to ever return to work.	I need to assess the different physical tasks of my job and see if the tasks might be modified to improve my ability to perform work activities. I may also need to try gradual re-entry.
I live on the sofa. I just can't do any housework anymore. All that carrying, lifting, and reaching is just too much. If the family wants meals, clean laundry, or vacuumed floors, they'd better do it themselves!	I should have a family meeting so we can decide how to divide household chores. I need to see how I can break down tasks into components that I can do. For example, I can't carry the laundry baskets, but I can sort and fold the wash.
I have no time to exercise or do relaxation techniques.	I can do my neck stretches while standing in the shower, or pelvic tilts while sitting in the office. I can do floor exercises while watching the 6 o'clock news. Relaxation techniques might be a good way to help me wind down before bed.
My pain's so bad, I refuse to even talk on the phone.	Talking on the phone aggravates my neck pain because I tend to hold the phone by squeezing it between my ear and shoulder. If I use a headset, I should be able to use the phone comfortably.
There's no point in even getting out of bed. My pain is just debilitating.	I'm going to have pain if I stay in bed or get out of bed. I might as well get up, get dressed, and start getting back into my regular routine. Staying in bed certainly isn't helping my pain.

247

Box 4
Identifying and Resuming Normal Activities

Activity assessment:

1. Select desired target activity

   _____

   _____

2. List barriers to achieving target activity

   _____

   _____

3. Identify intermediate activity that can currently be accomplished

   _____

   _____

4. Develop short-term strategy for accomplishing intermediate activity

   _____

   _____

5. Develop long-term strategy for accomplishing desired target

   _____

   _____

---

strategy helps remove patients from the role of sick and disabled and return them to being a contributing member of their social and work environment. Ms. Malone, for example, might change her impression that she no longer contributes to the family's household environment to an understanding that she and the family are now working effectively as a team to complete necessary household chores. CBT techniques can be used to help patients resume normal activity levels by first identifying a reasonable activity they wish they could do and developing a strategy plan for accomplishing it (*see* Boxes 4 and 5).

Benefits of CBT have been demonstrated across a broad range of chronic pain diagnoses and age groups, including both pediatric and geriatric patients with chronic pain *(26,27)*. Benefits include improved understanding of chronic pain, reduced pain severity, and resumption of functional activities. For example, in a study of adolescents with chronic pain and associated disability, completion of CBT resulted in improved school attendance in 64%, with 40% returning to school full time *(26)*.

5. SUMMARY

Psychological distress commonly accompanies chronic pain. Individuals with depression or anxiety are more likely to develop chronic pain and less likely to respond to pain treatment. Patients with comorbid pain and psychological distress typically require both pain management and treatment targeting psychological symptoms.

Box 5
Example of Completed Activity Assessment

---

1. Select desired target activity.
   - Shopping at an outlet mall with my daughter.
2. List barriers to achieving target activity.
   - Unable to ride in the car for the 2 hours to get to the stores.
   - Unable to stay in one position, either standing or sitting, without changing position for more than 20 minutes.
   - Unable to walk more than 45 minutes without needing to sit and rest.
   - Unable to carry heavy packages.
   - Afraid daughter will become angry and disappointed if we leave before she's done shopping.
3. Identify intermediate activity that can currently be accomplished.
   - Shopping at one store in the local mall.
4. Develop short-term strategy for accomplishing intermediate activity.
   - Discuss strategy with daughter, including need to take breaks during shopping.
   - Use a lumbar support for the car ride.
   - Arrange to do some brief stretches that can be done while standing after arriving at the mall. Follow this with 15 minutes of walking in the mall before you start shopping.
   - Select only one store to visit and agree beforehand that you won't go to any other stores that day, even if there's a great sale.
   - Take a watch and agree to shop for only 1 hour before stopping.
   - Plan to get lunch after shopping to celebrate being together.
   - After arriving home, use relaxation techniques and do your stretching exercises, even if you feel tired.
5. Develop long-term strategy for accomplishing desired target.
   - Successfully complete several brief trips to the local mall.
   - Gradually increase shopping time, remembering to take breaks to sit, stretch, and use pain management skills.
   - Identify rest stops on route to the outlet malls. Use rest stops to walk and do stretching exercises.
   - Identify two to four stores you will visit at the outlet mall.
   - Take breaks in between visiting each store.
   - Allow daughter to carry bundles to the car between stores to minimize carrying.
   - Don't be discouraged if your first attempt is not completely successful.

The use of psychological treatment techniques for chronic pain management is an important part of pain rehabilitation. Patients are most likely to improve when they combine medication, physical modalities, and psychological skills, rather than using just a single treatment modality.

REFERENCES

1. Aigner M, Bach M. Clinical utility of DSM-IV pain disorder. Compr Psychiatry 1999; 40:353–357.
2. McWilliams LA, Cox BJ, Enns MW. Mood and anxiety disorders associated with chronic pain: an examination in a nationally representative sample. Pain 2003; 106:127–133.
3. Gureje O, Simon GE, von Korff M. A cross-national study of the course of persistent pain in primary care. Pain 2001; 92:195–200.
4. Goldberg RT, Pachas WN, Keith D. Relationship between traumatic events in childhood and chronic pain. Disabil Rehabil 1999; 21:23–30.
5. Fransen M, Woodward M, Norton R, Coggan C, Dawe M, Sheridan N. Risk factors associated with the transition from acute to chronic occupational back pain. Spine 2002; 27:92–98.
6. Kopec JA, Sayre EC, Esdaile JM. Predictors of back pain in a general population cohort. Spine 2003; 29:70–78.
7. Nahit ES, Hunt IM, Lunt M, Dunn G, Silman AJ, MacFarlane GJ. Effects of psychosocial and individual psychological factors on the onset of musculoskeletal pain: common and site-specific effects. Ann Rheum Dis 2003; 62:755–760.
8. Raphael KG, Chandler HK, Ciccone DS. Is childhood abuse a risk factor for chronic pain in adulthood? Curr Pain Headache Rep 2004; 8:99–110.
9. Stein MB, Barrett-Connor E. Sexual assault and physical health: findings from a population-based study of older adults. Psychosom Med 2000; 62:838–843.
10. Golding JM. Sexual assault history and headache: five general population studies. J Nerv Ment Dis 1999; 187:624–629.
11. Green CR, Flowe-Valencia H, Rosenblum L, Tait AR. Do physical and sexual abuse differentially affect chronic pain states in women? J Pain Symptom Manage 1999;18:420–426.
12. Lampe A, Doering S, Rumpold G, et al. Chronic pain syndromes and their relation to childhood abuse and stressful life events. J Psychosom Res 2003; 54:361–367.
13. Marcus DA. Gender differences in chronic pain in a treatment-seeking population. J Gend Specif Med 2003; 6:19–24.
14. Pacak K, Palkovits M, Yadid G, Kvetnansky R, Kopin IJ, Goldstein DS. Heterogeneous neurochemical responses to different stressors: a test of Selye's doctrine of nonspecificity. Am J Physiol 1998; 275:R1247–R1255.
15. Wood PB. Stress and dopamine: implications for the pathophysiology of chronic widespread pain. Med Hypotheses 2004; 62:420–424.
16. Bair MJ, Robinson RL, Katon W, Kroenke K. Depression and pain comorbidity. a literature review. Arch Intern Med 2003; 163:2433–2445.
17. Currie SR, Wang J. Chronic back pain and major depression in the general Canadian population. Pain 2004; 107:54–60.
18. Suter PB. Employment and litigation: improved by work, assisted by verdict. Pain 2002; 100:249–257.
19. Blyth FM, March LM, Nicholas MK, Cousins MJ. Chronic pain, work performance and litigation. Pain 2003; 103:41–47.
20. Geisser ME, Roth RS, Robinson ME. Assessing depression among persons with chronic pain using the Center for Epidemiological Studies-Depression Scale and

the Beck Depression Inventory: a comparative analysis. Clin J Pain 1997; 13: 163–170.

21. Cano A, Sprafkin RP, Scaturo DJ, Lantinga LJ, Fiese BH, Brand F. Mental health screening in primary care: a comparison of 3 brief measures of psychological distress. Primary Care Companion J Clin Psychiatry 2001; 3:206–210.

22. Holroyd KA, France JC, Cordingley GE. Enhancing the effectiveness of relaxation-thermal biofeedback training with propranolol hydrochloride. J Consult Clin Psychol 1995; 63:327–330.

23. Evers AW, Kraaimaat FW, van Riel PL, de Jong AJ. Tailored cognitive-behavioral therapy in early rheumatoid arthritis for patients at risk: a randomized controlled trial. Pain 2002; 100:141–153.

24. Nielson WR, Weir R. Biopsychosocial approaches to the treatment of chronic pain. Clin J Pain 2001; 17(Suppl):S114–S127.

25. Astin JA. Mind-body therapies for the management of pain. Clin J Pain 2004; 20: 27–32.

26. Eccleston C, Malleson PN, clinch J, Connell H, Sourbut C. Chronic pain in adolescents: evaluation of a programme of interdisciplinary cognitive behaviour therapy. Arch Dis Child 2003; 88:881–885.

27. Reid MC, Otis J, Barry LC, Kerns RD. Cognitive–behavioral therapy for chronic low back pain in older persons: a preliminary study. Pain Med 2003; 4:223–230.

CME QUESTIONS—CHAPTER 15

1. Which of the following premorbid factors increases the risk for chronic pain?
    a. Sexual abuse in childhood
    b. Family violence during childhood
    c. Depression
    d. Anxiety
    e. All of the above

2. Which of the following statements is false?
    a. Work stress and a hectic schedule increase the likelihood of chronic pain.
    b. Depression and anxiety increase the risk for chronic pain.
    c. In most patients, chronic pain is really an acceptable way to describe feelings of work inadequacy and depression.
    d. Secondary gain often increases reports of pain severity and disability.

3. Which of the following statements is true?
    a. Screening for depression and anxiety should be reserved for patients with obvious symptomatology.
    b. Psychological symptoms rarely impact medical illnesses.
    c. Screening for depression should be done by referring patients to a psychiatrist.
    d. Brief, easy-to-administer screening tools for psychological symptoms are available for use in primary care practices.

4. Choose the correct statement:
    a. Psychological treatments, like cognitive–behavioral therapy and relaxation techniques, are only effective in patients with depression or anxiety.
    b. If depression or anxiety began after pain started, they will also go away once pain severity decreases.
    c. Cognitive–behavioral therapies encourage patients to become active participants in their pain management.
    d. None of the above
    e. All of the above

16

Obesity and Chronic Pain

CASE HISTORY

Ms. Jeffrey is a 47-year-old woman who complains of low back and knee pain for the last 10 years. This pain has been increasingly troublesome and limits her ability to perform laundry, cooking, and prolonged driving. On evaluation, her primary care physician (PCP) notes that she is obese. She is 5'7" tall, weighs 192 lbs, and has a body mass index (BMI) of 30.1 kg/m². She reports being slender most of her life, then gaining weight when she was in her mid 30s. Her weight has been stable for the last 5 years, and she reports no additional constitutional complaints. Ms. Jeffrey states that she's "too busy running her kids to their different school and sports events to exercise." She's tried numerous diets without success. Although she feels unattractive with her weight, she does not view her weight as a major concern and is primarily interested in pain control. Ms. Jeffrey's PCP tells her that her excess weight is causing her pain and the first thing she needs to do is lose weight. He suggests that Ms. Jeffrey lose about 15 lb then undergo a reassessment to see if any additional pain treatment will be necessary. Ms. Jeffrey becomes angry, feeling that her pain complaints are being ignored and she arranges to see a new doctor.

* * *

Obesity is a major health problem in the United States and has a significant influence on a wide variety of medical conditions, including chronic pain. Overweight and obese individuals do indeed have a greater risk for chronic pain in the neck, shoulder, back, and lower extremities. Weight reduction, even in modest amounts, can significantly reduce pain severity. Identifying excess weight and defining the need for weight reduction are important aspects of a comprehensive pain management program.

KEY CHAPTER POINTS

- More than half of adults in the United States are overweight or obese.
- Excess weight is associated with an increased prevalence of chronic pain in many body areas.
- Premorbid excess weight predicts chronic pain.
- Weight reduction results in reduced pain in many body areas.

From: *Chronic Pain: A Primary Care Guide to Practical Management*
Edited by: D. A. Marcus © Humana Press, Totowa, NJ

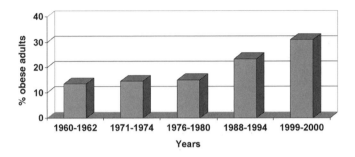

Fig. 1. Prevalence of obesity in the United States. (Based on ref. *1*.)

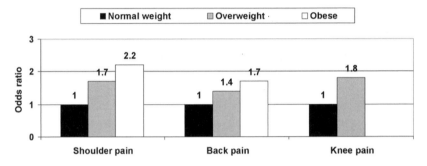

Fig. 2. Odds ratio for pain by weight category. (Based on refs. *3–5*.)

The prevalence of obesity has increased substantially in the United States over the last several decades (Fig. 1) *(1)*. According to the 1999–2000 National Health Examination Survey, 64.5% of US adults exceed their recommended weight, with 33.6% overweight (BMI range: 25–29.9 kg/m^2) and 30.9% obese (BMI $\geq$30 kg/m^2). Obesity is increasingly recognized as an important risk factor for a wide variety of health problems, including diabetes, cardiovascular disease, gallstones, and cancer *(2)*. As recognized by Ms. Jeffrey's doctor, excessive weight is also a risk factor for chronic pain.

1. OBESITY AND CHRONIC PAIN COMORBIDITY

The prevalence of chronic pain is higher in individuals with excess weight (Fig. 2) *(3–5)*. Pain impact is also negatively affected by increased weight. A study of 372 patients attending a specialty clinic pain revealed similar pain complaints in patients with different weight categories, although disability and depression were greater with increased weight (Fig. 3) *(6)*.

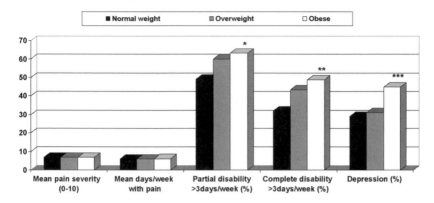

Fig. 3. Impact of obesity on pain, disability, and mood for patients with chronic pain. Significant difference among weight categories: $*p < 0.05$; $**p < 0.01$. Significant difference between normals and obese: $***p < 0.01$. (Based on ref. 6.)

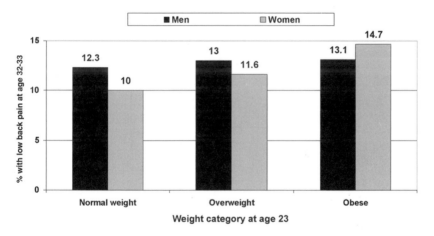

Fig. 4. Percentage of adults who develop new low back pain between ages 32 and 33 years, based on body mass index at age 23 years. Difference among weight categories for women is significant ($p = 0.02$). (Based on ref. 7.)

Obesity is linked to more significant pain risk and impact and also predicts new pain complaints. Early adulthood obesity predicted subsequent chronic back pain in women in a sample of almost 9000 adults (Fig. 4) *(7)*. In another study, the risk of an acute work injury developing into chronic pain qualifying the worker for workers' compensation benefits was increased in patients with excessive weight *(8)*. The odds ratio for the development of chronic, compensible pain was 1.00 in workers with a normal weight, 1.56 in overweight workers, and 1.85 in obese workers ($p = 0.01$).

Box 1
Calculating Body Mass Index (BMI)

BMI produces a number with the units kg/m^2. BMI can be calculated using English or metric units.

- Using pounds and inches

$$BMI = 703 \times \frac{\text{weight in pounds}}{\text{height in inches} \times \text{height in inches}}$$

- Using kilograms and meters

$$BMI = \frac{\text{weight in kilograms}}{\text{height in meters} \times \text{height in meters}}$$

- Using kilograms and centimeters

$$BMI = 10,000 \times \frac{\text{weight in kilograms}}{\text{height in centimeters} \times \text{height in centimeters}}$$

Box 2
Interpreting Body Mass Index

- Underweight <18.5 kg/m^2
- Normal 18.5–24.9 kg/m^2
- Overweight 25.0–29.9 kg/m^2
- Obese ≥30 kg/m^2

Obesity may influence pain by a variety of factors. Obesity negatively influences arthritis because of mechanical load on joints, particularly in the lower extremities *(9)*. In addition, obesity increases the release of proinflammatory cytokines that promote joint destruction *(10,11)*. Obesity has also been linked to depression, anxiety, and psychological disability, which are also linked to increased prevalence of chronic pain *(12–14)*.

2. OBESITY ASSESSMENT

Obesity assessment and management are important aspects of chronic pain care. Measures of obesity, including the BMI and percentage body fat, are influenced by both gender and age *(15)*. The BMI is recommended by a consensus panel from the National Heart, Lung, and Blood Institute (*see* Boxes 1 and 2). BMI is also an important weight marker because it accurately predicts health morbidity. For example, a BMI exceeding 24 kg/m^2 predicts an increased risk for hypertension, diabetes, and dyslipidemia *(16)*. A recent study showed the addition of waist circumference as an independent risk factor did not signifi-

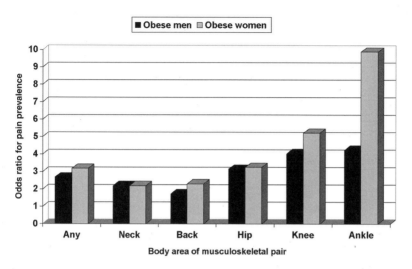

Fig. 5. Odds ratio for musculoskeletal pain in obese men and women. Odds ratios were adjusted for age, smoking, work status, and physical activity level. Prevalence of musculoskeletal pain in every body region was significantly higher in obese men and women compared with controls ($p < 0.001$). (Based on ref. *18*.)

cantly add to data obtained using the BMI to identify patients requiring treatment for obesity *(17)*.

3. OBESITY TREATMENT FOR PATIENTS WITH CHRONIC PAIN

Weight reduction reduces chronic pain affecting a wide variety of body regions. A longitudinal study of the relationship of obesity and musculoskeletal pain was conducted in 2460 men and 3868 women in Sweden *(18)*. The prevalence of musculoskeletal pain was significantly greater in obese individuals compared with controls for both men (58% of obese men vs 32% of controls) and women (68% vs 37%) (Fig. 5). Obese individuals were treated with either surgical or conventional therapy (diet, exercise, medications) and followed longitudinally. Weight reduction was significantly higher in obese individuals treated with surgery compared with nonsurgical methods for both men (–29.5 kg with surgery vs –0.4 kg with conventional treatment; $p < 0.001$) and women (–27.6 kg vs –0.3 kg; $p < 0.001$). Recovery from musculoskeletal pain after 2 years was significantly greater in both men and women after weight loss with surgery for every body area ($p < 0.05$) (Fig. 6). These data suggest that weight reduction may be an effective therapeutic intervention for patients with musculoskeletal pain. Several other studies have demonstrated a similar amount of pain reduction after weight loss, using surgical or nonsurgical techniques (Table 1) *(19–21)*.

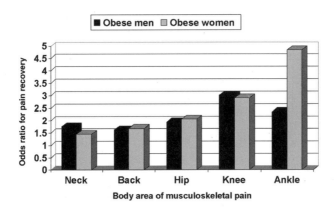

Fig. 6. Recovery from musculoskeletal pain after 2 years in obese individuals following surgical intervention . Odds ratios calculated by comparing 2-year recovery from musculoskeletal pain after surgical intervention (with significant weight loss of 27.6–29.5 kg) and nonsurgical weight intervention (with minimal weight loss of 0.3–0.4 kg). (Based on ref. *18.*)

Weight reduction is usually not successfully achieved or maintained through diet alone. Exercise offers therapeutic benefits for chronic pain and is the best predictor of successful weight loss *(22)*. Exercise capacity, however, is reduced in obese women because of complaints of musculoskeletal pain *(23)*. Therefore, alternative exercise programs in conjunction with weight reduction may be necessary for obese patients with chronic pain to maximize treatment compliance and benefit. Recommendations for initial exercise programs for overweight and obese individuals to improve success are shown in Boxes 3 and 4.

Many patients, like Mrs. Jeffrey, are discouraged about weight reduction, especially when numerous attempts have previously been unsuccessful. A study of middle-aged women participating in a 2-year weight-loss program identified poor self-motivation, numerous previous dieting attempts, dieting resulting in a weight loss of less than 4.5 kg during the previous 2 years, the number of years at current weight, and perceived barriers to exercise as independent risk factors for successful weight reduction *(24)*. These factors suggest that more aggressive and strictly monitored weight reduction will be necessary to achieve the desired weight reduction. Using daily exercise logs may improve the patient's understanding of exercise instructions and compliance (*see* Box 5A–C). By reviewing these logs, the health care provider can help the patient identify inadequate exercise (e.g., infrequent exercise sessions, failure to progress exercises, failure to elevate heart rate) or excessive exercise (e.g., too rapid progression of exercise, "crash-and-burn" patterns, excessive heart rate, or post-stretching exercise scores that suggest overstretching). Copies of these logs can also provide valuable chart documentation.

Table 1
Change in Pain After Weight Reduction

Study population (Reference)	Treatment	Average weight reduction	Change in pain
Knee osteoarthritis ($n = 84$); mean pretreatment weight = 77.2 kg (19)	Diet, exercise, and auricular acupuncture	12% after 8 weeks	Mean pain reduction = 39%. Pain was tolerable (2/10) in patients who achieved more than 15% weight reduction.
Musculoskeletal pain ($n = 43$) in obese women; mean pretreatment BMI = 37.8 kg/m² (18)	Diet	14% after 12 weeks; 10% at 64 weeks	Pretreatment increased prevalence of low back, knee, and foot pain. Low back pain occurred in 15 pretreatment and 11 after 12 and 64 weeks of dieting. Foot pain occurred in 13 pretreatment, 6 at 12 weeks and 5 at 64 weeks. Knee pain occurred in 15 initially, 9 at 12 weeks and 15 at 64 weeks. Back and foot pain decreased to prevalence seen in comparator, nonobese patients.
Morbidly obese with low back pain ($n = 29$); mean preoperative BMI = 48.0 kg/m² (20)	Vertical banded gastroplasty	42 kg (31%) after 2 years; Mean BMI at 2 years = 33.3 kg/m²	Complete pain resolution in 19 (66%)

BMI, body mass index.

259

Box 3

Exercise Initiation Recommendations for Overweight and Obese Adults

- Exercise program should be individualized and monitored by patient's health care provider.
  - Exercise recommendations need to be adjusted for patients with significant comorbid disease, such as cardiovascular or respiratory diseases.
- Aerobic exercise
  - Recommended low-impact exercises
    - Brisk walking
    - Bicycling
    - Swimming or pool exercise
  - Frequency: at least every other day
  - Duration: 30–45 minutes per exercise session
  - Intensity: 50% of heart rate reserve (*see* Box 4)
- Whole body stretching and flexibility exercises
  - Plus exercises targeted to specific pain area, as assigned by a physical therapist

Based on ref. *22*.

Box 4

Estimating Target HR Using HR Reserve Method

- Formula for calculation:

  Target HR=   [(maximal HR – resting HR) × 50%] + resting HR

  Maximal HR = 220 – age

  Target HR =   [(220 – age – resting HR) × 50%] + resting HR

- Example: 50-yr-old with a resting HR of 90 bpm

  Target HR =   [(220 – 50 – 90) × 50%] + 90

  Target HR =   130 bpm

HR, heart rate; bpm, beats/min.

---

3. SUMMARY

Ms. Jeffrey's doctor appropriately addressed weight reduction as an important treatment goal. Unfortunately, weight reduction is often neglected in general practice. A survey of 259 obese women revealed that their doctors had never provided weight control counseling to 28% of these women, and weight counseling was provided only "once in awhile" for an additional 39%

Box 5A
Sample Exercise Logs

Walking program:

Target goals are shown with dots. Place "X" in the boxes each day after you complete your walking program. Also count the number of times your heart beats in 60 seconds and record this as your heart rate each day that you exercise. Ideally, walk outside with a partner who walks at the same pace. If walking on a treadmill, listen to a television or music while walking.

Week 1:

	Sunday	Monday	Tuesday	Wednesday	Thursday	Friday	Saturday
1 mile	□	□	□	□	□	□	□
1/2 mile	□	□	□	□	□	□	□
1/4 mile	□	□	□	□	□	□	▣
1/8 mile	▣	□	▣	□	▣	□	□
Heart rate	____	____	____	____	____	____	____

Heart rate: record your heart rate at the end of your exercise session

Week 2:

	Sunday	Monday	Tuesday	Wednesday	Thursday	Friday	Saturday
1 mile	□	□	□	□	□	□	□
1/2 mile	□	□	□	□	▣	▣	□
1/4 mile	□	▣	▣	□	□	□	□
1/8 mile	□	□	□	□	□	□	□
Heart rate	____	____	____	____	____	____	____

Heart rate: record your heart rate at the end of your exercise session

Week 3:

	Sunday	Monday	Tuesday	Wednesday	Thursday	Friday	Saturday
1 mile	□	▣	□	▣	▣	▣	□
1/2 mile	▣	□	□	□	□	□	□
1/4 mile	□	□	□	□	□	□	□
1/8 mile	□	□	□	□	□	□	□
Heart rate	____	____	____	____	____	____	____

Heart rate: record your heart rate at the end of your exercise session

(25). In addition, 45% reported that their doctors never recommended standard weight-reduction techniques, such as diet, exercise, medications, or commercial weight-reduction programs.

Success with weight reduction can be improved by incorporating change in eating habits, including elimination of between meal snacking, reduction in

---

Box 5B
Sample Exercise Logs

Biking program:

Target goals are shown with dots. Place "X" in the boxes each day after you complete your biking program. Also count the number of times your heart beats in 60 seconds and record this as your heart rate each day that you exercise.

Week 1:

	Sunday	Monday	Tuesday	Wednesday	Thursday	Friday	Saturday
20 min	☐	☐	☐	☐	☐	☐	☐
15 min	☐	☐	☐	☐	☐	☐	☐
10 min	☐	☐	☐	☐	☐	☐	☒
5 min	☒	☐	☒	☐	☒	☐	☐
Heart rate	___	___	___	___	___	___	___

Heart rate: record your heart rate at the end of your exercise session

Week 2:

	Sunday	Monday	Tuesday	Wednesday	Thursday	Friday	Saturday
20 min	☐	☐	☐	☐	☐	☐	☐
15 min	☐	☐	☐	☐	☒	☒	☐
10 min	☐	☒	☒	☐	☐	☐	☐
5 min	☐	☐	☐	☐	☐	☐	☐
Heart rate	___	___	___	___	___	___	___

Heart rate: record your heart rate at the end of your exercise session

Week 3:

	Sunday	Monday	Tuesday	Wednesday	Thursday	Friday	Saturday
20 min	☐	☒	☐	☒	☒	☒	☐
15 min	☒	☐	☐	☐	☐	☐	☐
10 min	☐	☐	☐	☐	☐	☐	☐
5 min	☐	☐	☐	☐	☐	☐	☐
Heart rate	___	___	___	___	___	___	___

Heart rate: record your heart rate at the end of your exercise session

---

television viewing, and implementation of aggressive exercise *(26)*. Dieting without exercise is unlikely to achieve adequate and maintained weight reduction. Exercise also results in both direct cardiovascular and pain-relieving benefits. Patients with significant medical illness or deconditioning need to begin weight-reduction treatment with modest, regular exercise increased on a graded basis.

**Box 5C
Sample Exercise Logs**

Stretching exercise program:

Stretching exercises should be done twice a day for 15–20 minutes in each exercise session. Stretching should be completed at least 4 days/week. Log the time spent stretching, as well as your pain levels before and after exercise.

	Morning stretches			Evening stretches		
	Time (min)	Pain before	Pain after	Time (min)	Pain before	Pain after
Sunday	——	——	——	——	——	——
Monday	——	——	——	——	——	——
Tuesday	——	——	——	——	——	——
Wednesday	——	——	——	——	——	——
Thursday	——	——	——	——	——	——
Friday	——	——	——	——	——	——
Saturday	——	——	——	——	——	——

Do stretches in front of the television or with music playing.
Rate pain from 0 (no pain) to 10 (most severe pain imaginable).

REFERENCES

1. Flegal KM, Carroll MD, Ogden CL, Johnson CL. Prevalence and trends in obesity among US adults: 1999–2000. JAMA 2002; 288:1723–1727.
2. Field AE, Coakley EH, Must A, et al. Impact of overweight on the risk of developing common chronic diseases during a 10-year period. Arch Int Med 2001; 161: 1581–1586.
3. Miranda H, Viikari-Juntura E, Martikanien R, Takala EP, Riihimaki H. A prospective study of work-related factors and physical exercise as predictors of shoulder pain. Occup Environ Med 2001; 58:528–534.
4. Jinks C, Jordan K, Croft P. Measuring the population impact of knee pain and disability with the Western Ontario and McMaster Universities Osteoarthritis Index (WOMAC). Pain 2002; 100:55–64.
5. Webb R, Brammah T, Lunt M, Urwin M, Allison T, Symmons D. Prevalence and predictors of intense, chronic, and disabling neck and back pain in the UK general population. Spine 2003; 28:1195–1202.
6. Marcus DA. Obesity and the impact of chronic pain. Clin J Pain 2004; 20:186–191.
7. Lake JK, Power C, Cole TJ. Back pain and obesity in the 1958 British birth cohort: cause or effect? J Clin Epidemiol 2000; 53:245–250.

8. Fransen M, Woodward M, Norton R, et al. Risk factors associated with the transition from acute to chronic occupational back pain. Spine 2002; 27:92–98.
9. Sharma L, Lou C, Cahue S, Dunlop DD. The mechanism of the effect of obesity in knee osteoarthritis: the mediating role of malalignment. Arthritis Rheum 2000; 43:568–575.
10. Bastard JP, Jardel C, Bruckett E, et al. Elevated levels of interleukin 6 are reduced in serum and subcutaneous adipose tissue of obese women after weight loss. J Clin Endocrinol Metab 2000; 85:3338–3342.
11. Winkler G, Salamon F, Harmos G, et al. Elevated serum tumor necrosis factor-alpha concentrations and bioactivity in Type 2 diabetes and patients with android type obesity. Diabetes Res Clin Pract 1998; 42:169–174.
12. Sullivan M, Karlsson J, Sjostrom L, et al. Swedish obese subjects (SOS): an intervention study of obesity. Baseline evaluation of health and psychosocial functioning in the first 1743 subjects examined. Int J Obes Relat Metab Disord 1993; 17: 503–512.
13. Goldstein LT, Goldsmith SJ, Anger K, Leon AC. Psychiatric symptoms in clients presenting for commercial weight reduction treatment. Int J Eat Disord 1996; 20: 191–197.
14. Becker ES, Margraf J, Turke V, et al. Obesity and mental illness in a representative sample of young women. Int J Obes Relat Metab Disord 2001; 25(Suppl 1): S5–S9.
15. Jackson AS, Stanforth PR, Gagnon J, et al. The effect of sex, age, and race on estimating percentage body fat from body mass index: The Heritage Family Study. Int J Obes Relat Metab Disord 2002; 26:789–796.
16. Zhou BF. Predictive values of body mass index and waist circumference for risk factors of certain related diseases in Chinese adults: study on optimal cut-off points of body mass index and waist circumference in Chinese adults. Biomed Environ Sci 2002; 15:83–96.
17. Keirnan M, Winkleby MA. Identifying patients for weight-loss treatment: an empirical evaluation of the NHLBI obesity education initiative expert panel treatment recommendations. Arch Intern Med 2000; 160:2169–2176.
18. Peltonen M, Lindroos AK, Torgerson JS. Musculoskeletal pain in the obese: a comparison with a general population and long-term changes after conventional and surgical obesity treatment. Pain 2003; 104:549–557.
19. Larsson UE. Influence of weight loss on pain, perceived disability and observed functional limitations in obese women. Int J Obes Relat Metab Disord 2004; 28: 269–277.
20. Huang M, Chen C, Chen T, Weng M, Wang W, Wang Y. The effects of weight reduction on the rehabilitation of patients with knee osteoarthritis and obesity. Arthritis Care Res 2000; 13:398–405.
21. Melissas J, Volakakis E, Hadjipavlou A. Low-back pain in morbidly obese patients and the effect of weight loss following surgery. Obes Surg 2003; 13: 389–393.
22. McInnis KJ. Exercise and obesity. Coron Artery Dis 2000; 11:111–116.
23. Hulens M, Vansant G, Lysens R, et al. Exercise capacity in lean versus obese women. Scand J Med Sci Sports 2001; 11:305–309.

24. Teixeira PJ, Going SB, Houtkooper LB, et al. Weight loss readiness in middle-aged women: psychological predictors of success for behavioral weight reduction. J Behav Med 2002; 25:499–523.
25. Wadden TA, Anderson DA, Foster GD, Bennett A, Steinberg C, Sarwer DB. Obese women's perceptions of their physicians' weight management attitudes and practices. Arch Fam Med 2000; 9:854–860.
26. Coakley EH, Rimm EB, Colditz G, Kawachi I, Willett W. Predictors of weight change in men: results from the Health Professionals Follow-up Study. Int J Obes Relat Metab Disord 1998; 22:89–96.

CME QUESTIONS—CHAPTER 16

1. Obesity increased risk for developing:
    a. Heart disease
    b. Gallstones
    c. High cholesterolemia
    d. Chronic pain
    e. All of the above

2. Prevalence of which areas of chronic pain is/are increased in obese adults?
    a. Shoulder
    b. Back
    c. Knees
    d. All of the above

3. Which of the following statements is true?
    a. Pain reduction after weight reduction occurs only after patients achieve a normal body mass index (BMI).
    b. BMI is not associated with increased pain prevalence until patients reach a BMI ≥ 35 kg/m^2.
    c. Success at weight reduction is limited by long history of obesity, previous attempts at weight reduction, poor motivation to lose weight, and verbalized barriers to participating in exercise therapy.
    d. Obese women with comorbid depression should not be asked about weight, which may aggravate sense of low self-esteem.

4. Successful weight reduction in obese patients is maximized by utilizing:
    a. Graded exercise programs that begin with modest exercise.
    b. Patient-selected dietary therapy alone if they prefer to avoid exercise.
    c. Aggressive exercises initially, such as stair climbing or running programs.
    d. Infrequent monitoring of patient's progress to minimize discouragement as a result of slow progress.

VI
Opioids

17

Opioids in Chronic Pain

CASE HISTORY

Mr. Walter is a 55-year-old man with chronic low back pain. He underwent three back surgeries—including a fusion procedure, epidural steroid injections, facet blocks, and numerous medication trials—without benefit. He is a chef and restaurant owner, but his pain has prevented him from cooking in the restaurant or spending more than about 2 hours a day at work. He had been treated with nonsteroidal analgesics, but developed anemia from gastric ulcers. A trial of tramadol was unsuccessful. Mr. Walter's examination revealed pain with postural changes and restricted motion in his lumbar spine. He had no leg weakness, reflex changes, or numbness. His doctor diagnosed mechanical back pain and, after ensuring no history of drug or alcohol abuse, treated him with short-acting hydrocodone. Mr. Walter was instructed to take hydrocodone only when his pain was debilitating, and was given 30 pills. Mr. Walter called the clinic after 1 week, reporting good results from the hydrocodone, with mild constipation controlled by adding prune juice to breakfast and no cognitive effects. He requested a medication refill. The partner of Mr. Walter's treating physician authorized four refills. Mr. Walter returned to the clinic in 1 month and reported great satisfaction with his medication. He reported he could now grade his pain with a score of 6, on a scale of 1–10, instead of 9, and that he was sleeping better at night because his pain diminished and was able to spend 6 hours a day at the restaurant. He had even restarted cooking for some meals. In addition, he had resumed his stretching and flexion exercise program, now that his pain was better controlled. Although encouraged by this good report, Mr. Walter's doctor was surprised to see that in 1 month, Mr. Walter had used 150 tablets. The doctor angrily asked why Mr. Walter was using the medication so frequently, reminding Mr. Walter that he was instructed to use hydrocodone only for severe pain. Mr. Walter replied that his pain was always severe, and hydrocodone effectively relieved his pain, but only for approximately 4 hours. Therefore, Mr. Walter was taking hydrocodone four times daily. The doctor discontinued hydrocodone and requested consultation at a drug abuse facility.

* * *

From: *Chronic Pain: A Primary Care Guide to Practical Management*
Edited by: D. A. Marcus © Humana Press, Totowa, NJ

Infrequent, short-acting opioids, while effectively reducing Mr. Walter's pain, failed to provide the long-lasting relief he needed for his constant, severe pain. Mr. Walter discovered, as patients often do, that frequent dosing with a short-acting product would achieve longer lasting pain-relieving results. Failure of Mr. Walter to communicate the constant nature of his pain to the doctor and the doctor's failure to provide clear medication limits resulted in a dissatisfactory follow-up visit for both parties. Mr. Walter's frequent use of short-acting opioids appears to represent a legitimate attempt to achieve long-acting therapy results, rather than a typical pattern of abuse. Indeed, opioid therapy resulted in good achievement of treatment goals—both pain reduction and significant improvement in functional ability, with a marked increase in work hours.

KEY CHAPTER POINTS

- Long-term risk for gastric and renal toxicity with analgesics is minimized with opioid analgesics.
- Medication abuse behavior occurs in 25 to 30% of patients with chronic pain treated with opioids.
- Reasons for using opioid therapy include failure of other pain therapy, inability to tolerate other medications, and severe, disabling pain.
- Continued opioid treatment must be contingent on treatment compliance and achievement of functional improvement goals, such as increased household chores, return to work, or increased ability to participate in physical or occupational therapy.
- Reasons for selecting opioids, goals of treatment, goal attainment, and consideration of therapy adjustment must be clearly documented in patients' medical records.

Opioid treatment of chronic, nonmalignant pain remains controversial. Although expert opinion suggests that, in many circumstances, improved efficacy and reduced organ toxicity with opioids compared with non-opioid analgesics outweighs the risks for misuse and abuse *(1–3)*, many clinicians continue to be uncomfortable with an expanded role for opioids from malignant to nonmalignant chronic pain. This has resulted in marked differences in the prevalence of opioid prescriptions for chronic pain among medical practices (Fig. 1) *(4–6)*. In addition, although many doctors are concerned about risks for misuse and abuse in their patients, proper documentation of patients with chronic pain treated with opioids is poor. A recent survey of general medical clinic patients treated with opioids for chronic pain showed that the necessary documentation, including establishment of a treatment plan and demonstration of treatment response, was missing from most charts (Fig. 2) *(5)*. These studies support the need for additional education about risks and benefits of opioids, as well as development of practical guidelines for their use. This chapter is designed to provide a rational approach to the

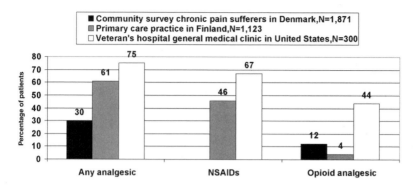

Fig. 1. Opioid prescribing habits. NSAIDs, nonsteroidal anti-inflammatory drugs. (Based on refs. *4–6*.)

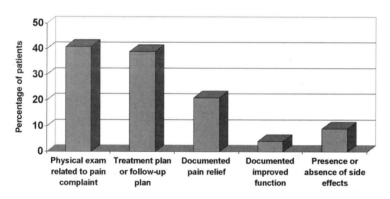

Fig. 2. Documentation in patients treated with analgesic opioids. (Based on ref. *5*.)

use of opioid analgesics in some patients with chronic pain, with a focus on reasons for treatment, typical treatment expectations, strategies to minimize drug misuse and abuse, and documentation tools.

1. RATIONALE FOR USING OPIOIDS IN CHRONIC PAIN

Some types of chronic pain, such as neuropathic pain and headache, can be effectively treated with nonanalgesic therapy, such as tricyclic antidepressants (TCAs) and some antiepileptic drugs (AEDs). These therapies, however, are much less effective for other common painful conditions, such as musculoskeletal pain. For severe pain complaints, analgesic medications are often needed, either as short-term therapy for management of pain flares or long-term therapy for persistent, constant, disabling pain. Choice between opioid and non-opioid analgesics requires a comparison of efficacy, safety, and tolerability.

Although both nonopioid and opioid analgesics can reduce pain complaints, prostaglandin effects of nonopioid analgesics contribute to significant organ toxicity, particularly with long-term use. Concern about long-term effects of chronic analgesic use are especially important in patients with chronic pain, due to expectations of long duration of pain complaints and requirements for analgesic therapy.

1.1. Risks of Non-Opioid Analgesics

An estimated 2% of adults in both Europe and the United States consume daily non-narcotic analgesics (7,8). Annual costs associated with toxicity from non-opioid analgesics in the United States approaches $1.9 billion (9). Nearly 75% of this cost is related to nonsteroidal anti-inflammatory drugs (NSAIDs), which result in an annual toxicity cost of $1.35 billion.

Chronic analgesic use results in significant gastrointestinal (GI) toxicity, with ulcers occurring in 15 to 30% of NSAIDs users. Gastroprotective agents are two to four times more likely to be used in patients with arthritis when they are treated with NSAIDs (10). Cyclooxygenase-2 (COX-2) inhibitors result in lower risk of GI side effects than nonselective NSAIDs. For example, overall incidence of GI adverse events was 19% for placebo, 26% with celecoxib, and 31% with naproxen in a comparative trial in patients with rheumatoid arthritis (11).

Nephrotoxicity also is associated with chronic analgesic use. Renal impairment occurs in 24% and renal papillary necrosis in 12% of patients with arthritis using chronic NSAIDs (12). Risks increase with analgesic overuse, with renal impairment in 65% and renal papillary necrosis in 27% of chronic analgesic overusers (13). Renal toxicity risks are not reduced with COX-2 inhibitors (14).

A recent analysis of female participants in the Nurse's Health Survey identified even infrequent analgesic use as an independent risk factor for developing hypertension (15). The survey followed 51,630 women with no history of hypertension or renal disease for 8 years. After adjustment for age, body mass index, sodium and alcohol intake, physical activity, family history of hypertension, diabetes, and smoking, risk for developing new-onset hypertension was increased similarly for women using aspirin, acetaminophen, or NSAIDs (Fig. 3). This risk is perhaps greater in elderly patients with established hypertension because NSAIDs reduce diuretic efficacy. For example, adding

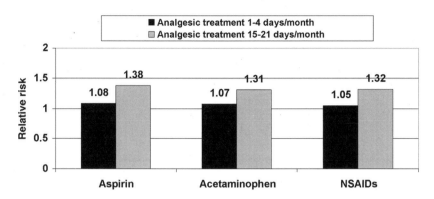

Fig. 3. Risk of new-onset hypertension in women treated with analgesics. NSAIDS, nonsteroidal anti-inflammatory drugs. (Based on ref. *15*.)

NSAIDs to diuretics doubled the risk for hospitalization from congestive heart failure in a large survey of more than 10,000 patients *(16)*.

1.2. Benefits of Opioid Analgesics

Opioids offer stronger analgesic potency, without prostaglandin-related adverse events. Superior long-term tolerability is perhaps the most significant benefit of opioid analgesics, as opioids typically offer only modest additional efficacy benefit in comparison to non-opioid analgesics. In a randomized, comparative study, 36 patients were treated with NSAIDs (maximum daily dose: 1000 mg naproxen), short-acting opioid (maximum daily dose: 20 mg oxycodone), or combined short- plus long-acting opioid (maximum daily dose: 200 mg morphine) *(17)*. The average dosage consumed in the short- plus long-acting opioid group was 41 mg of morphine per day. Pain control and tolerability were superior with opioids, although functional improvement (as measured by activity levels) was similar among all therapies (Fig. 4).

Pain relief efficacy can be maintained long-term when low doses of opioids are used. Pain was effectively reduced for 6 months in 58 patients with arthritis who were treated with sustained-release oxycodone (average daily dose: 40 mg) in a placebo-controlled study, without development of tolerance *(18)*. Pain and disability were similarly reduced a long-term study of 33 patients with low back pain followed for a mean of 32 months *(19)*. Five patients discontinued opioids after a short trial because of side effects. In the remaining 28 patients using long-term treatment, pain was reduced by 31% and disability by 42%. In addition, addictive behaviors or drug diversion occurred for none of these patients.

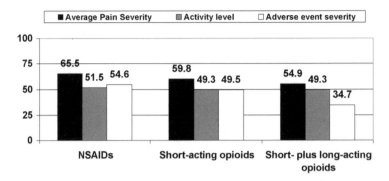

Fig. 4. Comparison of opioid and non-opioid analgesics for chronic back pain. Average pain and activity level scale: 100 = optimal; adverse event severity: 100 = extreme side effect. Differences among drugs were significant for pain ($p < 0.001$) and adverse events ($p < 0.0001$). NSAIDs, nonsteroidal anti-inflammatory drugs. (Based on ref. *17*.)

Box 1
Reasons to Consider Opioids for Nonmalignant Pain

- Analgesic overuse
- Inadequate response from other therapy
- Significant disability
- Severe pain that limits ability to participate in rehabilitation

---

1.3. Incorporating Opioids Into the Overall Management Plan

Opioids may be considered part of pain management for patients with disabling pain who have failed other therapy (*see* Box 1). Opioids should be incorporated into a comprehensive treatment plan, which may include physical therapy, occupational therapy, and psychological pain management skills. Additionally, pharmacological therapy does not need to be limited to either opioid or non-opioid therapies. Combining non-opioid medication with opioids can improve pain control for some patients. Eckhardt and colleagues evaluated experimental pain in healthy controls treated with placebo, gabapentin, morphine, and the combination of these medications *(20)*. Gabapentin alone was no more effective than placebo in improving pain tolerance. The addition of morphine to placebo increased pain tolerance by 41%, whereas the addition of both morphine and gabapentin increased pain tolerance by 76%.

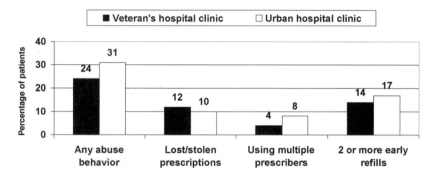

Fig. 5. Documented possible medication abuse behaviors in primary care outpatients prescribed opioids. Data obtained from 6-month chart review. (Based on ref. *22*.)

Constipation can become a treatment-limiting side effect with opioids, especially in patients concomitantly treated with other constipating medications, such as TCAs. Constipation can be reduced by adding an exercise program, fiber-rich foods, and stool softeners, as needed. Selection of opioid may also influence constipation. In a large study of more than 1800 patients with pain treated with opioids, constipation was more likely to occur with oxycodone (6.1%) or morphine (5.1%) in comparison with transdermal fentanyl (3.7%) *(21)*. Clinical experience supports reduction in constipation when patients are switched to fentanyl.

2. ABUSE AND MISUSE OF OPIOIDS

A major barrier to use of opioids in patients with chronic pain is the significant concern about medication misuse and abuse. A recent comparison of patients prescribed opioids for nonmalignant pain identified abusive behaviors in 24 to 31% (Fig. 5) *(22)*. Median time from initiation of opioids to first abusive behavior was 24 months.

Predicting which patients will develop abusive behaviors can be difficult. Pretreatment characteristics were evaluated in patients who used opioids chronically at a Veterans Administration Hospital pain clinic, almost 30% of whom developed features of abuse *(23)*. None of the baseline patient characteristics studied could be used to predict which patients would later develop abusive behaviors, including history of previous drug or alcohol abuse, abnormal scores on abuse screening tools, high pain severity, high perceived need

---

Box 2

Requirements for Prescribing Opioids for Chronic Pain

- Prescribe only for documented patients.
  - Never prescribe for patients before a full evaluation is completed.
  - Never prescribe for non-patients (yourself, relatives, employees, friends).
- Document evaluation and specific pain diagnosis.
  - Only prescribe opioids in patients with a clear pain diagnosis.
  - Never prescribe in the undiagnosed patient to "improve ability to cooperate with testing," unless the patient is acutely ill.
- Document reason for choosing opioid analgesic.
  - Failure or inability to tolerate non-opioid analgesics.
- Document specific treatment goals.
  - Minimize gastric/renal toxicity from non-opioid analgesics.
  - Improve functional ability.
  - Improve ability to participate in rehabilitative pain therapy.
- Document regular follow-up with identification of treatment efficacy and tolerability.
  - Specify goal targets that have been met or improved.
  - Document side effects, e.g., change in bowel habits or cognition.
- Document treatment plan at each visit.
  - Continue therapy owing to demonstrated efficacy/goal attainment.
  - Modify therapy because of failed goal attainment.
  - Medication discontinuation for non-efficacy or noncompliance.

---

for opioids, or depression. Identification of abusive behaviors in 25 to 30% of patients treated with opioids, along with lack of accurate predictors for abuse, suggests the need for pharmacological vigilance in all patients with chronic pain who are treated with opioids.

2.1. Minimizing Risks for Medication Misuse or Abuse

Risks for inappropriate opioid use are minimized by adhering to specific requirements for patient selection, treatment targets, and follow-up requirements (*see* Box 2). As with any medical therapy, opioids can only be prescribed to patients actively engaged in treatment, for whom a specific diagnosis that will be treated by the therapy has been established. Opioids must never be prescribed for non-patients, including patients referred but not yet evaluated. Therapy efficacy must be evaluated at regular intervals, with treatment plan modifications when efficacy targets, tolerability, or compliance is not achieved.

Box 3
Documentation Charting Sheets for Treatment of Chronic Pain

Pretreatment Assessment

Pain diagnosis: _____

Treatment recommendations (check all that apply):

☐ Medication
   ☐ Analgesic: _____
   ☐ Nonanalgesic: _____

☐ Nonpharmacological therapy:
   ☐ Physical therapy
   ☐ Occupational therapy
   ☐ Psychology
   ☐ Other: _____

Reason for selecting specific medication therapy (check all that apply):

☐ Diagnosis suggests benefit from a specific type of therapy
   (e.g., antiepileptics for neuropathic pain or migraine)
☐ Treatment of comorbid condition: _____
☐ Failure with non-opioid analgesics: _____
☐ Unable to tolerate non-opioid analgesics: _____
☐ Pain is disabling and/or precludes participation in rehabilitation

Treatment goals (check all that apply):

☐ Improve function
   ☐ Household chores
   ☐ Yard work
   ☐ Leisure activities
   ☐ School attendance
   ☐ Work
☐ Improve ability to participate in rehabilitation
☐ Provide safe, tolerated treatment
☐ Reduce pain to moderate severity level

Follow-up scheduled in _____weeks/months   *(Continued)*

Documentation in the medical record should clearly identify treatment goals, as well as goal attainment, treatment tolerability, and medication compliance. Charting sheets to be used at pretreatment assessment and in posttreatment follow-up are provided in Box 3. Box 4 shows these same sheets completed for our patient Mr. Walter based on his initial evaluation and response to hydrocodone.

Box 3 *(Continued)*
Documentation Charting Sheets for Treatment of Chronic Pain

Posttreatment Evaluation

Goal attainment (include specific targets achieved):

☐ Improve function

    ☐ Household chores: _____

    ☐ Yard work: _____

    ☐ Leisure activities: _____

    ☐ School attendance: _____

    ☐ Work: _____

☐ Improve ability to participate in rehabilitation: _____

☐ Provide safe, tolerated treatment: _____

☐ Reduce pain to moderate severity level: _____

Compliance with prescribed therapy:

☐ Yes

☐ No

Tolerability:

☐ Regular bowel movements (record frequency): _____

☐ Sedation/cognitive effects

☐ Weight change: _____

☐ Dry mouth

☐ Dizziness

☐ Nausea

☐ Other: _____

Treatment recommendations:

☐ Continue current treatment

☐ Change in therapy: _____

_____

_____

Follow-up scheduled in _____weeks/months

Risk for developing misuse or abuse behaviors can also be lessened by frankly discussing concerns with patients before therapy initiation. Providing pain medications on a strict treatment schedule, rather than as needed, lessens opportunities for misuse or overuse. Instructions for opioid dosing need to be specific and available to the patient in a written document. Opioid contracts can be useful tools to document treatment instructions, goals, and consequences for misuse (*see* Box 5).

Box 4
Documentation of Chronic Pain Treatment for Patient Mr. Walter

---

Pretreatment Assessment

Pain diagnosis: <u>Failed back syndrome, mechanical back pain</u>

Treatment recommendations (check all that apply):

☒ Medication
    ☒ Analgesic: <u>Hydrocodone, as needed for severe pain</u>
    ☐ Nonanalgesic: _____

☐ Nonpharmacological therapy:
    ☐ Physical therapy
    ☐ Occupational therapy
    ☐ Psychology
    ☐ Other: _____

Reason for selecting specific medication therapy (check all that apply):

☐ Diagnosis suggests benefit from a specific type of therapy
    (e.g., antiepileptics for neuropathic pain or migraine)
☐ Treatment of comorbid condition: _____
☒ Failure with non-opioid analgesics: <u>NSAIDs & tramadol</u>
☒ Unable to tolerate non-opioid analgesics: <u>anemia with NSAIDs</u>
☒ Pain is disabling and/or precludes participation in rehabilitation

Treatment goals (check all that apply):

☒ Improve function
    ☐ Household chores
    ☐ Yard work
    ☐ Leisure activities
    ☐ School attendance
    ☒ Work
☒ Improve ability to participate in rehabilitation
☒ Provide safe, tolerated treatment
☒ Reduce pain to moderate severity level

Follow-up scheduled in __1__ weeks/months   *(Continued)*

2.1.1. Establishing Goal-Contingent Therapy

As with all medical treatment, continuation of opioid therapy needs to be contingent on achieving specific goals. Although attaining no pain and no disability would be ideal goals for every patient, this level of complete relief is unlikely to occur in most patients and does not make an appropriate or readily attainable treatment target. Appropriate goals should be determined with patients prior to therapy initiation. Goal-setting is a joint project involving both

---

Box 4 *(Continued)*
Documentation of Chronic Pain Treatment for Patient Mr. Walter

---

Posttreatment Evaluation

Goal attainment (include specific targets achieved):

☒ Improve function

    ☐ Household chores: _____

    ☐ Yard work: _____

    ☐ Leisure activities: _____

    ☐ School attendance: _____

    ☒ Work: Working 6 h/d instead of 2 h/d; resumed cooking

☒ Improve ability to participate in rehabilitation: resumed exercise program

☒ Provide safe, tolerated treatment: _____

☒ Reduce pain to moderate severity level: Pain reduced from 9/10 to 6/10

Compliance with prescribed therapy:

☐ Yes

☒ No

Tolerability:

☒ Regular bowel movements (record frequency): daily BM if takes prune juice

☐ Sedation/cognitive effects

☐ Weight change: _____

☐ Dry mouth

☐ Dizziness

☐ Nausea

☐ Other: _____

Treatment recommendations:

☐ Continue current treatment

☒ Change in therapy: Discontinue hydrocodone. Begin sustained-release morphine 15 mg
twice daily

Follow-up scheduled in ___4___ weeks/months

---

health care provider and patient. These goals should be clearly documented in the patient's chart and opioid contract. Specific goals need to be individualized for each patient (Table 1). These goals will later serve as treatment outcome measures to determine treatment efficacy (Table 2). Although some treatment targets—such as improvement in mood, marital relationships, and sleep—are indeed important treatment targets for many patients with chronic pain, they are not the goals of opioid therapy and will require additional types of therapy, such as management with antidepressants and psychological services.

Box 5
Opioid Contract

Your doctor has diagnosed you with: _____

You have been prescribed the following opioid analgesic: _____

Opioid analgesics are strong pain relievers. They may cause constipation, nausea, and confusion. Therefore, you should not drive or operate machinery when adjusting to opioid therapy or if these effects occur. In addition, opioid analgesics are habit-forming. Patients using opioid analgesics regularly for 2 to 3 weeks usually develop medication habituation. This means that you may have withdrawal symptoms, like diarrhea, irritability, sleep disturbance, agitation, and runny nose, if you abruptly discontinue opioid therapy. Sometimes, patients can begin to crave the medication and develop serious problems with drug abuse. Some people also find that they build up a tolerance to opioid analgesics. Tolerance means that the medication becomes less and less effective the longer you use it. In that case, your opioid analgesic will need to be tapered and discontinued. Your doctor will help you minimize risks with your medication by establishing strict guidelines for medication use and requiring regular follow-up to assess treatment response and any side effects.

You have been prescribed opioid analgesic therapy for treatment of chronic pain because:
- ☐ You cannot take other non-opioid analgesics
- ☐ You have failed to respond to non-opioid analgesics and other therapy
- ☐ Your pain is disabling

Opioids analgesics are NOT expected to completely relieve your pain or treat non-pain problems, like depression, sleep disturbance, and anxiety. The goals of taking an opioid analgesic are:
- ☐ Improve function
- ☐ Improve your ability to participate in pain rehabilitation therapy
- ☐ Provide a safe pain-relieving treatment
- ☐ Reduce your pain to a moderate pain severity level

Continued prescription of this medication requires demonstration of:
- ☐ Improved function: _____
- ☐ Improved ability to participate in therapy: _____
- ☐ Pain reduction to moderate pain severity: _____

Your doctor will need to ensure that you are taking your medication correctly by requiring you to:
- ☐ Take your medication on a regular schedule and not adjust the dosage without written instructions from your doctor.
- ☐ Obtain prescriptions only at one pharmacy: _____
- ☐ Regular follow-up visits: _____
- ☐ Not request early medication refills.
- ☐ Not obtain any additional pain-relieving medications from any other healthcare provider.

Misuse or abuse of opioid analgesics occurs in about 25 to 30% of chronic pain patients. Failure to comply with these requirements or the development of medication tolerance may result in discontinuation of therapy and/or referral to a drug abuse counselor.

I have read the above contract with my treating physician and agree to its terms. In addition, I agree to allow my doctor and his staff to share this contract and communicate with my pharmacy and my other healthcare providers.

_____   _____
Consenting patient signature   Date of contract

_____   _____
Prescribing healthcare provider's signature   Date

Table 1
Treatment Goals for Opioid Therapy

End point goal	Appropriate goal	Inappropriate goal
• Pain relief	• Pain reduction to moderate severity • Reduction in number, severity, or duration of pain flares • Development of techniques to treat pain flares	• Complete relief of all pain • To become free of all pain • Elimination of any pain flares
• Functional improvement	• Increase tolerance for sitting, standing, or walking by specific amount: sit or stand 1 hour; walk 1/2 mile • Increase household chores: laundry 2 days/week, dinner preparation 3 nights/week, grocery shopping once weekly • Resume yard work • Return to school or reduce school absences from pain to no more than once a month • Return to work, e.g., return to work part time or at modified duties with a strategy to increase toward baseline work level • Participate in retraining or education to improve work readiness • Increase social/leisure activities: resume walking program, biking, swimming, or other sport; attend movies, concerts, or children's performances	• Feel comfortable while maintaining significant disability • Resume aggressive sports in which patient participated in youth • Return to regular work with no need to modify routine or work simplification
• Other	• Develop pacing skills and work simplification to assist in increasing activity level without intolerable increase in pain flares	• Improve anxiety, mood, marital strife, relationship issues • Improve sleep disturbance

282

Table 2
End Points Achieved With Opioids: Identification of Effective Therapy

End point goal	Response suggests effective therapy: realistic goals achieved	Response suggests ineffective therapy: realistic goals not achieved
• Pain relief	• My pain is now more tolerable, with moderate pain severity.	• My pain was about 50% better with the medication, so I doubled the dose to try to totally get rid of my pain. • My pain is really well controlled. Now when I lay on the sofa watching television all day, I'm really comfortable.
• Functional improvement	• I have been able to do my walking program every other day now and my stretching exercises each morning. • I have gone back to work part time. • I have started doing more household chores: laundry, cooking, mowing the yard. • I get out of bed every morning and fix breakfast for the kids instead of laying in bed all day.	
• Other		• I take my pain pills at night and it knocks me out for a good night's sleep. • When I really want to over-do activities, I just double up on my pain medication to control the pain before it starts. • If I know it's going to be a stressful day, I take a couple extra pain pills to keep things under better control. • I don't seem to worry so much, now that I'm taking the pain pills. I'm a lot calmer.

283

2.1.2. Requiring Patient Responsibility

Patients must be informed that the significant risk for misuse or abuse with opioids requires them to exercise considerable responsibility over their medications. Patients must know the policy for medication adherence before beginning opioids and understand that these rules represent a strict policy of the clinic and are not applied on a case-by-case basis. Repeated reports of misplaced, stolen, or damaged medications demonstrate poor patient responsibility and should result in the strong consideration for discontinuing medications. All patients with chronic pain should be asked about current, recent, and remote abuse of alcohol and drugs. Patients with current addiction problems should be referred to a drug rehabilitation facility before any pain management is attempted. Patients with recent problems with abuse or addiction should be managed by a pain specialist, ideally in conjunction with an abuse counselor.

The reasons for a lack of responsible behavior are not important. Whether the patient launders pain pills or spills them into the toilet, or whether the pills are stolen by a neighbor or consumed by a pet, the patient has not displayed responsible behavior. Many practices allow patients to have a single occasion of irresponsible behavior; however, if this recurs, the medications will not be continued. For example, if opioids were laundered in March and then stolen by the neighbor in April, the health care provider must let the patient know that while sympathetic to the patient's chaotic life, he or she cannot, in good conscience, continue to prescribe a therapy that requires strict monitoring when that appears to be impossible in the patient's life. Doctors should never argue with patients about the credibility of the stories about missing medications: "Your poodle couldn't possibly have eaten 80 Percocets and be fine," or "How could 40 pills possibly have fallen into the narrow opening of a nail polish remover bottle?" Without great effort, these stories cannot be proven to be false and discussions about excuse veracity encourages patients to develop more plausible stories for next time. Doctors need to accept the face-value validity of their patients' stories and present them as examples of lack of medication responsibility.

Medication use must be vigilantly monitored. Opioid prescriptions should be limited to a single health care provider. Prescriptions must be logged in the patients' records, with new prescriptions written on schedule to avoid medication overuse. In addition, random urine drug screens should be performed periodically on all patients using opioids to ensure appropriate medication use, confirm lack of abuse of nonprescribed habit-forming substances, and to prevent drug diversion. It is important to remember, however, that most laboratories set limits for drug detection that are designed to identify common levels of drugs of abuse. These levels may be too high to detect low levels used in patients prescribed opioids for chronic pain. If a routine drug screen is negative in a patient prescribed an opioid analgesic, repeat testing with a comprehensive screen designed to report even low levels of drugs should be performed.

Table 3
Opioid Dose Equivalents

Short-acting opioid dosage	Long-acting opioid dosage
4–8 (5 mg) hydrocodone or oxycodone	10 mg oxycodone twice daily
	15 mg morphine twice daily or 30 mg once daily
10 (5 mg) hydrocodone or oxycodone	25 μg fentanyl patch every 48–72 hours
	5 mg methadone twice daily
16 (5 mg) hydrocodone or oxycodone	40 mg oxycodone twice daily
20 (5 mg) hydrocodone or oxycodone	50 μg fentanyl patch every 48–72 hours
	10 mg methadone twice daily
	50 mg morphine twice daily or 100 mg once daily

It is often helpful to let the laboratory know the specific compound that the patient is prescribed and that even low levels of this drug are of interest to the doctor ordering the test. In addition, some commonly prescribed medications crossreact with drugs of abuse on standard drug screening tests, and may produce a false-positive. For example, with routine drug-screening testing, the NSAIDs oxaprozin may crossreact with benzodiazepines and ketorolac with cocaine. Comprehensive drug-screening tests identify specific compounds identified as possible substances of abuse, rather than general drug categories. Increased cost with comprehensive testing limits its use to patients with unexplained abnormalities on routine screening.

2.1.3. Determining Appropriate Dosing

Opioid therapy needs to be matched with pain characteristics. Patients with constant, disabling pain are best managed with low doses of a long-acting opioid. Intermittent pain flares may be treated with short courses (2–4 days) of short-acting opioids. Frequent pain flares that occur daily or several times daily should be managed with self-administered physical therapy modalities (such as heat, ice, oscillatory movements, or trigger-point therapy) and psychological pain management techniques (such as relaxation).

If opioids are utilized for chronic pain treatment, patients should be treated with low doses. Lack of familiarity with sustained-release opioid dosages may result in use of excessive quantities. Both patients and health care providers benefit from understanding the equivalency of a long-acting medication with short-acting medications that have been used previously. Table 3 provides a comparison between comparable doses of short- and long-acting opioid analgesics. Although opioids do not have a ceiling dose to set the maximum dose that may be prescribed, general practitioners should probably seek consultation with a pain specialist before escalating opioid doses to high levels (e.g., doses exceeding 50 μg fentanyl or 50 mg morphine twice daily or 40 mg oxycodone three times daily).

Maintenance of low opioid dosage limits development of tolerance and opportunities for medication abuse in the clinic. This practice is also supported by basic science research. Numerous experiments in rodents have convincingly shown that chronic exposure to high doses of opioids alters neurotransmitter activity in pain-provoking pathways, resulting in a paradoxical hyperalgesia or increased sensitivity to pain *(24)*. Therefore, lack of long-term efficacy with high doses of opioids may occur from the combination of lowering of the pain threshold and medication tolerance.

3. SUMMARY

Patients with musculoskeletal pain often require treatment with analgesics for pain flares or constant, disabling pain. Risks of gastric and renal toxicity with long-term use of non-opioid analgesics are minimized with opioid analgesics. Opioid therapy may also be considered when patients have failed to achieve benefit from other pain therapies, are unable to tolerate non-opioid analgesics, or have severe, disabling pain. Although prostaglandin-related adverse events do not occur with opioids, medication abuse behavior occurs in 25 to 30% of patients with chronic pain treated with opioids. Both patients and clinicians must be cognizant of this risk. Treatment strategies to reduce likelihood of misuse and abuse include establishing specific treatment targets, requiring strict medication schedule compliance, and arranging regular follow-up assessments.

REFERENCES

1. Friedman DP. Perspectives on the medical use of drugs of abuse. J Pain Symptom Manage 1990; 5(Suppl):S2–S5.
2. Shannon CN, Baranowski AP. Use of opioids in non-cancer pain. Br J Hosp Med 1997; 5:459–463.
3. Savage SR. Opioid use in the management of chronic pain. Med Clin North Am 1999; 83:761–786.
4. Mantyselka P, Ahonen R, Kumpusalo E, Takala J. Variability in prescribing for musculoskeletal pain in Finnish primary health care. Pharm World Sci 2001; 23: 232–236.
5. Clark JD. Chronic pain prevalence and analgesic prescribing in a general medical population. J Pain Symptom Manage 2002; 23:131–137.
6. Eriksen J, Jensen MK, Sjøgren P, Ekholm O, Rasmussen NK. Epidemiology of chronic non-malignant pain in Denmark. Pain 2003; 106:221–228.
7. Kromann-Andersen H, Pedersen A. Reported adverse reactions to and consumption of nonsteroidal anti-inflammatory drugs in Denmark over a 17-year period. Dan Med Bull 1988; 35:187–192.
8. Matzke GR. Nonrenal toxicities of acetaminophen, aspirin, and nonsteroidal anti-inflammatory agents. An J Kidney Dis 1996; 28 (1 Suppl 1):S63–S70.
9. McGoldrick MD, Bailie GR. Nonnarcotic analgesics: prevalence and estimated economic impact of toxicities. Ann Pharmacother 1997; 31:221–227.

10. Lapane KL, Spooner JJ, Pettitt D. The effect of nonsteroidal anti-inflammatory drugs on the use of gastroprotective medication in people with arthritis. Am J Manag Care 2001; 7:402–408.
11. Simon LS, Weaver AL, Graham DY, et al. Anti-inflammatory and upper gastrointestinal effects of celecoxib in rheumatoid arthritis. A randomized controlled trial. JAMA 1999; 282:1921–1928.
12. Segasothy M, Chin GL, Sia KK, et al. Chronic nephrotoxicity of anti-inflammatory drugs used in the treatment of arthritis. Br J Rheumatol 1995; 34:162–165.
13. Segasothy M, Samad SA, Zulfigar A, Bennett WM. Chronic renal disease and papillary necrosis associated with the long-term use of nonsteroidal anti-inflammatory drugs as the sole or predominant analgesic. Am J Kidney Dis 1994; 24:17–24.
14. LeLorier J, Bombardier C, Burgess E, et al. Practical considerations for the use of nonsteroidal anti-inflammatory drugs and cyclo-oxygenase-2 inhibitors in hypertension and kidney disease. Can J Cardiol 2002; 18:1301–1308.
15. Deider J, Stampfer MJ, Hankison SE, Willett WC, Speizer FE, Curhan GC. Nonnarcotic analgesic use and risk of hypertension in US women. Hypertension 2002; 40:604–608.
16. Heerdink ER, Leufkens HG, Herings RM, et al. NSAIDs associated with increased risk of congestive heart failure in elderly patients taking diuretics. Arch Int Med 1998; 158:1108–1112.
17. Jamison RN, Raymond SA, Slawsby EA, Nedeljkovic SS, Katz NP. Opioid therapy for chronic noncancer back pain: a randomized prospective study. Spine 1998; 23:2591–2600.
18. Roth SH, Fleischman RM, Burch FX, et al. Around-the-clock, controlled-release oxycodone therapy for osteoarthritis-related pain. Placebo-controlled trial and long-term evaluation. Arch Intern Med 2000; 160:853–860.
19. Schofferman J. Long-term opioid analgesic therapy for refractory lumbar spine pain. Clin J Pain 1999; 15:136–140.
20. Eckhardt K, Ammon S, Hofmann U, et al. Gabapentin enhances the analgesic effect of morphine in healthy volunteers. Anesth Analg 2000; 91:185–191.
21. Staats PS, Markowitz J, Schein J. Incidence of constipation associated with long-acting opioid therapy: a comparative study. South Med J 2004; 97:129–134.
22. Reid MC, Engles-Horton LL, Weber MB, Kerns RD, Rogers EL, O'Connor PG. Use of opioid medications for chronic noncancer pain syndromes in primary care. J Gen Intern Med 2002; 17:173–179.
23. Chabal C, Erjavec MK, Jacobson L, et al. Prescription opiate abuse in chronic pain patients: clinical criteria, incidence, and predictors. Clin J Pain 1997; 13:150–155.
24. Ossipov MH, Lai J, Vanderah TW, Porreca F. Induction of pain facilitation by sustained opioid exposure: relationship to opioid antinociceptive tolerance. Life Sci 2003; 73:783–800.

CME QUESTIONS—CHAPTER 17

1. Short-acting, immediate-release opioids should be considered in patients with:
   a. Frequent pain flares, occurring three times weekly
   b. Infrequent pain flares, occurring once per week or less
   c. Constant, disabling pain
   d. Constant, mild pain

2. Choose the correct statement:
   a. Abusive behaviors occur in approximately 4–9% of chronic pain patients treated with opioids.
   b. Medication abuse is unlikely to occur in patients with no personal or family history of abuse, depression, or anxiety.
   c. Opioids may be continued in patients who repeatedly report missing medications as long as they provide valid police reports of theft or other documentation.
   d. All of the above
   e. None of the above

3. Opioids may be prescribed for:
   a. Active patients
   b. Patients who have been referred for consultation but not yet evaluated when they will run out of their medications before the consultation appointment
   c. Close relatives
   d. Employees with no abuse history

4. Opioid dosage should be adjusted to achieve:
   a. Complete pain relief
   b. Complete relief of disability
   c. Improvement in sleep
   d. All of the above
   e. None of the above

Appendices
Patient Educational Materials

CONTENTS

CASE HISTORY

Ms. Stoll, a 47-year-old nurse's aide with chronic low back pain, complains:

I just don't know what to do. My doctor told me not to do activities that aggravate my pain, but he also told me to return to work, even though my pain started with a work injury. He also gave me a booklet of exercises. Whenever I do the exercises, my pain gets worse and he yelled at me when I told him I don't do them.

From: *Chronic Pain: A Primary Care Guide to Practical Management*
Edited by: D. A. Marcus © Humana Press, Totowa, NJ

Ms. Gray, a 23-year-old mother of a toddler, gets migraine headaches and grumbles:

Everybody seems to give me headache advice. My mother-in-law insists that most headaches are caused by foods and that I should avoid drinking coffee, eating chocolate and peanuts. My cousin says her headaches are relieved when she drinks coffee and to try that. One friend tells me she takes over-the-counter pain killers every day for her headache, while another claims her doctor told her that pain pills actually cause headaches. I'm too busy running around after my son to try everything. Wish I knew what was really likely to be helpful.

KEY POINTS

- Patients with chronic pain are very interested in education about pain.
- Receiving basic information significantly improves physical and emotional symptoms in patients with chronic pain.
- Effective education delivery systems include brief instruction by a health care provider, written handouts, and multimedia aides.

The inability of the medical profession to provide clear diagnoses, explanations, and treatment courses for patients with chronic pain may result in the worsening of sickness behavior and dependence on the health care system *(1)*. Patients understand this relationship and, like Ms. Stoll and Ms. Gray, they are usually eager to receive useful education from their health care providers. For example, an analysis of a survey asking pain specialists and patients with chronic headache about important aspects of care revealed that education was the top priority for patients *(2)*, but was considered important by only a minority of doctors. Additionally, 86% of the patients rated the receipt of answers to their questions as important compared with only 15% of doctors. Similarly, educating patients about headaches and teaching patients how to treat attacks were rated important by 72% of patients and 15% of doctors. Thus, although patients understand the importance of education, clinicians have only recently become aware of the valuable therapeutic effect education has on the outcome of patient care.

The education of patients with chronic pain effectively reduces fear of pain and pain-related disability. A single education session with a physical therapist, during which pain physiology or spine anatomy is explained, resulted in significant improvements in pain catastrophizing, disability perception, and range of motion ($p < 0.01$) *(3)* (*see* Fig. 1). The ability of patients to demonstrate significant improvements in attitude and physical limitations after this single intervention suggests that brief education administered during the course of a routine primary care office visit would also be beneficial. In one study, the addition of a single, 30-minute educational session about migraine and medication use with an allied health care worker plus three follow-up telephone

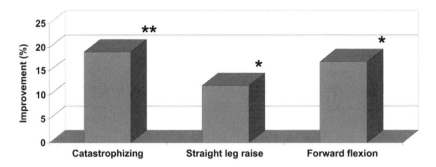

Fig. 1. Benefits of brief education about pain physiology for patients with chronic low back pain. Seventy-five patients with chronic low back pain (average pain duration: 3.9 years) were tested before and after a single informational session about pain physiology. Time between assessments was 3.5 hours. Improvements were significant (*$p < 0.01$; **$p < 0.001$). (Based on ref. *3*.)

calls resulted in a 47% reduction in headache activity compared with an 18% headache reduction in patients receiving only the doctor visit without supplemental education *(4)*.

Effective education can be delivered within the clinical environment or through outside resources. For example, a multimedia educational program consisting of pain education and relaxation delivered through written materials, television, and radio programs to 164 individuals with headache over 10 weeks decreased headache days by 50% and analgesic use by 30% *(5)*. In addition, work absence decreased by 45% and doctor visits decreased by 61%. Headache education administered via the Internet similarly improved headache, with a 31% reduction in headache activity *(6)*.

The appendices that follow provide a variety of educational tools that can be utilized in clinical practice. Providing written materials for patients to take home strongly reinforces the educational messages doctors provide during an office visit. The use of these materials can also reduce the face-to-face time required to deliver education in the busy office.

REFERENCES

1. Glenton C. Chronic back pain sufferers: striving for the sick role. Soc Sci Med 2003; 57:2243–2252.
2. Lipton RB, Stewart WF. Acute migraine therapy: do doctors understand what patients with migraine want from therapy? Headache 1999; 39(Suppl 2):S20–S26.
3. Moseley GL. Evidence for a direct relationship between cognitive and physical change during an education intervention in people with chronic low back pain. Eur J Pain 2004; 8:39–45.

4. Holroyd KA, Cordingley GE, Pingel JD, et al. Enhancing the effectiveness of abortive therapy: a controlled evaluation of self-management. Headache 1989; 29:148–153.

5. de Bruijn-Kofman AT, van de Wiel H, Groenman NH, Sorbi MJ, Klip E. Effects of a mass media behavioral treatment for chronic headache: a pilot study. Headache 1997; 3:415–420.

6. Andersson G, Lundström P, Ström L. A controlled trial of self-help treatment of recurrent headache conducted via the Internet. J Consult Clin Psychol 2000; 68: 722–727.

Appendix A
Rationale Behind Pain Management

WHY DO PAIN MANAGEMENT SKILLS WORK?:
THE GATE THEORY

Pain management skills are designed to block pain messages by sending other signals through the nerves and spinal cord that "fill up" the nervous system circuits, thereby blocking access to pain messages. For example, walking requires a great deal of effort from the nervous system, which has to judge muscle contraction, joint angles, and balance systems. Performing activities that "tie up" the transmission of nervous energy—such as relaxation techniques and exercising—help prevent pain messages from traveling along these same pathways.

Scientists have identified different types of nerves: small nerves that send pain messages and large nerves that send messages that do not cause concern. If the large nerves are busy, messages being sent by the small pain nerves are blocked. This is the basis for the gate theory.

Gate Theory

Pain starts with the activation or signaling of nerves in the skin. For these signals to reach the brain, they must first pass through a gating mechanism at the spinal cord. When pain nerves are activated, the pain gate opens and allows pain messages to reach the brain, at which time we become aware of the pain. When large nerves are activated by nonpainful changes in touch or temperature, the pain gate closes and messages other than pain messages travel to the brain. When the pain gate is closed, we are not aware of pain. There are pain gates in both the spine and brain (*see* Fig. 1).

Everyday pain experiences can be used to illustrate gate theory in action. For example, if your hammer slips and hits your finger, a pain message is formed in the nerves in the skin of the finger. This opens the pain gate in the spine and you became aware of a painfully smashed finger. To block that pain, you may pop your finger into your mouth and suck on it. Your tongue creates a touch signal that stimulates the large nerves and closes the pain gate. After a few seconds, however, you may pull the finger out of your mouth to look at it.

From: *Chronic Pain: A Primary Care Guide to Practical Management*
Edited by: D. A. Marcus © Humana Press, Totowa, NJ

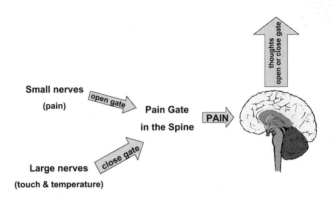

Fig. 1. Gate theory. Pain signals small nerves to open the pain gate, sending pain messages through the spine to the brain. Pain gates in the spine can be closed by stimulating the large nerves with touch or temperature changes. If pain signals reach the brain, thoughts can open or close pain gates. When pain gates are closed, pain severity is reduced. When pain gates in the spine and brain are allowed to stay open, more severe pain will be felt.

However, because looking at the finger does not activate sensory nerves, the pain gate is no longer closed and the pain messages are again free to travel to the brain. The same process applies when bumping your funny bone and finding relief from gently rubbing the elbow.

Another way to activate the large, pain-blocking nerves is by using heat. If you've ever overdone a day of yard work or cleaning and felt sore and achy all over, you know you can find almost instant relief by soaking in a tub of warm water. As soon as you are immersed in the warm water, the pain will seem to disappear. That's because heat activates the temperature-sensitive nerves and closes the pain gates. Once you get out of the tub, you'll "stiffen up" and the pain will return because the trauma of the day was not cured by soaking, but rather the pain signals were blocked from traveling to the brain. You will also notice that after soaking for about 15 minutes, the pain will return, even if you stay in the hot tub. This is because your brain gets bored of repeatedly receiving the same message, and will begin to block the heat signal, just like you can ignore a phone ringing. Curiously, the brain does not seem to tire of pain messages.

The Brain Influences Pain Severity

Once pain signals reach the brain, the brain decides how much attention to give to them and responds by opening and closing pain gates in the brain. If the brain is focused on other important tasks, it may ignore the pain. If the brain is not distracted, pain severity will be maximized. For example, people often complete their day's work while they have pain, only to find that the pain becomes intolerable once they get home at the end of the day. The work activities helped distract the brain from the pain messages. Also, there's a natural tendency to want to go to bed when pain starts, hoping that, by resting quietly, the pain will go away. However, this may cause the pain to become magnified. The brain has nothing else to divert attention away from the pain, so the pain signals will be felt at their maximum severity. Many activities can distract the brain from pain, including walking, biking, exercising, or practicing relaxation techniques.

How one thinks about pain can also affect how strongly one experiences pain signals. When children get bumps and bruises, parents can often "kiss it and make it better." This doesn't mean the children were faking their pain. They believe their parents have the power to take their pain away. For children, kissing a boo-boo is believed to be effective therapy. The same process works in adults. For example, have you ever noticed that pills for the heart are tiny and white or pastel colored, whereas pain pills are big and red or orange? Most people are afraid of heart pills, so these pills are designed to appear gentle and harmless. People don't want a gentle pain pill, but a strong one. Research shows that patients will achieve better pain relief if they take a big red pain pill ("I'm big and strong and can wipe out that pain") rather than taking the exact same medication packed in a tiny white pill ("I'm the gentle, wimpy pill"). This does not mean that people make up their pain. Instead, it shows that adults can also change how much pain travels through pain gates by thoughts about pain.

Pain management skills work because the brain can moderate pain severity. When one feels hopeless about pain ("There's nothing I can do to help"), the pain gates open and the severity of the pain increases. Having positive thoughts about one's ability to cope with the pain ("There are techniques I can use to help control my pain"), helps close pain gates and reduces pain severity. Although no one can just "think their pain away," knowing you have skills and medications to help control your pain helps close pain gates to reduce pain severity and help the treatments work even better.

Using Gate Theory in Pain Management

Different physical and mental conditions influence the pain gates.

Open pain gates: increase pain	Close pain gates: decrease pain
• Fatigue	• Feeling energetic, happy, and calm
• Boredom	• Being relaxed
• Depression	• Being in good physical shape
• Anger, frustration, or stress	• Being distracted or occupied with
• Being out of shape	non-pain topics
• Dwelling on pain	• Having positive pain expectations:
• Having negative pain expectations:	"I can help control my pain."
"There's nothing I can do to help my pain."	

A variety of techniques you can practice to help close pain gates are as follow:

- Distract the brain with non-pain messages: take a walk outside and look at the scenery, listen to soothing music, do stretches in the shower.
- Exercise to keep yourself fit.
- Practice relaxation and biofeedback techniques.
- Manage your mood and reaction to stress.
- Use heat or ice in a moist towel.

The brain gets bored of repeatedly hearing the same message. Ever notice how you'll stop hearing a fan hum or even a toddler whine after a few minutes? The same is true for strategies that close pain gates. These strategies usually work for about 15 to 20 minutes. So, instead of just soaking in a hot tub or resting under a heating pad, once the pain lessens, do some stretching exercises or relaxation skills to help keep those pain gates closed. Combining techniques (e.g., doing stretching exercises while practicing relaxation or watching a television program, or walking outdoors rather than on a treadmill) improves effectiveness in closing pain gates.

Using gate theory techniques will not eliminate all of your pain. However, by combining these techniques with medications and other therapies you may significantly improve the effectiveness of those other of those therapies.

So get up from your chair, escape from your boredom, and close those pain gates!

Appendix B
Exercise and Pain Management

WHY DO EXERCISES?
HOW CAN EXERCISE HELP REAL PAIN?

About 10 years ago, I injured my back while participating in an aerobic exercise class. I was diagnosed with a herniated disc and had to have surgery. After surgery, it was really hard to convince myself to exercise again, because that's what caused my pain in the first place. A couple of weeks after surgery, the pain started getting worse and I figured I better try something. Once I started exercising, I was surprised that the exercising actually made the pain better. Now, 10 years later, if I stop my exercise program, the pain comes back. Also, I can tell my back and all of my body are much stronger and I don't feel I get injured as easily as I did before.

—Dr. Marcus

Exercise is a vital part of pain management that provides two essential benefits: pain reduction and protection.

Pain Reduction

Pain causes an involuntary muscle spasm. If you twist your ankle, the muscles around the ankle become stiff, forming a natural cast around the injury that helps stabilize the injured joint while it heals. People with back pain sometimes notice this, saying, "I bent over and the pain was so bad I couldn't stand up." When you have chronic pain, your muscles develop a pattern of muscle spasm that no longer is helpful for protecting a newly injured area. The muscle spasm itself is also painful.

It's easy to see what happens to these structures when we don't exercise. If you've ever spent a couple of days in bed rest, due to illness or your pain, you probably noticed that your whole body felt stiff and achy once you started getting out of bed. Our muscles and joints expect to be used, and if we don't use them, our pain usually becomes worse.

Pain management exercises begin with gentle stretching. This helps relieve the muscle spasm. When you start exercising, you should notice that after a few repetitions, the stretching exercises feel soothing. After the exercise session is over, however, the muscles will probably go into spasm again. That's

From: *Chronic Pain: A Primary Care Guide to Practical Management*
Edited by: D. A. Marcus © Humana Press, Totowa, NJ

why you need to do stretching exercises a couple of times each day. As you perform a consistent routine of stretching, your muscles get used to being stretched and are less likely to go into spasm. This will result in longer lasting pain relief.

If you do stretching exercises too vigorously or overstretch the muscle, the muscles react by increasing muscle spasm. For this reason, you need to work with a therapist while beginning an exercise program, especially if you notice pain aggravation with exercise. The therapist will encourage you to stretch muscles just to the point that you first feel them stretching and not to the point that you've stretched as far as you possibly can.

Pain Protection

Muscles and connecting structures, like tendons and ligaments, provide important protection for the rest of the body. In order to provide protection, they must be in shape and strong. We keep our muscles, tendons, and ligaments in good shape by exercise.

After we've been injured once, there's a natural tendency to try to avoid future injuries. For example, when I hurt my back exercising, I was scared to start exercising again. It's natural to think, "I'll just sit quietly in the chair and that way I'll never be hurt again." Unfortunately, the more inactive we become, the more out of shape our protective muscles, ligaments, and tendons become. This puts us at high risk for injury, from even slight trauma. When these tissues are out of shape, minor incidents, like twisting our ankles, carrying small bags of groceries, or bending, can result in major pain flares. Future injury from these minor events is reduced when the supporting and protective structures of our bodies are strong and flexible.

How Do You Get Started?

Forget the "no pain, no gain" motto. Pain exercise first concentrates on stretching and later works on muscle strengthening. Stretching exercises are very boring, but very important. Try to do them while watching a television program or listening to the radio, so you don't dread doing them and find excuses for not stretching. You will need to do stretches for the whole body and also stretches that target your pain areas.

Body reconditioning exercises—such as walking, swimming, and biking—are also essential. Your doctor can help you decide which exercise is right for you. Begin this program gradually and slowly increase exercise duration and intensity after you have become comfortable at each exercise level. Don't increase the exercise intensity too quickly, otherwise you'll cause muscle spasm and increased pain. Don't exercise too little, or you won't achieve exercise benefits.

GENERAL PRINCIPLES OF STRETCHING EXERCISE

- Perform stretches twice daily, in the morning and before bed.
- Begin stretches after taking a warm shower or using a heating pad over your most painful area for 15 minutes.
  - ○ Perform deep-breathing exercises or relaxation techniques while warming the painful area before exercises.
- Perform exercises while listening to music or television to provide distraction
- Perform each stretch slowly. Stretch until the first sensation of stretching is reached, then hold the stretch for 5 seconds. Relax and repeat 3 to 10 times.
- When pain flares up, do your exercise program, but reduce intensity and number of repetitions.
- If pain levels are higher after stretching, apply ice wrapped in a towel to the most painful area for 10 minutes.
  - ○ If pain levels are consistently high after stretching, reduce the extent of the stretch and review your exercise program with your physical therapist.

WHOLE-BODY STRETCHES

Lay down on the floor on your back, with your legs stretched out on the floor. Perform each stretch slowly. Stretch until the first sensation of stretching is reached. Then hold stretch for 5 seconds. Relax for 10 seconds and repeat three times.

Exercise description	Exercise drawing

Neck rotation

Rotate your neck slowly to the left, trying to place your left ear flat on the floor. Hold for 5 seconds. Return to the center and relax. Then rotate to the right and hold for 5 seconds. Return to center and relax.

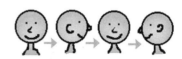

Shoulders and arms

Hold each arm out at the shoulder so your body makes a giant cross. Keeping your arms on the floor, bend your elbows to make a 90-degree angle, keeping your arm on the floor. This is your starting position. Keeping your arms on the floor between the shoulder and elbow, rotate your forearms up and over, so your fists become level with your waist. Rotate back to the starting position.

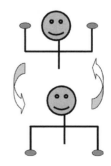

Raise both arms back over your head. Breathe out and reach out with your arms in a half circle, first up toward the ceiling then down to your sides. Breathe in and reach overhead again. If this is uncomfortable in your back, try bending your knees when you do this exercise.

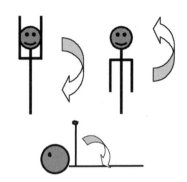

Lift both arms toward the ceiling. Hold. Lower both arms to your sides. If this is uncomfortable in your back, try bending your knees when you do this exercise.

Back

Lift your left arm up to the ceiling. Grab your left wrist with your right hand. Keeping your left arm straight (do not bend the left elbow), pull the left arm across your chest to the right. Turn chin to the left. Hold. Then raise right arm to the ceiling, grab the right wrist with left hand, and pull the right arm across the chest to the left. Turn chin to the right. Hold.

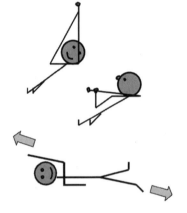

Stretch your right arm over your head. At the same time, point your left toe and stretch your leg. The arm and leg should be reaching in opposite directions. Hold. Repeat with the left arm and right leg.

Pelvis

Squeeze and tighten buttock muscles. Hold. Tighten muscles in the stomach and buttocks, pressing the small of your back flat onto the floor. Hold.

Bend your knees. Keep knees together and your shoulders on the floor. Slowly lower your knees to the floor at the right, causing a rotation of your pelvis. Turn your head to the left, away from your knees. Hold. Return knees and head to the center. Then lower your knees to the left and look right. Keep your head and shoulders on the floor to allow your pelvis to rotate.

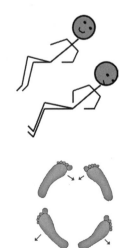

Legs

Spread your feet apart by about 2 feet. Turn both feet in toward the middle. Hold. Turn both feet out so your arches are turned toward the ceiling. Hold.

FLARE MANAGEMENT

Even if you practice your exercises and pain management techniques consistently, you will probably experience times of increased pain or pain flares. If the increased pain has the same characteristics as your typical pain, flare management techniques are often helpful. If you develop a new pain, see your doctor.

Flare management techniques are used when chronic pain increases to help minimize pain. Several techniques may be used together:

- Apply heat or ice (whichever you find more soothing) for 20 minutes to the painful area.
- Begin relaxation techniques: deep breathing, imagery, or biofeedback.
- Perform stretching exercises that stretch your painful area. Be sure to stretch slowly, and only to the point of first feeling a stretching sensation.
- Do oscillatory movements (small, rhythmic, side-to-side movements of the painful area). For example, for neck pain, turn the head through about 25% of its full range of motion. Starting with your head facing forward, first turn your head away from the painful side and back. Repeat at a rate of about one per second, for a total of 30 seconds. Rest for 30 seconds; then repeat until no further relief is noted. Then switch to turning the head toward the painful side, and proceed as above. Your therapist can describe oscillatory movements for your painful area.
- Trigger-point compression: you may notice certain spots on your muscles that aggravate your pain when you press them. These are called trigger points. If you identify trigger points, apply pressure to them with your fingers and hold for 12 to 60 seconds. Release the pressure, and proceed with your usual stretching exercises.

Appendix C
Psychological Pain Management

PSYCHOLOGICAL PAIN MANAGEMENT TECHNIQUES

Many effective pain management techniques are taught by psychologists. These techniques are designed to help reduce muscle spasm and the number of pain messages sent by the brain. These techniques are effective for most people with chronic pain. Pain improvement after use of these techniques does not mean that the pain was "imaginary" or "psychological." Additionally, these techniques are not designed to treat serious psychological problems, such as depression and anxiety. Relaxation training, biofeedback, and stress management are among the many techniques taught by psychologists. Patients achieve the most benefit from these techniques when they receive some formal training from an experienced therapist.

Relaxation

Relaxation techniques should be learned while sitting in a comfortable chair, with arms and legs uncrossed, feet flat on the floor, and eyes closed. Each practice session should last for about 15 to 20 uninterrupted minutes. Once you have regularly practiced and mastered these techniques, you will be able to use them whenever you feel yourself starting to tense or in anticipation of stress.

- Progressive muscle relaxation involves alternately contracting and relaxing muscles throughout your body. With your eyes closed, tense and then relax individual muscles in different parts of your body, starting at your feet and moving toward your neck and face. Hold the tension for 10 to 15 seconds, then release. Tense and release the muscles in your feet, then in other parts of the body in the following order: legs, abdomen, arms, shoulders, neck, jaw, eyes, and forehead. Focus on the sensations of the muscles when they are no longer tensed. With practice, you will begin to recognize when your muscles are tensed. For example, you may notice tension in your face, neck, and shoulders when sitting in traffic or waiting in a line at the store. Once you feel this tension, work to release it before your pain flares.
- Cue-controlled relaxation uses a combination of deep breathing and repetition of the word "relax." Begin this exercise with a slow, deep, abdominal breath. Place your hand over your abdomen to feel it moving in and out with each breath. After inhaling, hold the breath for 5 to 10 seconds then exhale, slowly repeating the word "relax." Repeat. After you are comfortable with this technique, you should be able to close your eyes and take a deep abdominal breath before confronting

From: *Chronic Pain: A Primary Care Guide to Practical Management*
Edited by: D. A. Marcus © Humana Press, Totowa, NJ

stressful situations, e.g., a doctor's visit, a meeting with the boss, or a discussion with your teenager. This will reduce the impact of stress on your pain.

Thermal Biofeedback

- Some people find it difficult to feel relaxed and use biofeedback as part of their relaxation training as an external monitor. To begin, place a handheld thermometer on your finger and measure the temperature. While practicing relaxation skills, check the temperature on your thermometer. When you are relaxed, the finger temperature should increase by about 2 to 3° Fahrenheit (probably to about 96°).
- An inexpensive finger thermometer and biofeedback audiotape may be obtained from Primary Care Network (1-800-769-7565).

Stress Management

Stress is one of the most common triggers for pain flares, aggravating pain in about 30% of people with chronic pain. Individuals usually notice that stress aggravates their usual health problems: people with heart disease experience chest pain; people with irritable bowel syndrome develop diarrhea, and patients with chronic pain have pain flares. Stress management does not mean avoiding or eliminating all of the stress in your life. Instead, you learn to have your body react differently when exposed to stress so that your pain is less likely to become flared. For example, many people feel stressed when stuck in traffic, reacting with anger, clenched teeth, and tightening of muscles in the neck and upper back. After learning stress management, you may still get stuck in traffic, but you will be able to respond by repeating soothing thoughts ("I will make my appointment. I am a responsible person.") or listening to music while practicing relaxation techniques (such as slow, deep breathing). In this way, your body will not release pain-provoking chemicals or cause muscle spasm, both of which may aggravate your pain condition. These same strategies can be used before attending a meeting with one's boss or a child's teacher, before beginning a discussion about family issues with spouse or child, or while waiting in a long line at the grocery store.

Most people experience stress symptoms when exposed to new environments and situations. Identify situations that are typically stress provoking for you, that cause you to feel your jaw or hands clench or begin to sweat. For some people, major events—such as taking an examination in school or giving a speech or a business presentation—will result in a stress response. For others, seemingly minor events—such as making a phone call, driving in traffic, meeting a child's teacher, or even meeting an old friend—may be stress provoking. Understanding your body's reaction to frequent situations allows you to plan to use relaxation techniques and stress management immediately before each event to minimize the stress response and the impact stress will have on your chronic pain.

Appendix D
Pain Medications

DOSING GUIDE FOR CHRONIC PAIN MEDICATIONS

Type of medication	Indication	Adult dosage

Antidepressants	Depression
	Neuropathic pain
	Headache
	Fibromyalgia
	Sleep disturbance
		Amitriptyline (Elavil®)
		  25–150 mg at bed
		Imipramine (Tofranil®)
		  25–150 mg at bed
		Paroxetine (Paxil®)
		  10–20 mg twice daily
		Sertraline (Zoloft®)
		  25–50 mg twice daily

Antiepileptics	Neuropathic pain
	Migraine
	Anxiety
	Sleep disturbance
		Gabapentin (Neurontin®) 100–300
		  mg two to three times daily
		Topiramate (Topamax®) 50–100 mg
		  twice daily
		Valproate (Depakote®; for migraine)
		  125–250 mg twice daily

Muscle relaxant	Myofascial pain Sleep disturbance	Tizanidine (Zanaflex®) 1–4 mg at bed or twice daily

Nonnarcotic analgesics	Pain flares
	Inflammation
		Ibuprofen (Motrin®) 400 mg every
		  6 hours
		Tramadol (Ultram®) 50–100 mg
		  every 6 hours

Opioids, short-acting	Disabling pain flared	Hydrocodone 5–10 mg every 6–8 hours
Opioids, long-acting	Disabling constant pain	Morphine 15–30 mg twice daily Methadone 5 mg twice daily

From: *Chronic Pain: A Primary Care Guide to Practical Management*
Edited by: D. A. Marcus © Humana Press, Totowa, NJ

Appendix E
Chronic Headache

MECHANISM OF MIGRAINE

Exposure to a variety of possible triggers—food, stress, change in sleep pattern, or hormonal medication—causes an imbalance in pain chemicals within the brain that results in stimulation of the trigeminal nerve. The trigeminal nerve supplies pain fibers to the head and face, as well as a variety of additional important functions. Activation of the trigeminal system results in tenderness of the scalp, so that brushing the hair is painful. Trigeminal nerves also signal blood vessels around the head, causing them to expand so that more blood can flow through them. Enlargement of these blood vessels can sometimes be seen at the temples. In addition, migraineurs notice a throbbing or pulsing sensation similar to that of the heartbeat. Trigeminal signals also go to parts of the brain to cause sensitivity to light, sound, and smell, as well as trigger cravings for certain foods, such as chocolate. Messages are also sent into the upper part of the cervical spinal cord, where they pass through the vomiting center, resulting in nausea during headache. In the cervical spinal cord, muscles in the back of the neck and shoulders may also become activated, causing muscle spasm and neck pain during migraine. Treatment of migraine is designed to eliminate possible triggers or change the balance of pain chemicals that are affected by these triggers (*see* Fig.1).

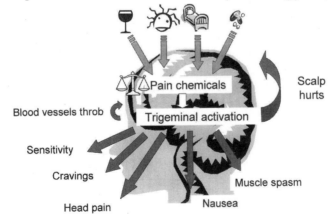

Fig. 1. *See* caption on p. 308.

From: *Chronic Pain: A Primary Care Guide to Practical Management*
Edited by: D. A. Marcus © Humana Press, Totowa, NJ

HEADACHE AS A BALANCING ACT

People with headaches can imagine that they have a scale in the brain that controls the balance between a headache occurring or not occurring on any given day. The left side of the scale contains brain chemicals that prevent headache activity, including serotonin, γ-aminobutyric acid (GABA), and endorphins. The right side of the scale contains chemicals that trigger headache, such as dopamine and norepinephrine. Exposure to certain foods or stress increases activity in the pain-producing chemicals in the right side of the scale and result in the increased likelihood of a headache occurring. Headache therapies work by increasing the activity of chemicals on the pain-prevention side. Triptans, such as Imitrex®, Maxalt®, Relpax®, and Zomig®, and antidepressant medications, such as Elavil® or Paxil®, increase serotonin activity. Interestingly, nonpharmacological therapies, such as relaxation and biofeedback, have also been shown to increase serotonin activity. Antiepileptic drugs, such as Depakote®, Neurontin®, and Topamax®, increase GABA activity. Pain pills increase endorphin activity. This increase in headache-protecting chemicals reduces the likelihood of headache (*see* Fig. 2).

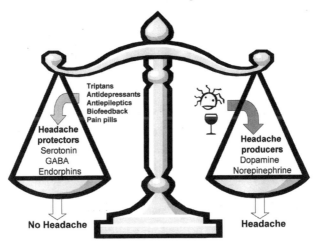

Fig. 2. Headache is a balancing act. Headache is caused by a change in the balance of brain chemicals. The headache protector chemicals serotonin, GABA, and endorphin protect against head pain. Dopamine and norepinephrine cause pain. Headache activity is reduced when the amount of headache protectors is high. Many headache therapies work by increasing activity or amounts of headache protectors. Headache triggers, like stress and some foods, increase activity or amounts of headache-producing brain chemicals.

Fig. 1. *(Previous page.)* Mechanism of migraine. Exposure to triggers (including foods, stress, changes in scheduling, or hormones) causes changes in pain chemical balance that triggers the trigeminal system. Activating the trigeminal system causes a variety of migraine symptoms: pain, nausea, cravings, and sensitivities to lights, noises, and smells.

DAILY HEADACHE RECORDING DIARY

Day	Severity (0–3)				Medication used	Menstrual
__/__/__	Morning	Noon	Evening	Bed	(Prescription and OTC [a])	days
Sunday						
Monday						
Tuesday						
Wednesday						
Thursday						
Friday						
Saturday						

[a] OTC, over-the-counter.

Instructions:

1. Record Sunday's date in the first column.
2. Record headache severity every day, four times daily (morning, noon, evening, and night) using the following severity scale:

   0 = no headache
   1 = mild headache (able to continue with routine activities)
   2 = moderate headache (activities restricted)
   3 = severe headache (unable to perform usual activities)

3. Record all medications used for headache: prescription and over-the-counter
4. Women: record any days with menstrual flow

[a] OTC, over-the-counter.

HEADACHE-FREE DIET

Only about 30% of headache sufferers can identify specific food triggers. This diet is designed to identify individual foods that may be a trigger for you. Specific foods are avoided to limit exposure to chemicals that can trigger headaches. Any food not listed in the "AVOID" column is allowed. Only a sample of allowed foods are listed.

Category	Avoid	Allowed	Chemical
Meats	Aged/cured meat: bacon, bologna, chicken liver, ham, pepperoni, salami, sausage Nuts: peanuts and peanut butter, pumpkin, sesame, and sunflower seeds Pickled herring, snails	Beef, poultry, fish, eggs	Nitrites Tyramine
Dairy	Buttermilk Ripened "stinky" cheese: bleu, brick, cheddar, emmentaler (Swiss), guyere, parmesan, provolone, brie, stilton, camembert, gouda Sour cream	Cheese: American, Velveeta®, cream cheese, cottage cheese, Ricotta Milk Yogurt (limit: 1/2 cup/day)	Histamine Phenylethylamine Tyramine
Fruit	Banana, fig, kiwi, mango, raisin, papaya, plum, strawberry	Apple, apricot, cherry, cranberry, nectarine, peach, pear, prune, watermelon Citrus (limit: 1/2 cup/day)	Tyramine
Vegetable	Avocado, corn, eggplant, olives, onion, pickles and pickled food, sauerkraut, spinach, snow pea, tomato Beans: broad, fava, garbanzo, lentils, lima, navy, pinto, soy	Artichoke, asparagus, beet, broccoli, carrot, cauliflower, lettuce, pea, potato, squash, string bean, zucchini	Histamine Tyramine
Bread and Cereal	Donuts, fresh homemade yeast bread and coffee cake, pizza, sourdough bread	Bagels, hot and cold cereal, crackers without cheese, commercial bread, English muffin, pasta, rice	Tyramine
Beverages	Alcohol Caffeinated beverages: chocolate, coffee, tea, Mountain Dew®, cola	Caffeine-free soda: 7-Up®, Sprite®, ginger ale Fruit juice (except citrus)	Histamine Phenylethylamine Tyramine

Continued

Category	Avoid	Allowed	Chemical
Desserts	Chocolate Mincemeat	Cakes and cookies without yeast or chocolate Gelatin Ice cream and sherbet	Phenylethylamine
Additives	Accent and seasoned salt, meat tenderizer. Monosodium glutamate (often listed as natural flavoring, hydrolyzed protein, carrageenan, or caseinate): this common food enhancer is found in many prepared foods. Avoid canned, frozen, and prepared foods; food in jars; weight-loss powders; dry soup/bouillon; potato chips; Chinese food. Nutrasweet: diet foods, Equal®		
Medicine and habits	Caffeinated: Anacin®, Aqua Ban®, diet pills, Excedrin®, Midol®, No Doz®, Norgesic®, Tussirex®, Vanquish®, Vivarin® Nicotine		

Diet instructions:

1. Follow a regular eating schedule. Don't skip meals or fast.
2. Read food and medicine labels.
3. Follow the diet strictly for 3 weeks. If headache improves, slowly add one food back into your diet each week. Food triggers should produce a headache within 12 hours. If your headache does not improve on this diet, food is not the trigger for your headache.

Adapted from American Council for Headache Education Tyramine-restricted Diet and Theisler CW. *Migraine Headache Disease: Diagnostic and Management Strategies.* Gaithersburg, MD: Aspen Publishers, Inc; 1990, pp. 111–112.

HEADACHE MEDICATION GUIDE
For Migraine and Tension-Type Headaches
Section I: Acute Care Medications

To be used for infrequent, severe headaches (less than 3 days/week).

Medication	Dosage	Common side effects

Analgesics
Aspirin,
Ibuprofen,
Naproxen,
Excedrin®
Tylenol®
	Aspirin: 650 mg (2 tabs) every
	  3–4 hours; daily maximum: 4 g/day
	Ibuprofen: 400 mg (2 Advil® tabs)
	  every 4–6 hours
	Naproxen: 440 mg (2 Aleve®)
	  every 8 hours
	Excedrin®: 2 tabs every 6 hours
	Tylenol®: 650 mg every 4 hours daily;
	  maximum: 3.5 g/day
		Stomach upset, dizziness, fluid
		  retention, bleeding, ringing in the
		  ears, hearing loss, kidney or liver
		  damage

Anti-nausea
Reglan®
Compazine®
Thorazine®
Tigan®
	Reglan®: 10 mg by mouth or
	  IM injection
	Compazine®: 25 mg rectally
		Drowsiness, dystonia, Parkin-
		  sonism; rarely tardive dyskinesia
		  or neuroleptic malignant syn-
		  drome

Isometheptene
Midrin®
	2 tabs initially, then 1 in 1 hour if
	  needed; no more than 5 pills/day
	  and 10 pills/week
	*Note: Avoid if taking MAO-I or uncontrolled
	high blood pressure or glaucoma.*
		Drowsiness, dizziness, rash

Dihydroergotamine
DHE-45®
Migranal®
	Nasal spray: 1 spray (0.5 mg) in
	  each nostril. May repeat in
	  15 min. Maximum: 4 sprays/day,
	  8 sprays/week.
	Note: Avoid with erythromycin.
		Nausea, chest tightness, leg cramps,
		  vomiting, increased blood
		  pressure

Triptans
Imitrex®
Maxalt®
Zomig®
Relpax®
Axert®
Amerge®
Frova®
	Available as injections, nasal
	  sprays, and oral pills.
	Imitrex pills: 50–100 mg; may
	  repeat once in 2 h
	*Note: Avoid if heart disease or uncontrolled
	high blood pressure*
		Tingling, anxiety, nausea, sedation,
		  weakness, chest/neck tightness

Remember:

1. Read the labels of your medicine to identify what you're taking.
2. Take acute care medicines at the beginning of a bad headache attack, when symptoms are still mild. If you have warning signs before a headache starts, use acute therapy when the warning signs occur.
3. Limit acute care medications to no more than 3 days/week to avoid medication overuse headache.

Section II: Preventive Medications

For prevention of frequent headache (more than 3 days/week).

Medication	Dosage	Common side effects
Anti-depressant Tricyclic: Elavil® Tofranil® SSRI: Paxil®	Elavil or Tofranil: 25–100 mg 2 hours before bed Paxil: 5–20 mg twice daily *Note: Avoid tricyclic if glaucoma.*	Sedation, dry mouth, dizziness, weight change, sexual dysfunction, blurred vision, urine retention
Antihypertensive Inderal® Calan®	Inderal 80–160 mg daily; long-acting form may be used once daily Calan: 240–480 mg daily; long-acting form may be used once daily	Depression, sedation, constipation, dizziness
Anti-epilepsy Depakote® Neurontin® Topamax®	Depakote: 125–250 mg twice daily Neurontin: 100–400 mg 2–3 times daily Topamax: 50–100 mg twice daily	Weight change, hair thinning, tremor, bleeding, nausea, dizziness, rash, sleepiness, numbness, nausea
Antihistamine Periactin®	Periactin: 4 mg 2–3 times daily *Note: Avoid if glaucoma or using MAO-I.*	Drowsiness, weight gain, dry mouth, constipation

Remember:

1. Don't expect headache reduction for at least 2–3 weeks after starting preventive medications.
2. Take preventive medications every day. Acute care medications can also be used for infrequent, severe headaches.
3. Once headaches are controlled, take preventive medications for 4–6 months before trying to taper the dose. If headaches return when the dose is tapered, resume the previously effective dose. Try to taper the dose again in 6 months.
4. Anti-inflammatory medications, such as naproxen 250–500 mg twice daily, may be used during the menstrual week for menstrual headache or taken for several weeks while tapering off pain killers in patients with medication overuse headache.

ACUTE MIGRAINE THERAPY TARGET GOALS

What Is Acute Migraine Therapy?

Acute migraine therapy is used to treat an individual headache episode. Acute migraine medications, which include analgesics and triptans, should effectively relieve the symptoms of migraine and disability that occur with the migraine.

Acute migraine medications should be limited to a maximum of 3 days per week on a regular basis. Regular use of any acute care medication for more than 3 days per week over several weeks to months can result in a worsening pattern of headache, called medication overuse headache.

If you have frequent headaches and need to use your acute care medication more often than 3 days per week, talk to your doctor about considering the addition of a migraine preventive therapy.

How Do I Use Acute Migraine Therapy?

In general, acute care medications are most effective when they are used before a migraine episode becomes severe or you have to reduce your activities because of your headache. Some medications, such as the triptans, are still effective when used to treat migraines that are already severe. Migraine relief, however, will be faster and more complete if any acute treatment, including triptans, is taken earlier during a migraine episode.

You have been prescribed the following specific acute migraine therapy:

Drug name and dose: _____
Route of administration:

- Oral tablet (take with water)
- Orally dissolving tablet (take without water)
- Nasal spray
- Injection

When a migraine begins, take _____ .
You may repeat the dose in _____ hours.

What Should I Expect?

Realistic target goals for acute care medication include:

- Rapid relief of all migraine symptoms
  - Relief should be obtained within 2 hours
  - Some treatments achieve faster relief
  - If relief is taking longer than 30–60 minutes, consider asking your doctor to adjust your treatment.

- Complete relief of all migraine symptoms
  - Within 2 hours, all symptoms of migraine should be gone.
  - Consider asking for a medication adjustment if you have persistent pain.
- After you initially treat your headache, the headache should not come back within 24 hours.
- You should not have any side effects that make you reluctant to use your medication.

ACUTE MIGRAINE THERAPY SATISFACTION ASSESSMENT

Try your new acute migraine therapy for three migraine episodes to accurately assess its efficacy. Keep track of how effectively your treatment goals were met by completing the chart below. Write down how long it took to achieve headache relief. Circle yes or no responses for the remaining questions.

	Headache 1 Date: __/__/__		Headache 2 Date: __/__/__		Headache 3 Date: __/__/__	
How quickly did you achieve relief of your migraine symptoms? (record minutes or hours)						
Was relief fast enough for you?	Yes	No	Yes	No	Yes	No
Did your migraine symptoms go away completely?	Yes	No	Yes	No	Yes	No
Is the formulation you're using (tablet, dissolving tablet, nasal spray, or injection) convenient and effective for you?	Yes	No	Yes	No	Yes	No
Are you having any troublesome side effects that make you hesitant to use your medication?	Yes	No	Yes	No	Yes	No

List any troublesome side effects or other comments:

_____

_____

_____

After treating three headaches, are you satisfied with this treatment?　　Yes　No

If No, why not? _____

HEADACHE MEDICATION GUIDE
For Cluster Headaches

Section I: Acute Care Medications

Medication	Dosage	Common side effects
Oxygen	100% oxygen at 7–8 L/minute for 10 minutes by face mask. May repeat up to 4 times daily.	Generally well tolerated.
Dihydroergotamine DHE-45® Migranal®	Nasal spray: 1 spray (0.5 mg) in each nostril. May repeat in 15 minutes. Maximum: 4 sprays/day, 8 sprays/week. *Note: Avoid with erythromycin.*	Nausea, chest tightness, leg cramps, vomiting, increased blood pressure.
Triptans: Imitrex®	Imitrex injection: 6 mg subcutaneously *Note: Avoid if heart disease or uncontrolled high blood pressure is present.*	Tingling, anxiety, nausea, sedation, weakness, chest/neck tightness.
Lidocaine	4% intranasal lidocaine: 1 mL in nostril on painful side. Lie with head extended for 1 minute. May repeat once.	Generally well tolerated.
Steroid Dexamethasone	Dexamethasone: 8 mg single dose	High blood pressure, increased blood sugar, confusion, tremor, stomach ulcers. More serious side effects include cataracts, bone thinning and necrosis.

Section II: Preventive Medications

Medication	Dosage	Side effects
Antihypertensive Calan®	Calan: 240–480 mg/day; long-acting form may be used once daily.	Constipation, diarrhea, dizziness, fluid retention
Anti-epilepsy Depakote® Neurontin® Topamax®	Depakote: 125–250 mg twice daily Neurontin: 100–400 mg 2–3 times daily	Weight gain, hair thinning, tremor, bleeding, nausea, dizziness, rash
Methysergide Not available in the United States	4–8 mg daily Drug holiday every 6 months. Check periodic CXR, IVP, abdominal CT	Leg cramps, leg swelling, numbness in fingers/toes, chest pain, nausea; rarely retroperitoneal fibrosis

Continued

Medication	Dosage	Side effects
Lithium Lithobid®	600–1200 mg daily to achieve blood level of 0.6–1.2 May combine with calcium channel blocker	Tremor, confusion, decreased thyroid function, increased urination, blurred vision, nausea, fatigue, weight gain, swelling. May treat tremor with Inderal®.
Indomethacin Indocin®	Indocin: 25–50 mg 2–4 times daily *Note: Used to rule out Chronic Paroxysmal Headache, a rare, cluster-like headache in women.*	Gastric irritation, dizziness, fatigue, ringing in ears
Triptan Imitrex® Maxalt® Zomig® Relpax® Axert® Amerge® Frova®	Imitrex pills: 25–50 mg at bed (used short-term for severe cluster period) *Note: Avoid if heart disease or uncontrolled high blood pressure.*	Tingling, anxiety, nausea, sedation, weakness, chest/neck tightness
Antihistamine Periactin®	Periactin: 4 mg 2–3 times daily *Note: Avoid if glaucoma or using MAO-I.*	Drowsiness, weight gain, dry mouth, constipation

CT, computed tomography; CXR, chest x-ray; IVP, intravenous pyelogram.

Occasionally used for prevention of cluster headaches: anti-nausea medications, anti-anxiety medications, antidepressants, propranolol, and anti-inflammatory medications. For doses and side effects, refer to migraine/tension-type medication sheets.

Discontinue alcohol intake and smoking during cluster: both aggravate cluster headaches and nicotine decreases medication effectiveness.

MEDICATION OVERUSE OR REBOUND HEADACHE

If you have frequent headaches, your doctor may talk to you about medication overuse or drug rebound headaches. People who get headaches often notice they develop more frequent and more severe headaches when they are regularly using acute care headache or pain medications (e.g., aspirin, ibuprofen, Tylenol®, Excedrin®, narcotics, or triptans) more than 3 days a week. Medication overuse headaches are generally a dull, everyday headache pain that seems to wax and wane throughout the day. Although taking headache or pain medication will make the headache temporarily better, frequent use of medication may actually be making the headache worse.

How Can a Pain Reliever Cause Pain?

Medication overuse headaches are similar to caffeine withdrawal symptoms. Coffee drinkers typically awaken with a morning headache and irritability, which are relieved after drinking a cup of coffee. After several hours, when the coffee is out of their system, the caffeine-withdrawal headache and irritability return. Coffee drinkers will "medicate" these symptoms with "doses" of coffee throughout the day. Because they don't wake up during the night for coffee, their symptoms are usually at their worst when they wake up in the morning, announcing, "Nobody better talk to me until I've had my cup of coffee." Coffee drinkers easily recognize these symptoms as caused by caffeine. They know that stopping caffeine for a few days will not improve their symptoms, and may even make them temporarily worse. Once they've avoided coffee for several weeks, though, they will no long have these cycling headaches and irritability.

This same pattern occurs in the medication overuser, who wakes early with a bad headache and takes a headache pill. When the headache returns in 3 or 4 hours, they take more pills, and may repeat this several times throughout the day.

How Are Medication Overuse Headaches Treated?

Medication overuse headaches must be treated by medication withdrawal. Under medical supervision, analgesics and triptans can be discontinued. Narcotics and barbiturate combinations (e.g., Fiorinol® or Fioricet®) are tapered. Sometimes people use medications during this withdrawal period that do not cause rebound headache, such as naproxen, Celebrex®, or Ultram®.

Improvement after medication withdrawal is usually not seen for several *weeks to months* after stopping the overused medication (*see* Fig. 3 *[1]*). Because medication overuse headache only occurs in people with an underlying headache disorder, like migraine or tension-type headaches, all headaches will not be cured by discontinuing daily medications.

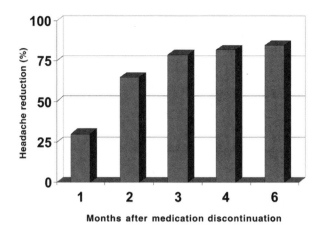

Fig. 3. Percentage of patients experiencing headache improvement after discontinuing overused medications. Improvement occurs in the majority of patients who discontinue medications, although early improvement 1 month after discontinuing occurs in only about 30% of patients.

Standard headache preventive medications (such as antihypertensives, anti-depressants, and anti-epileptics) tend not to work when people are also using daily pain killers. So you may want to talk to your doctor about a second trial of a medicine that was found to be ineffective while you were also using daily or near daily pain killers.

How Can I Avoid Medication-Overuse Headaches?

To avoid developing medication overuse headaches, don't regularly take acute care or pain medications more than 3 days per week. You need to have at least 4 days per week with no acute care medication. This means you cannot use aspirin 2 days, a triptan 3 days, and a narcotic 2 days each week. Maintaining a headache diary can help identify if you are overusing a single medication or a combination of several medications. If you regularly have headaches more than 3 days per week, talk to your doctor about preventive headache treatments.

REFERENCE

1. Rapoport AM, Weeks RE, Sheftell FD, Baskin SM, Verdi J. The "analgesic wash-out period": a critical variable in the evaluation of treatment efficacy. Neurology 1986; 36(Suppl 1):100–101.

CME QUESTIONS

1. Patients with chronic headaches rate which of the following as the most important doctor attribute?

    a. Doctor provides information and explains headache care.
    b. Doctor is recognized as a national expert in pain management.
    c. Doctor is knowledgeable about all the latest medications.
    d. Doctor is friendly to patients and staff.

2. Pain education results in which of the following benefit(s)?

    a. Decreased catastrophizing
    b. Decreased disability
    c. Improved motion
    d. All of the above
    e. None of the above

3. Which of the following education delivery systems is/are effective?

    a. Brief instruction by a health care provider
    b. Written materials, videos, and audio presentations
    c. Internet resources
    d. All of the above
    e. None of the above

4. Effective techniques for closing pain gates include:

    a. Exercise
    b. Relaxation
    c. Repeating positive messages
    d. All of the above
    e. None of the above

Index